Catherine Garel

MRI of the Fetal Brain

Normal Development and Cerebral Pathologies

Springer-Verlag Berlin Heidelberg GmbH

Catherine Garel

MRI of the Fetal Brain

Normal Development
and Cerebral Pathologies

With contributions by
Anne-Lise Delezoide · Laurent Guibaud
Guy Sebag · Pierre Gressens
Monique Elmaleh-Bergès · Max Hassan
Hervé Brisse · Emmanuel Chantrel

With 621 Figures and 82 Tables

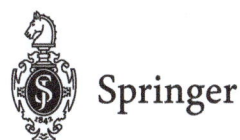

Springer

ISBN 978-3-540-40747-8   ISBN 978-3-642-18747-6 (eBook)
DOI 10.1007/978-3-642-18747-6

Original French Edition published by Sauramps
1. Garel, C.: Developpement du cerveau foetal
2. Garel, C.: Imagerie du cerveau foetal pathologique

Translated by V. Delezoide

CATHERINE GAREL, MD
Department of Pediatric Imaging
Hôpital Robert Debré
48 Boulevard Serrurier
75935, Paris Cedex 19
France

Library of Congress Cataloging-in-Publication Data
Garel, Catherine, 1959– [Développement du cerveau foetal.
English] MR imaging of the fetal brain: normal development
and cerebral pathologies/Catherine Garel. p.; cm. Originally
published in 2 v. entitled: Le développement du cerveau foetal,
and: Imagerie du cerveau foetal pathologique. Includes bibli-
ographical references and index. Contents: Pt.1. Development
of the fetal brain – Pt.2. Imaging of the pathological fetal brain.
ISBN 3-540-40747-2 (alk. paper) 1. Fetal brain–Magnetic resonance imaging. 2. Fetal brain–Abnormalities–Magnetic resonance imaging. I. Garel, Cathérine, 1959– Imagerie du cerveau
foetal pathologique. English. II. Title. [DNLM: 1. Brain-
embryology. 2. Fetal Diseases–diagnosis. 3. Magnetic Resonance Imaging–methods. WL 141 G229d 2004] RG629.B73G3713
2004 612.6'40181–dc22

© Springer-Verlag Berlin Heidelberg 2004
Originally published by Springer-Verlag
Berlin Heidelberg New York in 2004

Cover design: F. Steinen, eStudio Calamar, Spain
Product management and layout: B. Wieland, Heidelberg
Typesetting: AM-production, Wiesloch

21/3111 – 5 4 3 2 1   SPIN 11820673
Printed on acid-free paper

Foreword

It is becoming increasingly clear that many developmental disorders of childhood have a prenatal basis, either resulting from abnormal programming of development or from some sort of in utero injury. It is less clear how to determine the cause of the brain abnormality, at what stage it can be determined, and how this knowledge can be used to benefit our patients. Prenatal imaging is clearly an important component of all of these steps. Although prenatal ultrasound has been in use for more than two decades and its strengths are well understood, prenatal MRI is newer and its capabilities are only beginning to be appreciated. This book and others like it are helping attain that insight.

In this book, Dr. Garel and her co-workers present the basic elements of proper use and interpretation of fetal cerebral MRI. The book starts with a description of the optimal techniques used for the studies. It continues to describe normal fetal brain development, as assessed by pathology and MRI. Finally, it describes and illustrates many abnormalities of the fetal brain, both developmental and acquired (destructive). Of note, the authors do not merely list abnormalities of the brain; instead, they explain the relevant embryology or pathogenesis of the disorder, describe sonographic findings, and discuss what adds to the assessment. This approach helps physicians understand what they are seeing and reduces the chances for misdiagnosis.

In short, this book is an excellent and important addition to the growing field of prenatal diagnosis.

A. James Barkovich, MD

Professor of Radiology, Neurology, Pediatrics, and Neurosurgery
University of California, San Francisco

Acknowledgements

We would like to warmly thank all the contributors to this book:

- Professor Max Hassan who, from the opening of the hospital in 1988, has worked at establishing close co-operation with the gynaecology-obstetrics department and has, from the very beginning, brought his knowledge, enthusiasm and human warmth.
- Professor Guy Sebag, whose expertise in MRI techniques has encouraged the constant development of ever more precise image acquisition sequences, and hence furthered the parallel development of this new symptomatology.
- Doctor Anne-Lise Delezoide and her valuable knowledge of neurofetopathology, without which this book could not have been made. The present work is indeed based on the constant comparisons we make between the data provided in this field by our two disciplines.
- Professor Laurent Guibaud, with his characteristic rigour, has contributed his no less valuable knowledge of the pathology of the posterior fossa.
- Doctor Pierre Gressens, whose knowledge of fetal brain development is extremely valuable in our weekly multidisciplinary meeting. We extend our thanks to him along with Professor Guy Sebag, both of whom consented to read this work and have enriched it with their highly beneficial advice.
- Doctor Monique Elmaleh-Bergès, who carried out a large number of the fetal cerebral MRI examinations presented here, and whose competence in the neuroradiology field is essential in our line of work.
- Doctor Hervé Brisse, for his significant contribution to the development of this activity during his postgraduate studies and later as a fellow in the department.
- Doctor Emmanuel Chantrel who collected biometry, gyration and myelination data at the basis of the first part of this book.

Moreover, we wish to thank:

- Professor Gabriele Benz-Bohm for her constant support in promoting the idea of an English version of the French original.
- Doctor Patricia Terdjman, in remembrance of all the Tuesday mornings we spent together interpreting fetal MR images.
- The MRI technicians (Katia Bourlois, Christelle Dos Santos, Sophie Duret, Christine Guégan, Thierry Lefèvre, Catherine Nicelli, Nelly Scimia and Corine Tavernier) who combine rigour and good humour in their daily work.
- Magali Nater, who looked after the preparation of the manuscript as well as the archiving of fetal MR images.

In addition to A. L. Delezoide, the fetopathological examinations were interpreted by the following doctors: M. Bucourt, M. Catala, L. Choudat, F. Daïkha-Dahmane, M.C. Dauge-Geoffroy, C. Fallet-Bianco, C. Fondacci, P. Georges, J.C. Larroche, E. Le Galloudec, F. Menez and F. Razavi. Without the great precision of their examination protocols, the comparison with MRI data would not have been so fruitful.

We are also indebted to the entire gynaecology-obstetrics team at the Hôpital Robert Debré, without whose collaboration this atlas could not have been made, and particularly:

- Professor Philippe Blot, whose constant concern when he was at the head of department was to encourage these multidisciplinary collaborative efforts.
- Professor Jean-François Oury (now of department head) and Doctor Dominique Luton, who work in the same spirit of rigour and openness.
- Doctor Edith Vuillard who conducted a great number of the US examinations presented in this atlas.
- The antenatal diagnosis midwives' team, who looked after the coordination between our two units with efficiency and unfailing dedication.

Finally, we wish to address a word of sincere thanks to the doctors in the neonatology (Prof. Aujard's department), intensive care (Prof. Beaufils's department), neurology (Prof. Evrard's department) and medical genetics (Dr Baumann's and Prof. Verloes's department) teams, who take an active part in our weekly multidisciplinary meetings.

Contributors

C. GAREL, MD
Hospital Consultant
Medical imaging specialist
Department of Pediatric Imaging
Hôpital Robert Debré
Paris, France

A.-L. DELEZOIDE
University Lecturer, Hospital Consultant
Development Biology Department
Hôpital Robert Debré
Paris, France

L. GUIBAUD
University Professor, Hospital Consultant
Pediatric and Fetal Imaging
Hôpital Debrousse
Lyon, France

G. SEBAG
University Professor, Hospital Consultant
Pediatric Imaging Department
Hôpital Robert Debré
Paris, France

P. GRESSENS
Research Scientist
INSERM E9935 and
Pediatric Neurology Department
Hôpital Robert Debré
Paris
Experimental Imaging Laboratory
UFR Lariboisière, Saint-Louis
Université Paris VII, Denis Diderot
Paris, France

M. HASSAN
Professor, Hospital Consultant
Pediatric Imaging Department
Hôpital Robert Debré
Paris, France

M. ELMALEH-BERGES
Hospital Consultant
Pediatric Imaging Department
Hôpital Robert Debré
Paris, France

H. BRISSE
Physician, Medical Imaging Specialist
Institut Curie
Paris, France

Contents

List of Abbreviations

AD	Atrial diameter
APDV	Anteroposterior diameter of the vermis
BPD	Biparietal diameter
TCD	Transverse cerebellar diameter
DV3	Lateral diameter of the third ventricle
DV4	Anteroposterior diameter of the fourth ventricle
FOD	Fronto-occipital diameter
HV	Height of the vermis
IHD	Interhemispheric distance
IOPD	Interopercular distance
LCC	Length of the corpus callosum
SV	Surface of the vermis
WG	Weeks of gestation

Introduction

This book is meant for all those whose work brings them to imaging the fetal brain, particularly for the radiologists who conduct magnetic resonance imaging (MRI) of the fetal brain, but also for neurofetopathologists who wish to compare radiological images with their own data. It is also aimed at obstetric sonographers, with the goal of improving knowledge of the brain in all three spatial dimensions and of the different cerebral pathologies, and hence seeks to improve the conditions of sonographic observation of the fetal brain.

Cerebral anomalies at birth account for approximately 9% of all isolated anomalies and are present in 15.9% of cases of multiple malformations. They therefore constitute a critical element of antenatal diagnosis. In France, termination of pregnancy enjoys a very specific judicial framework, since in some cases it is authorized as late as the end of pregnancy. Some major anomalies can be screened in the first trimester of pregnancy. Other more subtle abnormalities, whether they are systemic malformations or acquired (ischaemic, infectious, etc.), are only detectable at a later stage and are sometimes missed by ultrasonographic diagnosis. The screening of such abnormalities has greatly benefited from the development of fetal MRI and has become the main field of investigation. The role held by fetal MRI has continued to grow in importance during the past few years, and this examination is now part of the arsenal of every major centre of antenatal diagnosis, in view of optimizing the reliability of the prognostic and diagnostic information given to the parents. However, we often come up against a lack of established standards. Now, in this area as in others, only thorough knowledge of the normal condition and its variations can allow us to grasp what a pathological state is. This is the purpose of the first part of this book, which is an MRI atlas of the fetus's cerebral development.

Morphological knowledge of the human fetal brain has until now been dependent on only fetopathological studies which, it should be remembered, can only concern a limited number of fetuses. The fetal brain has also been widely studied with ultrasonography, but some steps in development remained difficult to evaluate, particularly myelination and cerebral gyration, whose value as an indicator of cerebral maturation is well known. The poor visibility of cerebral sulci in sonography can be explained by the fineness of pericerebral spaces, the artefacts of reverberation on the calvaria, and the impossibility of obtaining a constant three-dimensional study of the brain. Furthermore, some biometric sonographic values, such as the biparietal diameter, are based on measurements of the skull, and not of the cerebral parenchyma. Other biometric values, notably those concerning the posterior cranial fossa, cannot be consistently obtained whatever the stage of pregnancy or the position of the fetus's head.

The second part of the book is dedicated to fetal cerebral pathologies. It is essential to know how to detect such pathologies, analyse them and know their prognoses. This second part reflects the experience of the prenatal diagnosis centre at the Hôpital Robert Debré in postnatal paediatric imaging and in fetal imaging. The paediatric imaging (obstetrical ultrasonography, fetal MRI and postnatal imaging), gynaecology-obstetrics, neurofetopathology, paediatric neurology, neonatology, intensive care and medical genetics teams have all taken an active part in the centre's study of cerebral pathologies. Year after year, this experience has been regularly enriched through the multidisciplinary collation of prenatal imaging data with data obtained from postnatal imaging or neurofetopathological examination.

For the study of abnormalities of the posterior fossa, the staff of this Paris centre was completed by the contribution of Professor Laurent Guibaud, who is in charge of prenatal imaging in the Paediatric and Fetal Imaging Department of the Hôpital Debrousse in Lyons.

For purposes of didactic efficiency, the seven chapters in this second part are all built on the same structure: a brief overview of the fundamental data – embryology, mechanism and/or current genetics data – to place the abnormality assessed within the wider context of morphogenesis. The symptomatology of imaging – the very core of each chapter – is systematically doubly illustrated by ultrasonographic and MR images. Indeed, it would be unwise to artificially overvalue the complementary contribution of MRI by underexploiting the possibilities of ultrasonography, whether such underexploitation results from incomplete knowledge of cerebral malformation pathologies, insufficient practice of prenatal ultrasonography or even an extensive and excessive application of the precaution principle.

Neurofetopathology and/or postnatal imaging slices, presented as much as possible in planes identical to those of the prenatal images, are intended to clarify the abnormalities studied as fully as possible. Finally, each chapter ends with a brief perspective of the data currently available on the prognosis for the disorder studied.

The current uncertainties are, however, also addressed. Fetal neurology is indeed a rapidly evolving discipline, in which our knowledge is still incomplete, particularly regarding the imaging of a few very rare pathologies. However, some unknowns paradoxically remain in the study of some of the more common pathologies because of a lack of studies conducted on a large cohort of fetuses that would allow us to evaluate the contribution of MRI and to determine a long-term prognosis: ventricular dilatation is the perfect illustration (see Chap. 11).

PART I

Development of the Fetal Brain

Technique

Since the first report of MRI in pregnancy in 1983 [1], the technique used has considerably evolved. Nowadays, fetal MRI should be performed on a high-field unit (1.5 T) with a phased-array surface coil to achieve optimal imaging quality. The problem of fetal motion has been significantly diminished by the development of ultrafast imaging techniques and a consequent decrease in acquisition time. However, the problem has not been entirely solved and even if many sequences are much faster than they used to be, T1-weighted sequences still require a long time and motion artefacts are therefore still worrying. Fetal sedation is not universally used. In our institution, we continue using a sedation by maternal oral administration of flunitrazepam (1 mg) 30 min before the beginning of the examination.

Let us remember that the innocuousness of MRI has yet to be proved, although clinical and experimental research [2, 3] has not shown any deleterious effects on the fetus induced by MRI.

In the United States, the National Radiological Protection Board recommends not using MRI during the first trimester, the morphogenesis period, unless pregnancy is interrupted [4]. Axial, coronal and sagittal images should be acquired orthogonal to the fetal brain. A variety of T1- and T2-weighted sequences are available.

The purpose of this chapter is to detail the contribution of the different sequences in the evaluation of fetal cerebral anatomy and pathology and to analyse their advantages and drawbacks.

T2-Weighted Sequences

Technique

T2-weighted sequences are the most frequently used and make up the basis of fetal MRI. Ultrafast T2-weighted sequences such as HASTE (half-Fourier acquired single-shot turbo spin-echo) or RARE (half-Fourier single shot rapid acquisition with relaxation enhancement) sequences can also be acquired. For both sequences, a half-Fourier algorithm is used to reconstruct the images. Images are acquired on a slice-per-slice basis. Therefore, motion artefacts are limited to the slices in which the motion occurred.

The acquisition time per image is approximately 400 ms with a 1- to 3-s time interval between slices to allow a full relaxation of the excited spins.

With the newest generation of MRI units, 3D T2-weighted single-shot sequences such as a 3D true Fast Imaging Steady Precession (true FISP, b.FFE, Fiesta) can be acquired, considerably reducing the acquisition time. The true FISP is a gradient-echo technique with fully refocused transverse magnetization [5–9].

Advantages and Drawbacks

These heavily T2-weighted sequences provide a good signal-to-noise ratio with excellent T2-weighted contrast resolution of fetal tissues, due to the high water content of fetal brain and therefore its long T2 relaxation time.

However, some data acquired in HASTE for the outer portion of the K-space come from the last echoes. Therefore, this sequence suffers from a T2 decay during data collection that causes blurring of the images along the phase-encoding direction. This is responsible for a decrease in the signal-to-noise ratio and signal-to-contrast ratio and is particularly pronounced for tissues with a relatively short T2, causing possible loss of these tissues on the image [5–14].

Compared with T2 fast spin-echo sequences, there are limitations with HASTE in the detection of small (<5 mm) hyper- and hypointense lesions. Conversely, small markedly hyperintense lesions may be well detected. In infants and children [12], sensitivity for the detection of myelination and migration disorders is rather low compared with T2-weighted turbo spin-echo sequences, which better differentiate grey from white matter. In another postnatal series [13] the flow void effect of an aneurysm was observed with HASTE but the nidus of an arteriovenous malformation was missed; this might be related to the limited spatial resolution caused by blurring.

Comparing HASTE and true FISP [11] for the analysis of the fetal brain, point-spread function blurring in HASTE occurs slightly during the second trimester because myelination is still poorly developed and there is not a significant difference between both techniques. However, the delineation of early myelination in the tegmentum of the pons by HASTE is degraded by the blurring effect. Moreover, the nature of true FISP, which affords equal K-space weighting (and hence no blurring artefacts), is responsible for a better delineation of the multilayer cellular migrational process with true FISP than with HASTE.

During the third trimester, significant blurring of the myelinated white matter is observed along the phase-encoding direction in the HASTE images but not in the true FISP images. Thus this sequence is more conspicuous at this stage. Moreover, true FISP provides high-quality images at a significantly lower specific radiofrequency absorption rate. Its sensitivity to field heterogeneity should be improved by shimming technology and the banding artefacts should decrease with improvements in gradient coil design (thus reducing TR) [5–14].

Applications

These ultrafast T2-weighted images are essentially used to delineate the fetal brain and hence to accurately evaluate biometry and sulcation (see Chap. 4).

Moreover, the high contrast resolution of heavy T2-weighted sequences makes them useful in the evaluation of brain structures such as the corpus callosum, cavum septi pellucidi, ventricles, vermis and cerebellar hemispheres. Consequently, whenever a pure anatomical survey of the brain is necessary, this type of sequence is recommended.

Conversely, the evaluation of the cerebral parenchyma is incomplete with this type of sequence. Ac-

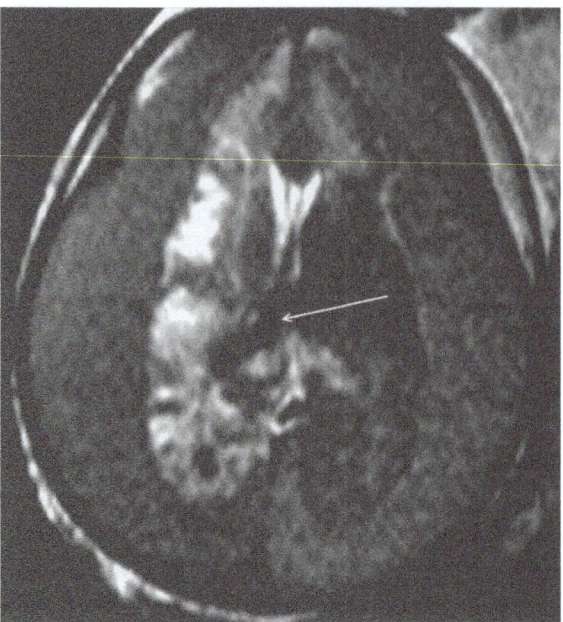

a

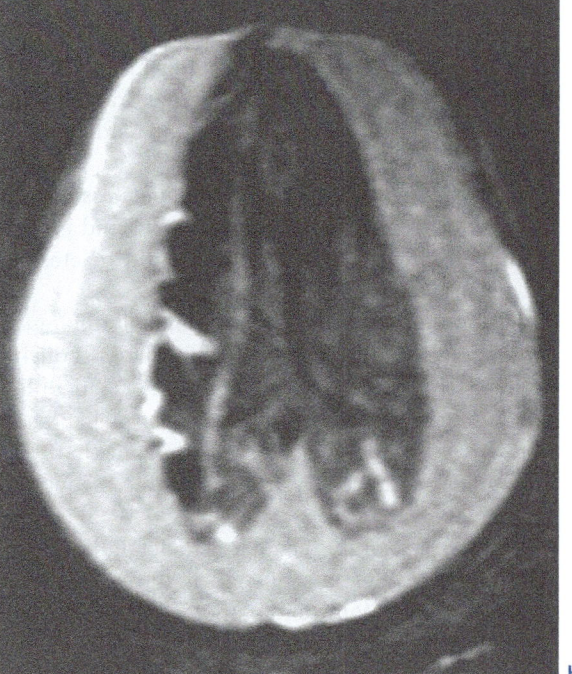

b

◀ **Fig. 1 a,b.** A 34-week-old fetus. Subdural haematoma with laminar necrosis, intraventricular bilateral haemorrhage and diffuse ischaemic lesions of cerebral parenchyma. T2- (a) and T1- (b) weighted transverse slice at the level of the lateral ventricles. The subdural haematoma is hyperintense on T1-weighted images and has an intermediate signal on T2 images. A clot (hypointense on T2 image) is visible in the right ventricle (*arrow*). The parenchyma is hyperintense and heterogeneous on the T2 image in the right hemisphere and the frontal part of the left one. The hyperintense cortical signal of the right hemisphere on the T1 image is related to laminar necrosis and was not discernible from ischaemic deeper lesions on T2 images. The hyperintensity of the posterior part of the left hemisphere is related to calcified ischaemic lesions which were not depicted on T2 images

tually, as mentioned above, for technical reasons, some lesions, especially small lesions with a short T2, cannot be depicted by ultrafast T2 sequences.

Myelination is not as clearly shown as on T1-weighted images. Calcifications, some types of haemorrhagic lesions, subependymal nodules in tuberous sclerosis (see Chaps. 9, 14) may be completely overlooked by this type of sequence (Fig. 1). Therefore, whenever not only the anatomy of the brain but also the parenchyma has to be evaluated, which is nearly always, it is indispensable not to rely on ultrafast T2 images but to add other sequences.

T1-Weighted Sequences

Technique

Fast gradient-echo sequences with low flip angles (fast low-angle shot: FLASH sequence) are used to obtain T1-weighted images. Spoiler gradients are applied to reduce residual transverse magnetization. In this type of sequence, all images are acquired simultaneously over the entire duration of the sequence so that all images can be altered if fetal motion occurs during the data acquisition.

In addition, the acquisition time is markedly longer than for ultrafast T2-weighted sequences and may reach 1 or 2 min. Therefore, fetal sedation is recommended for this type of sequence to reduce fetal motion [5–7].

Advantages and Drawbacks

T1-weighted imaging becomes increasingly valuable with the progression of pregnancy because developing myelination shortens T1-relaxation [5]. It has been proved that this type of sequence is valuable for evaluation of fetal brain maturation (see Chap. 4).

Moreover, T1-weighted imaging has proved to be valuable for detecting intra- or pericerebral haemorrhage [15]. However, some chronic small haemorrhagic lesions may be overlooked (Fig. 2): microcalcifications (in laminar necrosis, calcified leucomalacia) (see Chap. 14) (Fig. 1), fat in pericallosal lipomas (see Chap. 8) or subependymal nodules in tuberous sclerosis (see Chap. 9) that are detected as hyperintense foci on T1-weighted images in fetuses and infants.

However, fetal neuroanatomy is less well depicted by T1-weighted images than by ultrafast T2-weighted images, and there is sometimes little difference in intrinsic signal intensity between the different cerebral structures. Moreover, as mentioned above, fetal and maternal motion artefacts are still a problem with this type of sequence.

Applications

T1-weighted sequences are recommended as soon as a precise study of the fetal cerebral parenchyma is necessary, that is in most of the following cases: suspicion of haemorrhagic and/or ischaemic lesions in the context of ventriculomegaly (the most frequent indication for fetal MRI), intrauterine growth retardation with Doppler abnormalities, cytomegalovirus (CMV) or toxoplasmosis seroconversion, a twin-twin transfusion or follow-up of in utero death of a monozygotic twin, cerebral arteriovenous malformation, etc.

This list is not exhaustive, and as already mentioned, lipomas and subependymal nodules in tuberous sclerosis are also well depicted with T1-weighted images.

Besides these two types of sequences (ultrafast T2 images and T1-weighted images), other sequences may also be added.

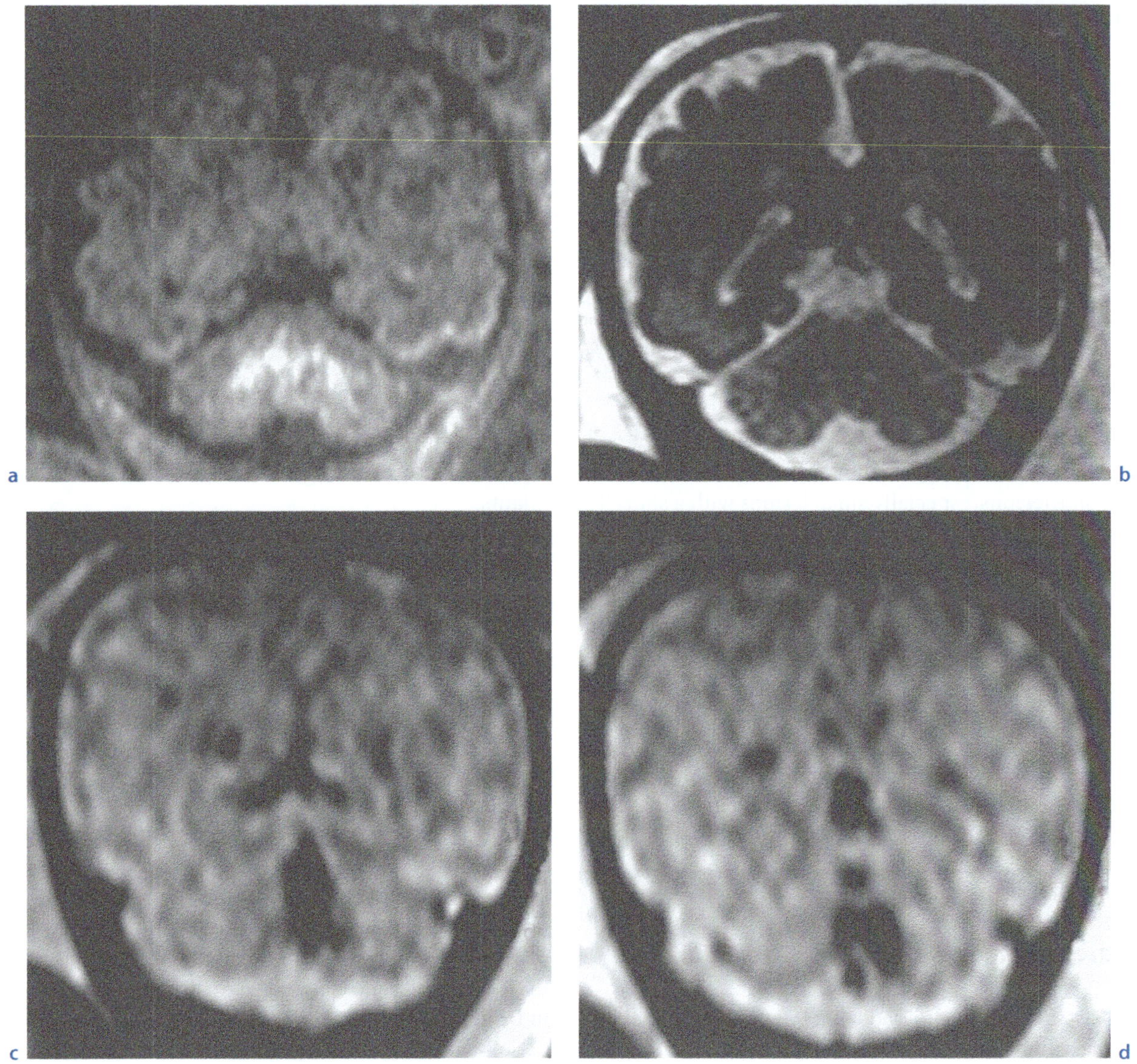

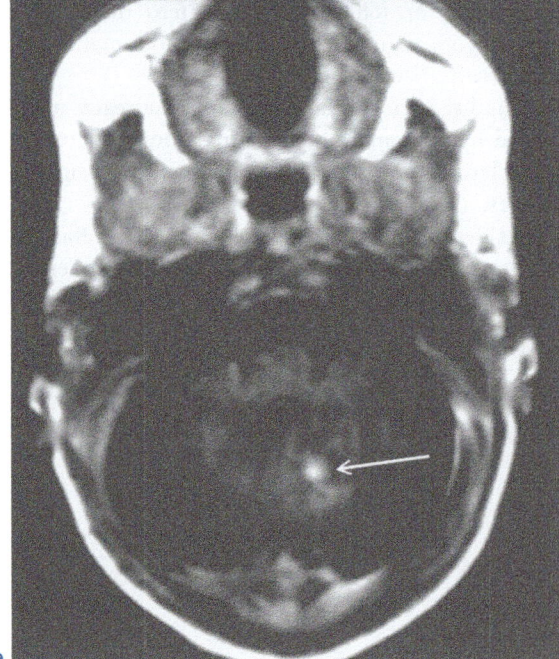

Fig. 2a–e. A 33-week-old fetus. Capillary telangiectasia angioma of the cerebellum (**a–c**). Coronal T1 (**a**), T2 (**b**) and T2* (**c, d**) slice at the level of the atria. No abnormality is detected on T1- and T2-weighted slices. On T2* images, a marked hyposignal is visible in the vermis and the medial part of the left cerebellar hemisphere. It is related to silent microbleeds in a capillary telangiectasia which is visible (*arrow*) on the T1-weighted transverse slice (**e**) acquired after birth after gadolinium injection

Gradient-Echo T2-Weighted Sequences

Technique

Gradient-echo T2* imaging is applied with a long TE and/or a gradient echoplanar technique. Haemosiderin deposits or calcifications create a magnetic dipole that generates an interference on intravoxel parameters and is responsible for a signal loss.

The longer the TE, the more easily haemosiderin deposits are detected [16].

Advantages and Drawbacks

This type of sequence assesses the skull, facial osteocartilaginous structures and the spine. Moreover, it is very accurate for detecting chronic haemorrhagic lesions or silent cerebral microbleeds with haemosiderin deposits (Fig. 2) and calcifications. Conversely, it has a low signal-to-noise ratio and provides a poor depiction of cerebral anatomy and parenchyma.

Applications

Gradient-echo T2-weighted sequences are indicated when there is a suspicion of haemorrhagic lesions or calcifications (in some ischaemic lesions). They must necessarily be combined with ultrafast T2-weighted and T1-weighted images.

Diffusion Tensor Imaging

Technique

The goal of diffusion tensor imaging is to study the diffusion of water in the cerebral parenchyma, which is evaluated by measuring the apparent diffusion coefficient (ADC) and the anisotropy fraction (AF) in the cerebral parenchyma.

Transverse slices of the fetal brain are acquired with a multishot echo planar imaging (EPI) sequence with diffusion gradient (amplitude: 30 mT/m, b: 600 s/mm^2) applied in six noncolinear axes (acquisition time ~1 min).

ADC and AF are measured in different anatomical regions that are easily spotted so that the measurements are reliable: basal ganglia, frontal white matter, corpus callosum, cerebral peduncles.

Applications

Diffusion tensor imaging has been evaluated in neonates [17, 18] but is not currently used in fetuses. It could assess microstructural changes of fetal cerebral white matter related to maturation and myelination. Normal data have been established in a small series [19]. Our preliminary results [20] indicate significantly different ADC values in different anatomical locations [frontal white matter (1.8 μm^2/ms), genu corpus callosum (1.3 μm^2/ms), peduncular pyramidal tract (1.2 μm^2/ms)]. A significant ADC decrease and FA increase is observed with progression of pregnancy in relation with progressing myelination.

In the future, evaluation of such data could be useful in the detection of ischaemic lesions that could be overlooked by classic fetal imaging sequences (see Chap. 14). It could also be useful in the assessment of white matter microstructure and myelination, and in the assessment of oedema (intra- versus extracellular oedema). Moreover, in the future, some parenchymal lesions due to abnormal metabolism or limited blood supply could also be detected by proton MR spectroscopy because of alteration of fetal cerebral metabolism.

Gadolinium Injection

Gadolinium crosses the placenta, enters the fetal circulation and is excreted by the fetal kidneys into the bladder and then into the amniotic fluid. It is then swallowed by the fetus and these repeated cycles of excretion and reabsorption lengthen the half-life of gadolinium. Adverse effects (retarded development, skeletal and visceral abnormalities) have been observed in rats after high doses of gadolinium [5]. Consequently, even if no proof of any deleterious effect of gadolinium in pregnant women exists, it is recommended not to use it for fetal MRI. However, it has been used to evaluate placental abnormalities [21, 22].

Conclusion

Fetal MRI techniques are currently undergoing rapid development and provide more and more information about the fetal brain. The development of ultrafast T2-weighted sequences has certainly contributed enormously to extending the applications of fetal MRI and spreading this technique. However, the limits of the different sequences must be kept in mind in order to use them properly in the evaluation of the fetal brain.

Materials

Screening of cerebral abnormalities is the main field of investigation of fetal MRI [23–49]. However, unlike ultrasonography, fetal MRI is currently not a routine examination in antenatal diagnosis. In our antenatal diagnosis reference centre, the indications for fetal MRI examinations are decided during our weekly multidisciplinary staff meetings. In view of establishing standards, we selected 225 examination results concerning fetuses aged from 22 to 38 weeks of gestation among the 600 fetal cerebral MRI examinations our institution has carried out from 1991 to 2000. Gestational age was determined in each case by a precocious sonography at 12 weeks of gestation.

Some of these MRIs were carried out on a suspicion, based on sonographic observations, of a cerebral malformation that was not confirmed by MRI study. Most fetuses, however, were deemed to have normal brains by sonographic examination, both in terms of biometric data and morphological study. The MRI examinations of these fetuses were carried out as part of exploration protocols of risk situations possibly involving cerebral pathologies: cleft lip and/ or palate, decrease in the fetuses' movements, bilateral clubfoot, antecedents of cerebral anomalies in the sibship, hydramnios, and observation of cardiac rhabdomyomas. Cerebral MRIs of these fetuses were considered normal. In the cases where the pregnancy was medically terminated because of an extracerebral pathology, the fetuses' neurofetopathological examinations were normal. In the other cases, the postnatal follow-up revealed no neurological particularities, whether the follow-up was clinical (ranging from 1 to 3 years in length), sonographic (by transfontanellar sonography), or by MRI.

The examinations with too many artefacts were left out of the study. Sometimes, however, only one sequence had artefacts. We then kept the rest of the examinations for our study, which accounts for the variations in the number of cases, notably for the analysis of sulci. All cases of ventriculomegaly, however mild (AD between 10 and 15 mm), were excluded.

We also voluntarily excluded twin pregnancies from the study. Indeed, a delay in gyration ranging between 2 and 3 weeks was described in fetuses aged between 19 and 32 weeks of gestation in comparison with monofetal pregnancies [50]. Thus, it was not possible to include these fetuses in a study destined to establish a reference atlas of normal fetal cerebral MRI. Moreover, the study took into account neither the fetuses' sexes nor the side of the brain (left or right hemisphere). In his study [50], Chi noticed a clear left–right asymmetry in the development of some sulci, but did not point out any difference between the brains of male and female fetuses.

Examinations carried out on fetuses at 22–23 weeks of gestation, 24–25 weeks of gestation and 37–38 weeks of gestation were grouped because of insufficient numbers in these age groups and the absence of significant progression from one week to another of the data collected in these subgroups. Single examinations on each fetus studied aged between 35 and 36 weeks of gestation were only grouped for the biometric study.

The population studied was distributed as follows: eight fetuses in the 22- to 23-gestational-week period, seven fetuses at 24–25 weeks of gestation, five fetuses at 26 weeks of gestation, 16 fetuses at 27 weeks of gestation, 11 fetuses at 28 weeks of gestation, 18 fetuses at 29 weeks of gestation, 24 fetuses at 30 weeks of gestation, 21 fetuses at 31 weeks of gestation, 25 fetuses at 32 weeks of gestation, 20 fetuses at 33 weeks of gestation, 24 fetuses at 34 weeks of gestation, 17 fetuses at 35 weeks of gestation, 11 fetuses at 36 weeks of gestation and 18 fetuses for the last 2 weeks (37–38 weeks of gestation). The distribution of the number of fetuses as a function of the gestational age is represented in the histogram below.

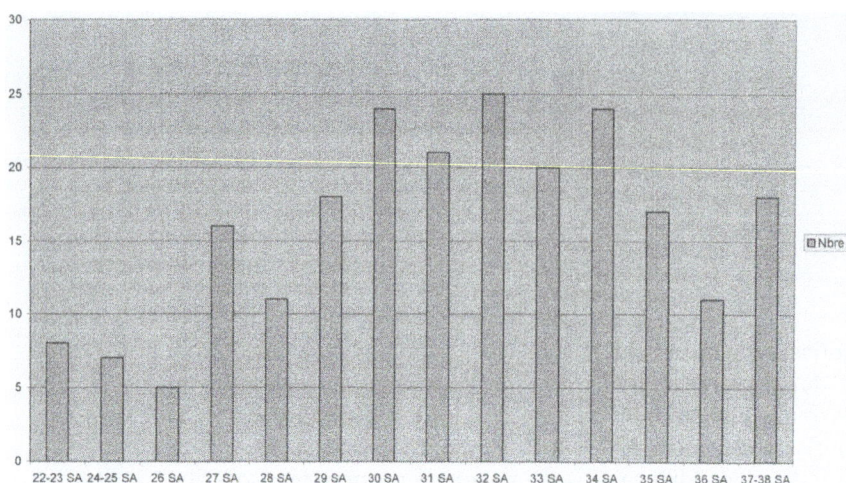

Graph. 1. Number of fetuses studied

Methodology

Examination Protocol

Because this is a cohort study, the fetal MRIs have always been carried out according to a precise standardized protocol, with the slices either parallel or perpendicular to the brain stem.*

Most examinations ($n = 180$) were done on a Gyrex Elscint 0.5-Tesla MRI with a spine coil. Two types of sequences were used: a gradient-echo T1-weighted sequence (parameters: TR, 300 ms; TE, 15 ms; angle, 90°; thickness, 5 mm; field of view, 320 × 320 mm; matrix, 200 × 200; four excitations) preferably in the axial plane, and a T2-weighted sequence of the E-short T2 type (TR, 20 ms; TE, 9.2 ms; angle, 70°; thickness, 5 mm; matrix 200 × 200; 12 excitations). These two sequences form the basis for this atlas (for biometry, chronology of the appearance of sulci, and myelination); they were therefore used in nearly all the examinations. Other sequences have also been used, notably thick E-short-weighted sequences, which give a surface image.

Furthermore, 45 examinations were carried out on a Philips Intera 1.5-Tesla unit, essentially using T2-weighted sequences with single-shot acquisition: T2-SSh-TSE (TR, 24,617 ms; TE, 100 ms; angle, 90°; thickness, 3 mm; field of view, 280 × 280 mm; matrix, 256; one or two excitations; turbo factor, 84 mm; synergy abdomen or surface coil, 25 slices in 19–24 s). This type of sequence is now the most widely used, as the reliability, resolution and contrast are better. Since these last examinations were of better quality than the previous ones, it is essentially these that were used to illustrate the T2-weighted slices in this atlas.

Reference Slices

The fetuses' brains were explored in the three spatial planes (sagittal, coronal and axial). Our study is based on the analysis on each fetus of nine slices we consider as the most representative of the fetal brain:

- Two sagittal slices:
  - A T2-weighted midline sagittal slice (no. 1)
  - A T1-, or more frequently T2-weighted parasagittal slice, at the level of the sylvian fissure (no. 3)
- Four T2-weighted coronal slices parallel to the axis of the brain stem:
  - An anterior slice, at the anterior part of the frontal lobes (no. 4)
  - A slice at the level of the third ventricle (no. 5)
  - A slice at the level of the lateral ventricles' temporal horns (no. 6)
  - A slice at the level of the ventricular atria (no. 7)
- Three axial slices perpendicular to the axis of the brain stem:
  - A T1-weighted slice at the level of the fourth ventricle (no. 8)
  - A T1-weighted slice at the level of the third ventricle (no. 9)
  - A slice at the level of the vertex, most frequently T2-weighted (no. 10)

For some fetuses, a few slices were not interpretable regarding either biometry or the analysis of gyration or myelination. This explains the fluctuations in the number of cases from the study of one parameter to another.

---

* For each examination, fetal sedation was obtained by oral administration of flunitrazepam (1 mg) approximately 20 min before the examination so as to decrease fetal movement. This type of sedation is the most commonly used. It must be remembered that in this domain fetal MRI raises the question of innocuousness. Currently, clinical and experimental research [2, 3] has not demonstrated harmful effects to the fetus brought on by MRI. However, in the United States, the National Radiological Protection Board recommend that MRI should not be used during the first trimester. In addition, usage dictates that gadolinium should not be injected until it has been proved that it is innocuous during pregnancy. (See chapter 1)

Moreover, we have added a parasagittal slice (no. 2) at the level of the lateral ventricle, nearly always T2-weighted. This slice was not systematically studied for all fetuses but seemed valuable for studying gyration of the convexity.

An example of each one of these slices is laid out in the following pages, facing the corresponding neuropathological slice. The various anatomical structures recognizable on those slices that were used in the making of this atlas are indicated.

Fetopathology: MRI Correlation of the Ten Reference Slices

Figs. 1–20. Slices 1–10

Fig. 1. Slice 1. Fetopathological slice at 39 weeks of gestation

1 Secondary cingular sulci

2 Cingular sulcus

3 Marginal sulcus

4 Internal parieto-occipital fissure

5 Calcarina fissure

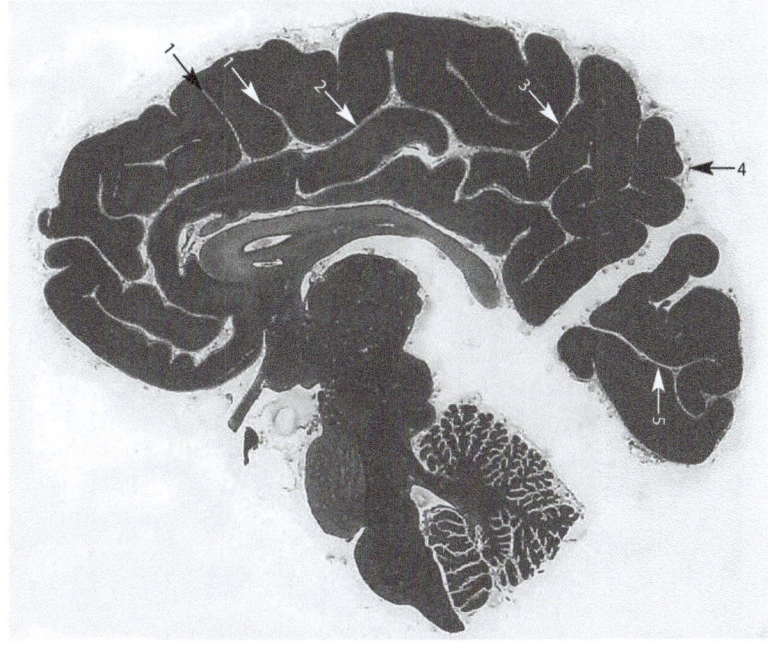

Fig. 2. Slice 1. MRI slice at 34 weeks of gestation

1 Cingular sulcus

2 Marginal sulcus

3 Internal parieto-occipital fissure

4 Calcarina fissure

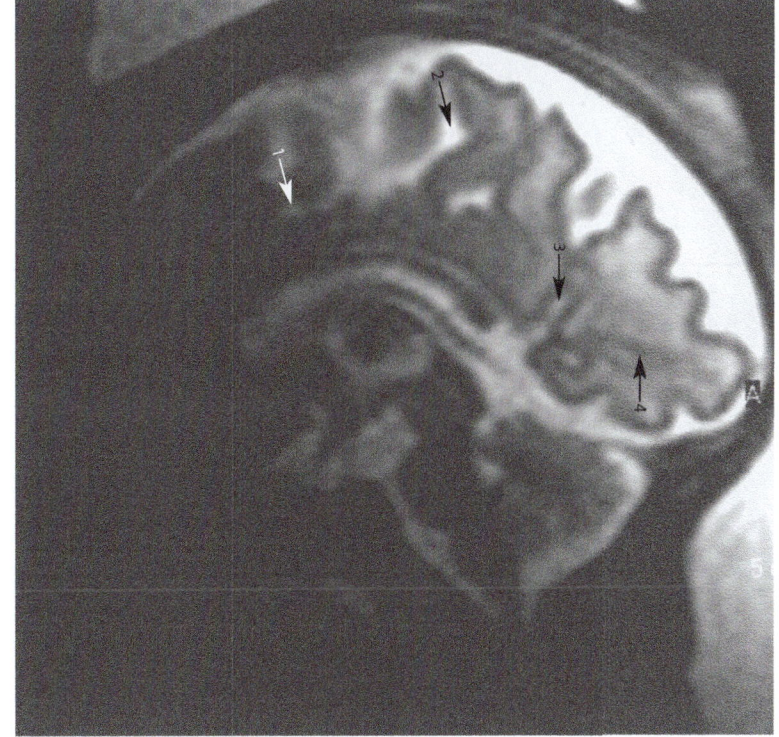

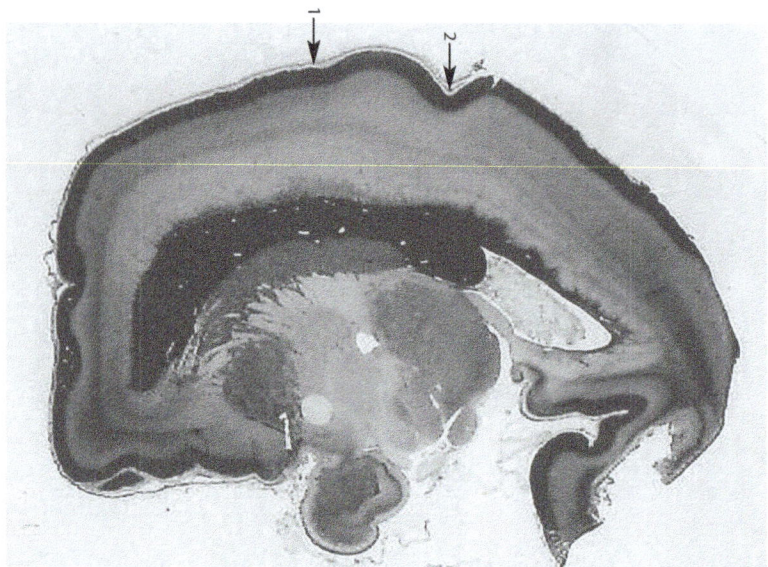

Fig. 3. Slice 2. Fetopathological slice at 24–25 weeks of gestation

1 Central sulcus

2 Postcentral sulcus

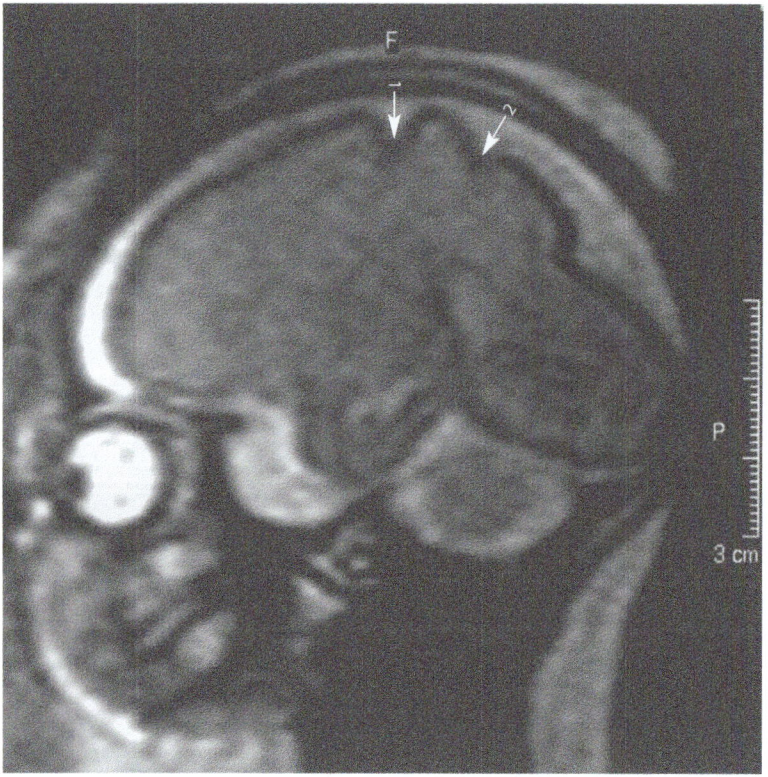

Fig. 4. Slice 2. MRI slice at 26 weeks of gestation

1 Central sulcus

2 Postcentral sulcus

Fig. 5. Slice 3. Fetopathological slice at 24–25 weeks of gestation

1 Lateral sulcus (whose banks delimit the sylvian fissure)

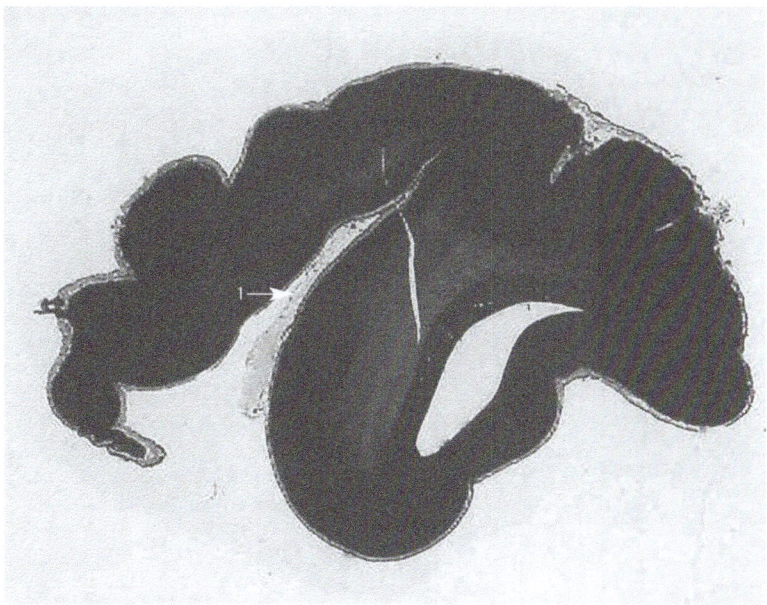

Fig. 6. Slice 3. MRI slice at 24–25 weeks of gestation

1 Lateral sulcus (whose banks delimit the sylvian fissure)

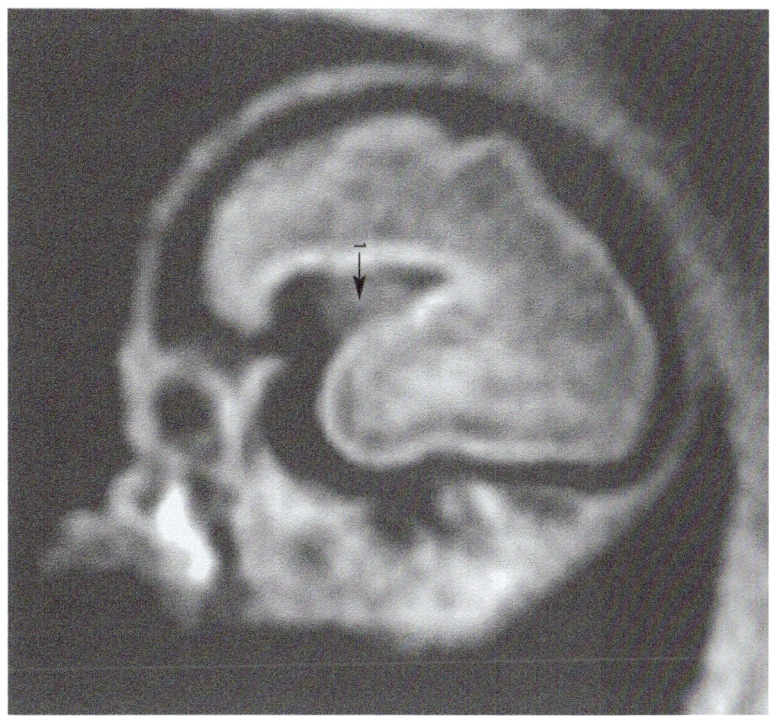

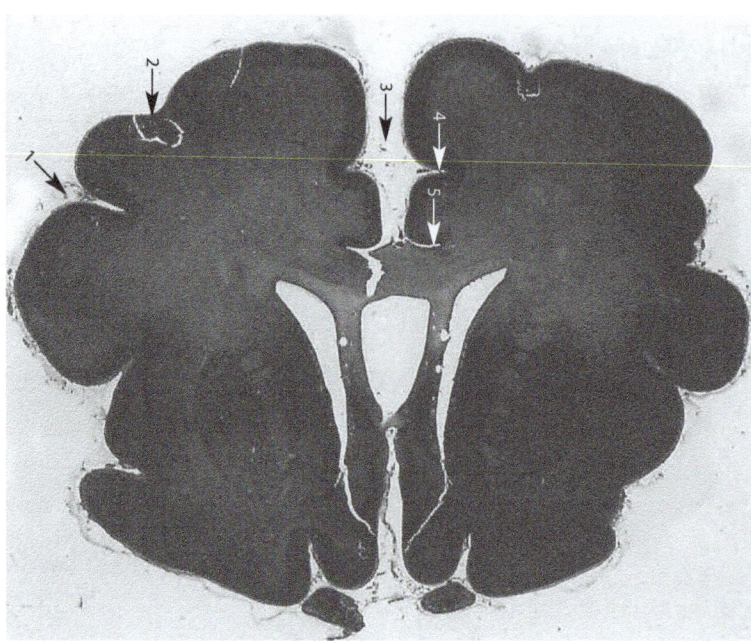

Fig. 7. Slice 4. Fetopathological slice at 27 weeks of gestation

1 Inferior frontal sulcus

2 Superior frontal sulcus

3 Interhemispheric fissure

4 Cingular sulcus

5 Callosal sulcus

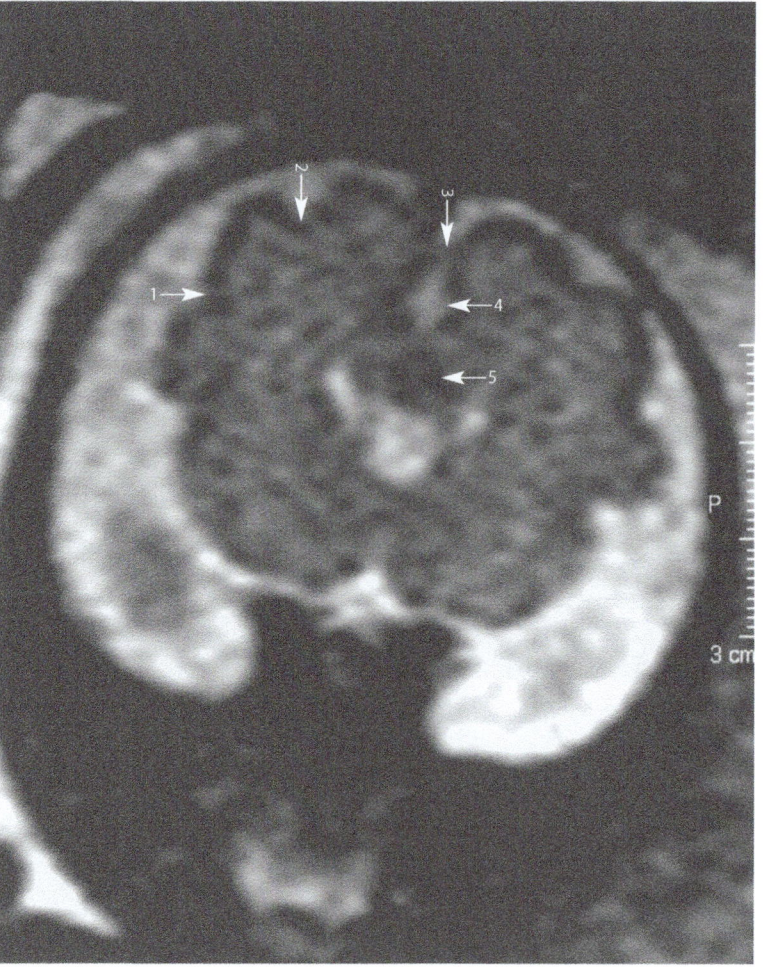

Fig. 8. Slice 4. MRI slice at 29 weeks of gestation

1 Inferior frontal sulcus

2 Superior frontal sulcus

3 Interhemispheric fissure

4 Cingular sulcus

5 Callosal sulcus

Fig. 9. Slice 5. Fetopathological slice at 32 weeks of gestation

1 Callosal sulcus

2 Cingular sulcus

3 Superior temporal sulcus

4 Inferior temporal sulcus

5 External occipitemporal sulcus

6 Hippocampal fissure

7 Third ventricle

8 Collateral sulcus

9 Lateral sulcus

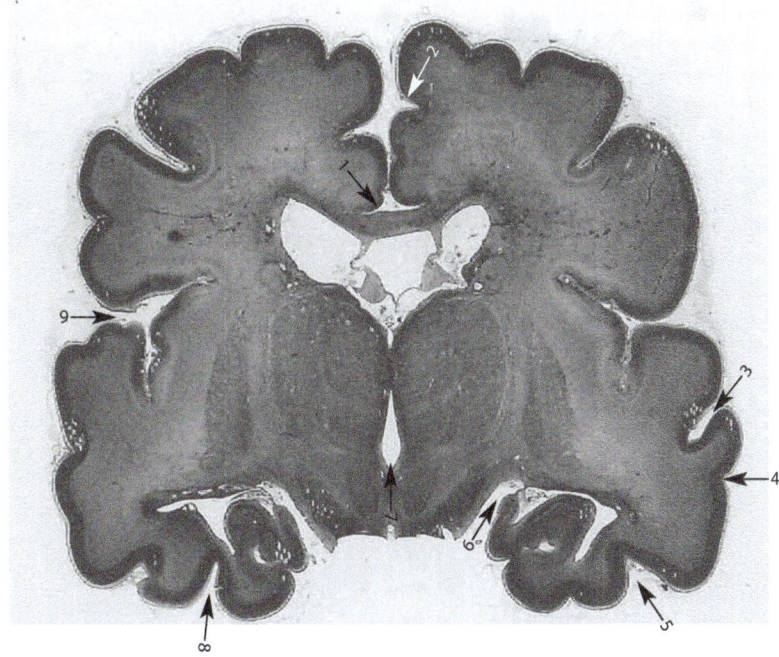

Fig. 10. Slice 5. MRI slice at 33 weeks of gestation

1 Callosal sulcus

2 Cingular sulcus

3 Superior temporal sulcus

4 Inferior temporal sulcus

5 Hippocampal fissure

6 Third ventricle

7 Collateral sulcus

8 Lateral sulcus

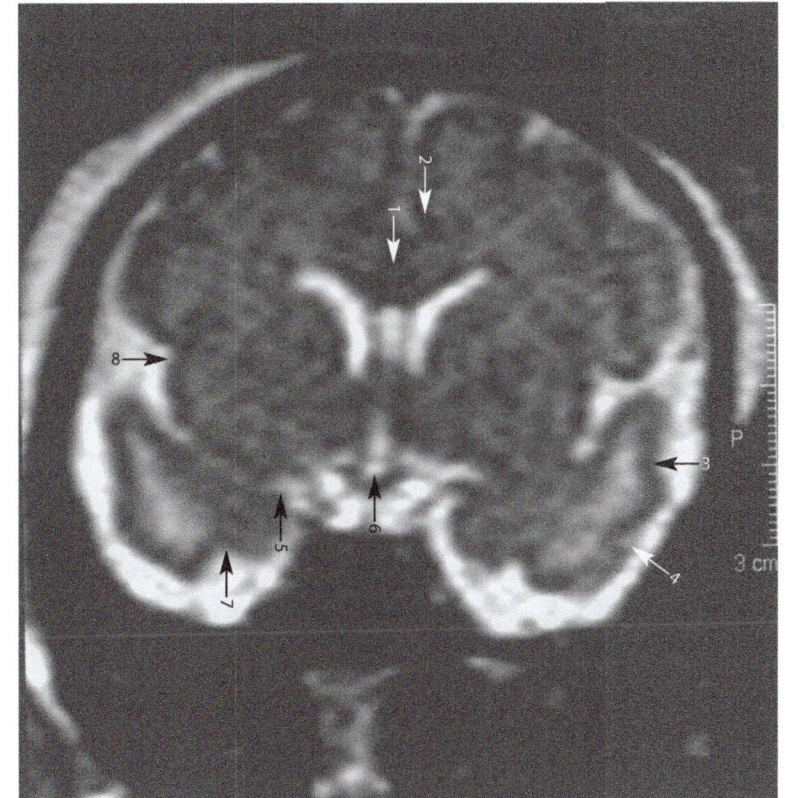

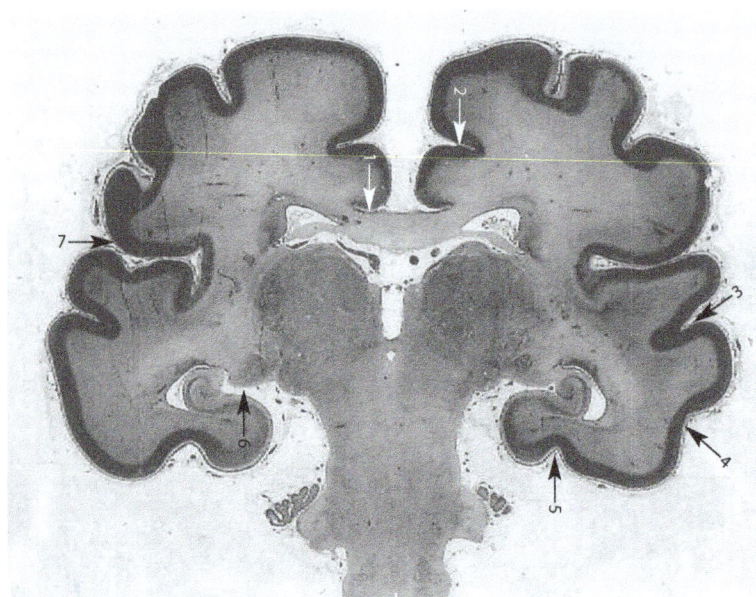

Fig. 11. Slice 6. Fetopathological slice at 30 weeks of gestation

1 Callosal sulcus

2 Cingular sulcus

3 Superior temporal sulcus

4 Inferior temporal sulcus

5 Collateral sulcus

6 Hippocampal fissure

7 Lateral sulcus

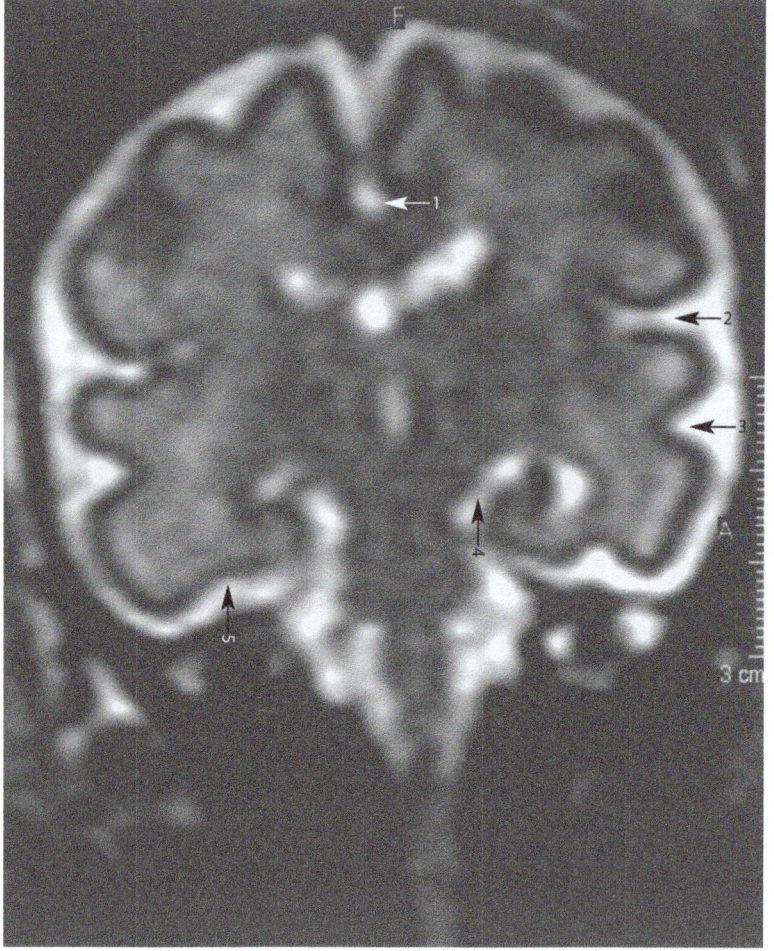

Fig. 12. Slice 6. MRI slice at 31 weeks of gestation

1 Cingular sulcus

2 Lateral sulcus

3 Superior temporal sulcus

4 Hippocampal fissure

5 Collateral sulcus

Fig. 13. Slice 7. Fetopathological slice at 30 weeks of gestation

1 Intraparietal sulcus

2 Atrium

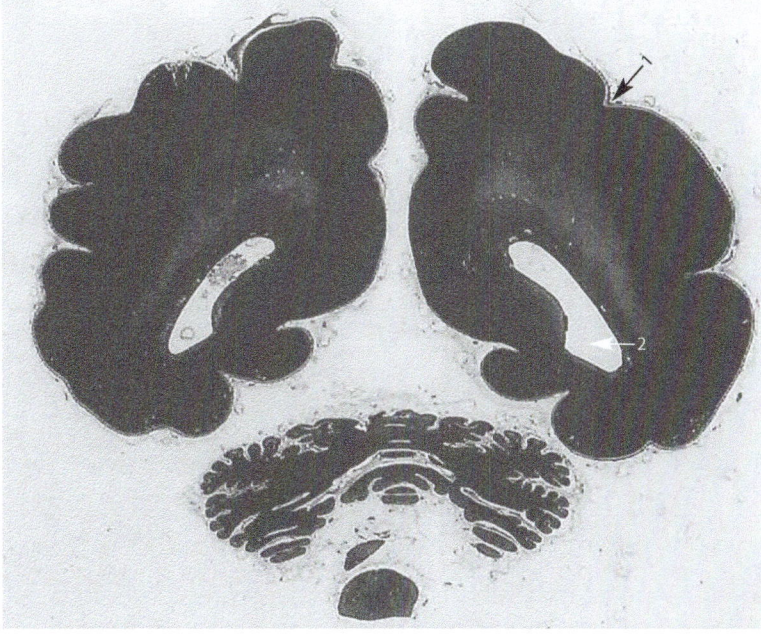

Fig. 14. Slice 7. MRI slice at 31 weeks of gestation

1 Intraparietal sulcus

2 Atrium

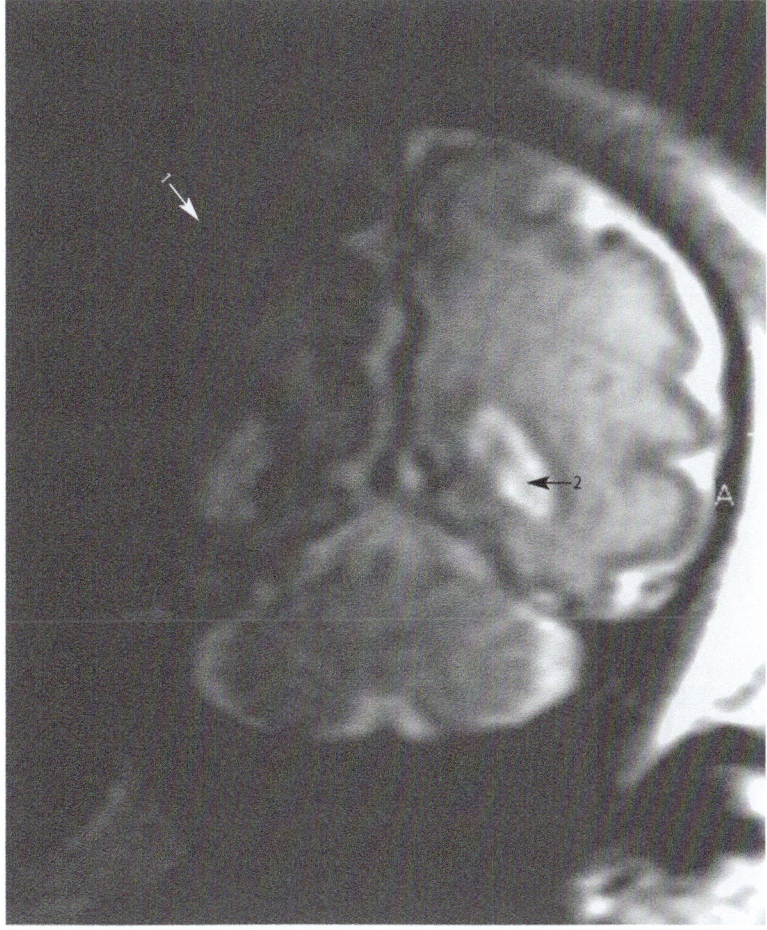

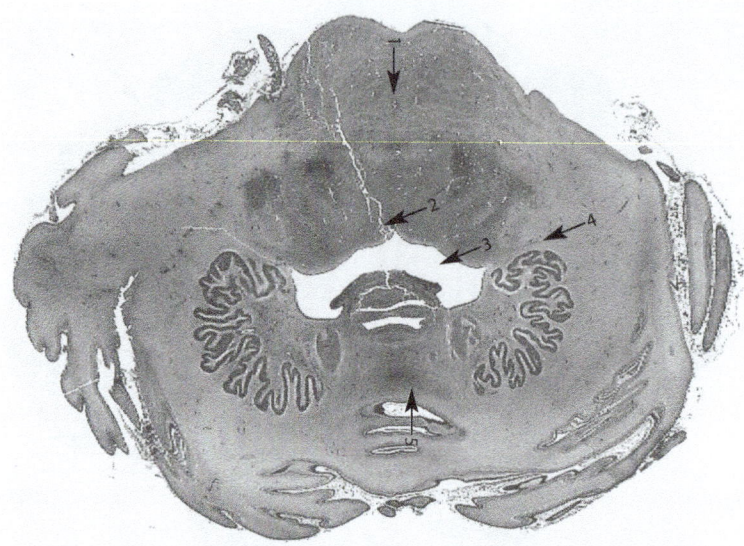

Fig. 15. Slice 8. Fetopathological slice at 27 weeks of gestation

1 Pons

2 Tegmentum

3 Fourth ventricle

4 Middle cerebellar peduncle

5 Vermis

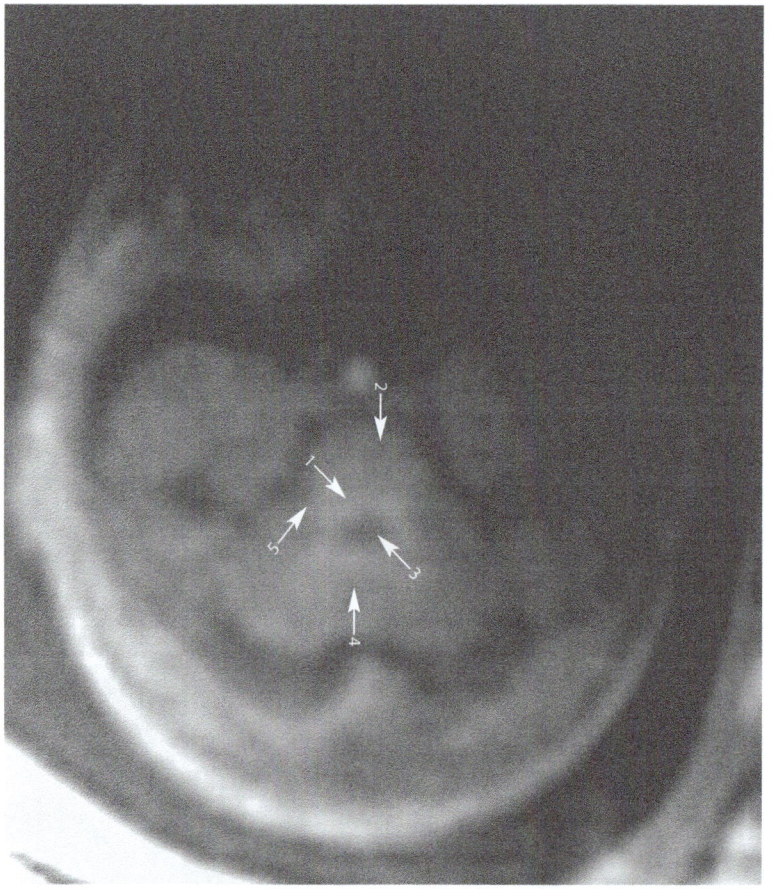

Fig. 16. Slice 8. MRI slice at 27 weeks of gestation

1 Tegmentum

2 Pons

3 Fourth ventricle

4 Vermis

5 Middle cerebellar peduncle

Fig. 17. Slice 9. Fetopathological slice at 39 weeks of gestation

1 Internal capsule, anterior limb

2 Internal capsule, posterior limb

3 Thalamus

4 Globus pallidus

5 Putamen

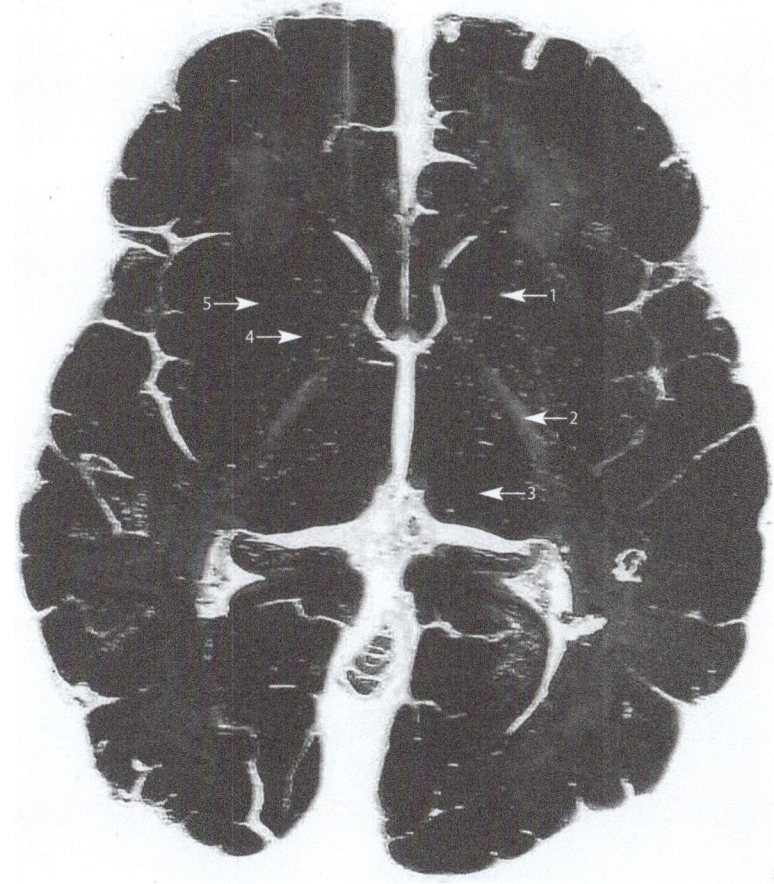

Fig. 18. Slice 9. MRI slice at 37–38 weeks of gestation

1 Globus pallidus

2 Thalamus

3 Internal capsule, posterior limb

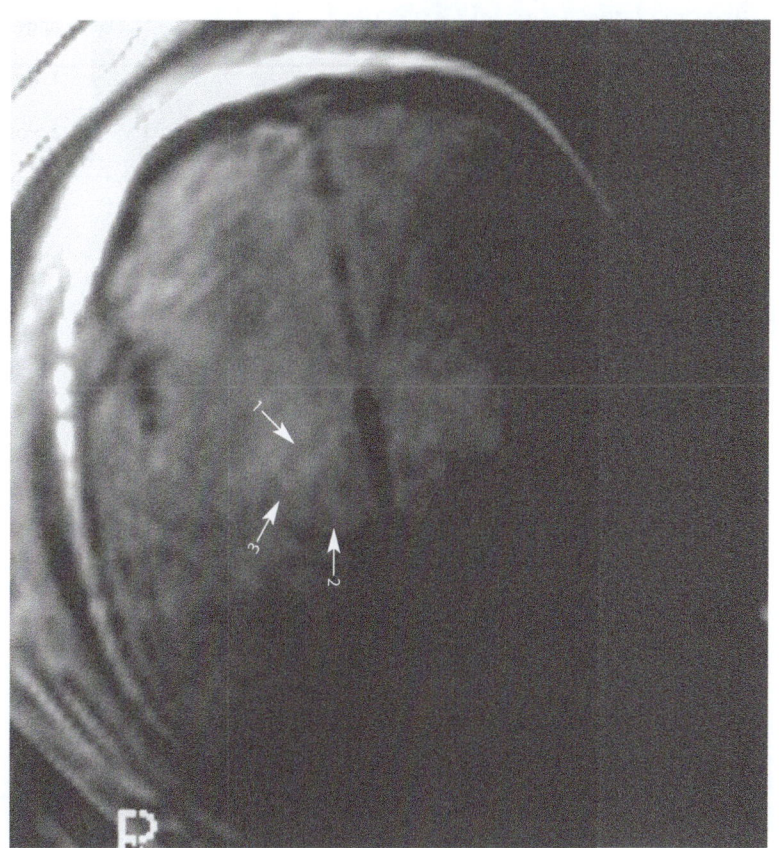

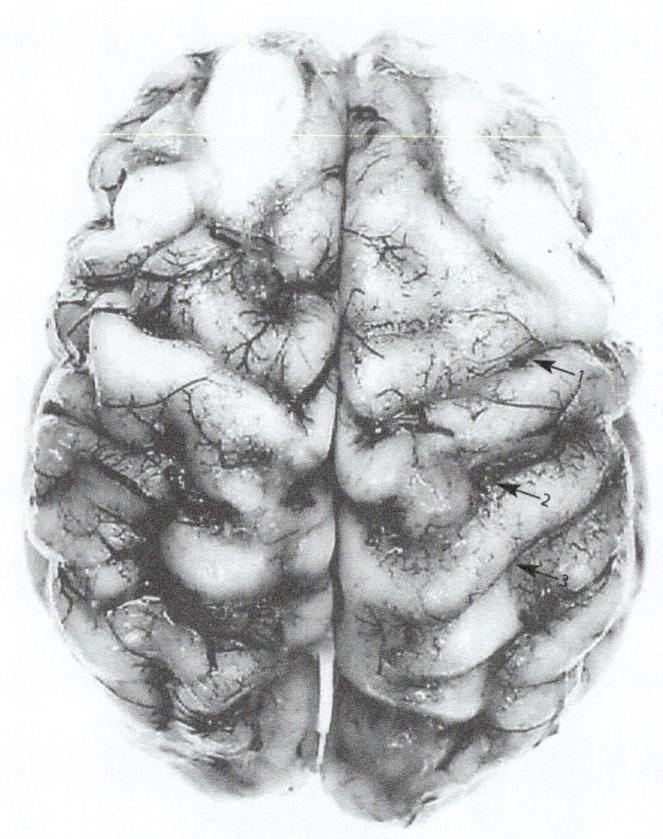

Fig. 19. Slice 10. Fetopathological slice at 29 weeks of gestation

1 Precentral sulcus

2 Central sulcus

3 Postcentral sulcus

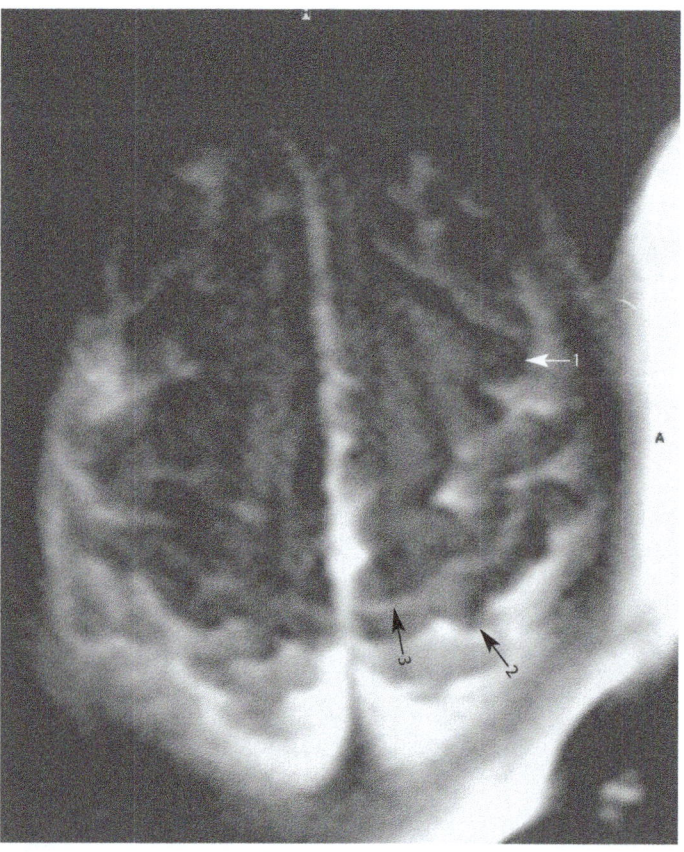

Fig. 20. Slice 10. MRI slice at 33 weeks of gestation

1 Precentral sulcus

2 Postcentral sulcus

3 Central sulcus

Biometric Study

The biometric study involves measurements of various cerebral structures. Most of these measurements were made on the examination console, systematically for all fetuses. Other measurements were taken a posteriori from films: these are the older examinations, or measurements that were not systematically made in each examination (diameters of the 3rd and 4th ventricles, interopercular distances, and interhemispheric distance).

The statistical study of biometrical data was conducted under the supervision of Doctor J. Bloch, senior reader in the Public Health and Biostatistics Department at the Hôpital Robert Debré. It comprises a calculation of the mean (accurate to one decimal place), the standard deviation (to two decimal places), and the 10th, 25th, 50th, 75th and 90th percentiles (to the unit). The minimum and maximum values are also shown. The choice of this statistical method is based on the relatively limited number of cases studied for each week of gestation. Out of concern for precision, we did not want to use smoothing methods; we opted instead for presenting the results in their raw state. The subjects of analysis and reading of these results will be widely addressed in Chap. 5.

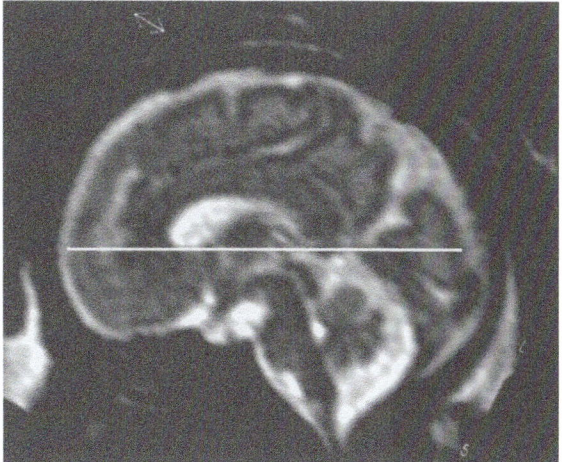

Fig. 21

Fronto-occipital Diameter (Fig. 21)

Fronto-occipital diameter (FOD) is measured on the midline sagittal slice (slice no. 1) as the distance between the extreme points of the frontal and occipital lobes.

Measurement of the FOD is an undeniable asset of fetal MRI when compared to antenatal ultrasonography. Indeed, when associated with measurement of the cerebral biparietal diameter, it enables a proper valuation of the fetal brain, since, unlike sonography, it eliminates the measurement errors linked with the broadening of pericerebral space. The joint estimation of these two measurements makes it possible to take into account possible variations in cerebral shape linked with the contours of the skull (notably by dolicho- or brachycephaly).

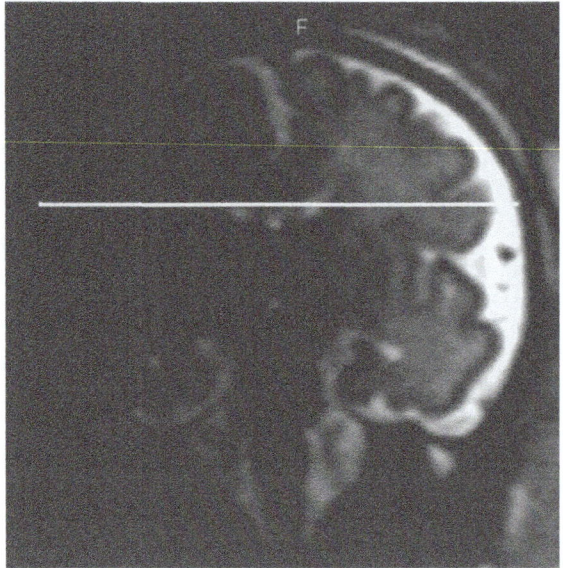

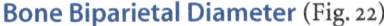

Fig. 22

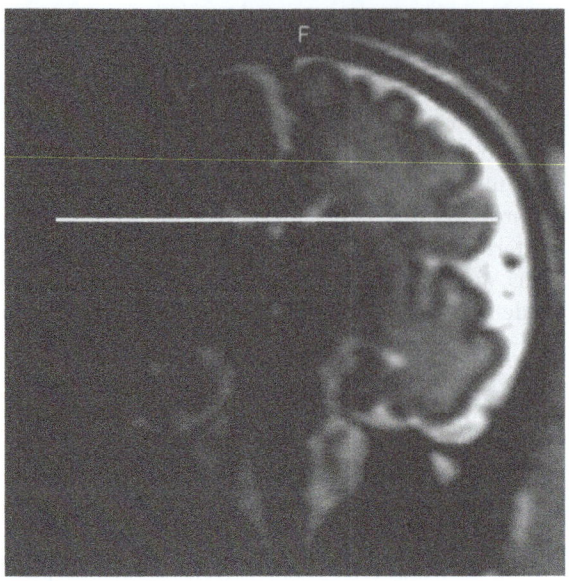

Fig. 23

Bone Biparietal Diameter (Fig. 22)

Bone biparietal diameter (bone BPD) corresponds to the greatest diameter of the skull. It is measured on the coronal slice at the level of the temporal horns of the lateral ventricles (slice no. 6) as the distance between the two internal tables of the skull.

The measurement of the bone BPD corresponds to the BPD in antenatal ultrasonography, and has the same shortcoming: it is an evaluation of the skull rather than of the brain itself. Thus, measurements of the cerebral BPD and the FOD are generally preferred. The difference between the bone and cerebral BPDs, however, is a useful value: the size of pericerebral space, which progressively decreases during pregnancy.

Cerebral Biparietal Diameter (Fig. 23)

Cerebral biparietal diameter (cerebral BPD) is the actual measurement of the greatest transversal diameter of the brain on the coronal slice at the level of the temporal horns of the lateral ventricles (slice no. 6).

Like FOD, it is an undeniable asset of fetal MRI over antenatal sonography. It too enables a good evaluation of the fetal brain by avoiding the measurement errors linked with the broadening of pericerebral space.

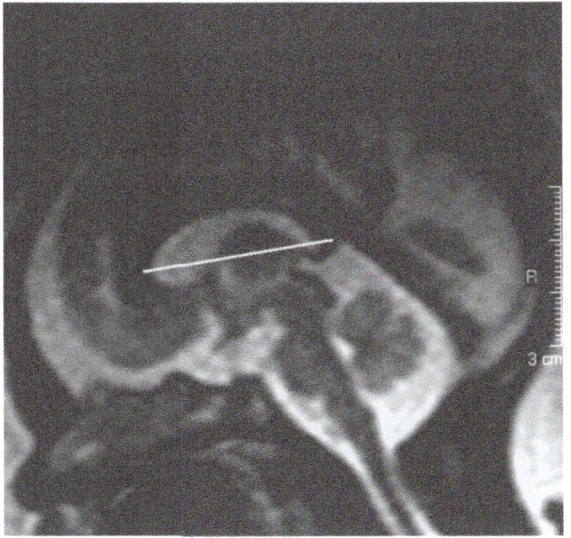

Fig. 24

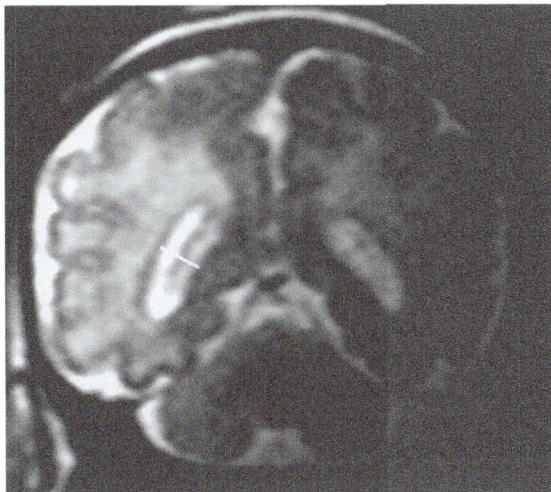

Fig. 25

Length of the Corpus Callosum (Fig. 24)

The corpus callosum is hypointense on T2-weighted sequences. Its length is measured on the midline sagittal slice (slice no. 1), from the genu to the posterior extremity of the splenium.

The LCC/FOD index was calculated to appreciate the relative growth of these two entities.

Due to the limitations of MRI spatial resolution, it is currently impossible to evaluate the corpus callosum's thickness with any reliability.

Lateral Ventricles (Fig. 25)

The transversal diameter of lateral ventricles, or atrial diameter (AD), is measured on the coronal slice at the level of the atria (slice no. 7). It is measured on an axis perpendicular to that of the ventricle, at mid-height of the ventricle's slice.

After the first trimester of pregnancy, the lateral ventricles' size remains stable until term. In common practice, the 10-mm threshold is considered pathological. Ventricular dilatation is deemed mild under 15 mm, and severe beyond 15 mm. The lateral ventricles' frontal horns, which are physiologically thin, are only measured when they broaden.

The AD/cerebral BPD index shows the size of the lateral ventricles relative to the brain.

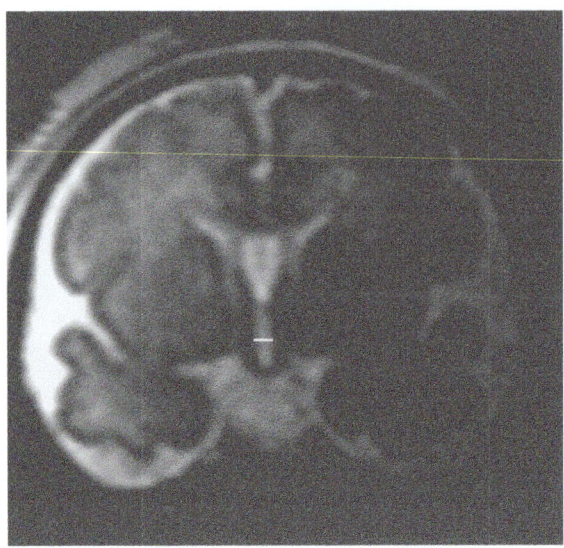

Fig. 26

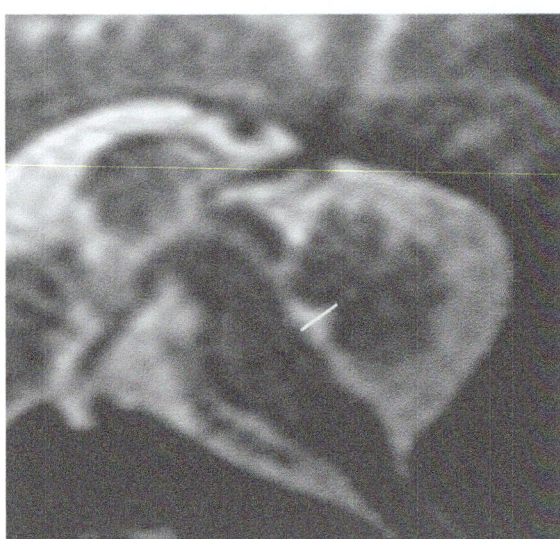

Fig. 27

Third Ventricle (Fig. 26)

The lateral diameter of the third ventricle (DV3) is measured on the coronal T2-weighted slice at the level of this structure (slice no. 5).

The DV3/cerebral BPD index was calculated to assess the relative size of this ventricle in proportion to the brain.

Fourth Ventricle (Fig. 27)

The fourth ventricle of the anteroposterior diameter (DV4) is evaluated on the midline sagittal slice (slice no. 1), between the median parts of its roof and its floor.

The DV4/FOD index was calculated to assess the relative size of the fourth ventricle in proportion to the brain.

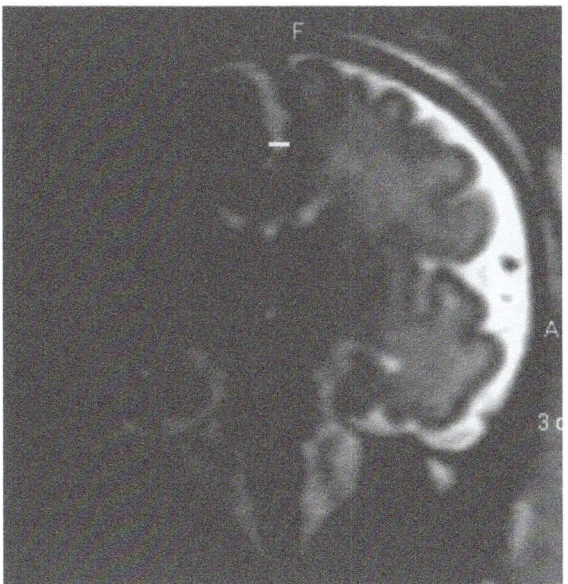

Fig. 28

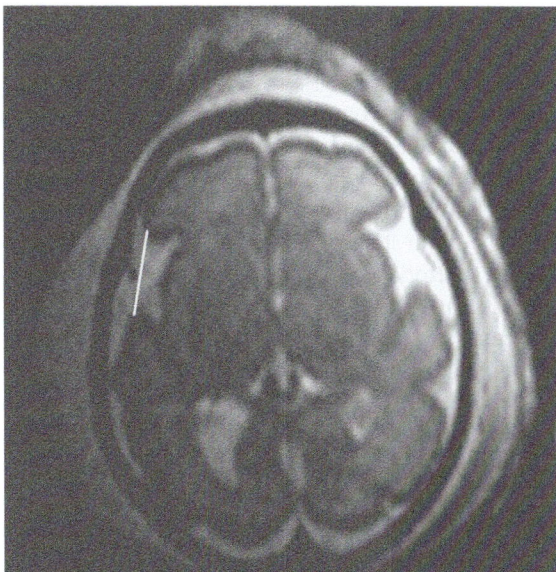

Interhemispheric Distance (Fig. 28)

Interhemispheric distance (IHD) is measured on the coronal slice at the level of the two temporal horns (slice no. 6) between the internal edges of the hemispheres, at an equal distance from the vertex and the corpus callosum, directly above the cingular sulcus.

Along with the measurement of the difference between the bone and cerebral BPDs, it contributes to the evaluation of the pericerebral spaces. The IHD/cerebral BPD ratio shows the size of median pericerebral space in proportion to that of the brain.

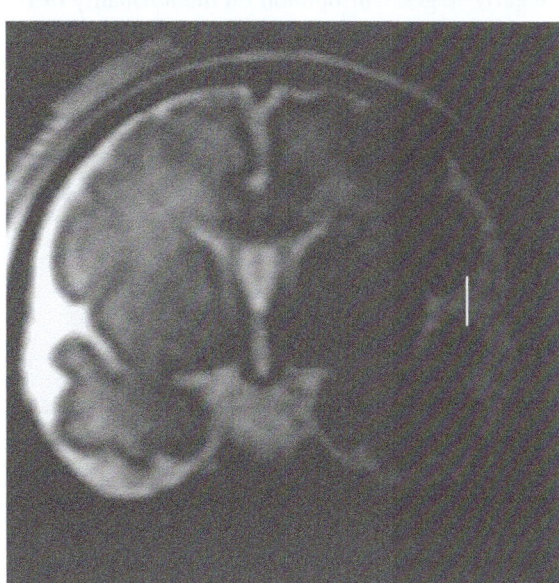

Anteroposterior and Craniocaudal Interopercular Distances (Figs. 29, 30)

Figs. 29, 30

Anteroposterior and craniocaudal interopercular distances (IOPD) are measured on the axial (slice no. 9) and coronal (slice no. 5) slices, respectively, at the level of the third ventricle.

On the axial slice, the distance between the anterior edge and the posterior edge of the sylvian fissure was measured at its most external point.

On the coronal slice, the distance between the superior edge and the inferior edge of the sylvian fissure was measured at its most external point.

Height and Anteroposterior Diameter of the Vermis (Figs. 31, 32)

Height and anteroposterior diameter of the vermis are measured on the midline sagittal slice (slice no. 1).

HV corresponds to the greatest height of the vermis, which is generally more or less parallel to the axis of the brain stem.

The anteroposterior diameter of the vermis (APDV) goes from the median part of the fourth ventricle's roof and corresponds to the greatest anteroposterior diameter.

Because of the vermis's small size, the spatial resolution of fetal MRI cannot currently check the integrity of the vermis by counting its nine lobes. A relatively crude morphological study showed that the visibility of the primary, secondary and horizontal fissures remains somewhat inconsistent, particularly in early stages. Our opinion on the normality of the vermis is therefore mainly based on biometric data: height, anteroposterior diameter and surface.

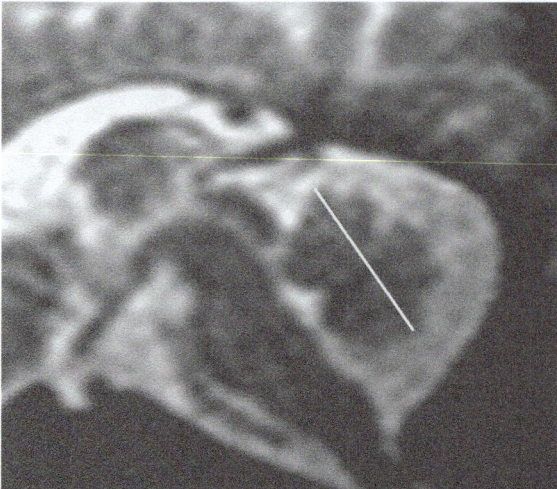

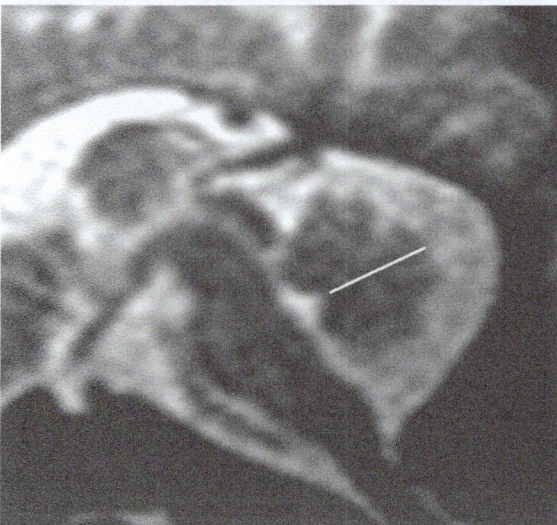

Figs. 31, 32

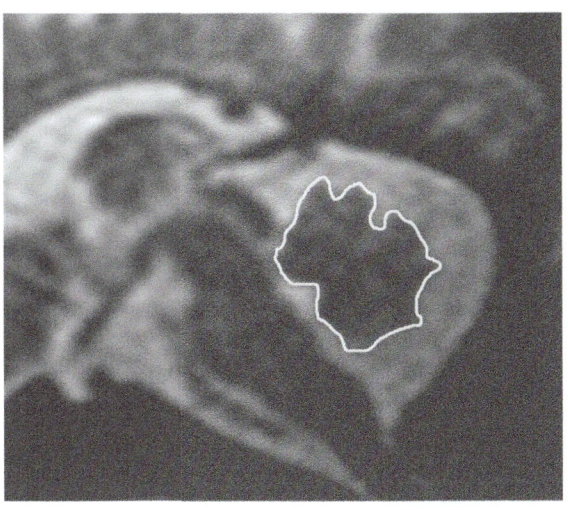

Fig. 33

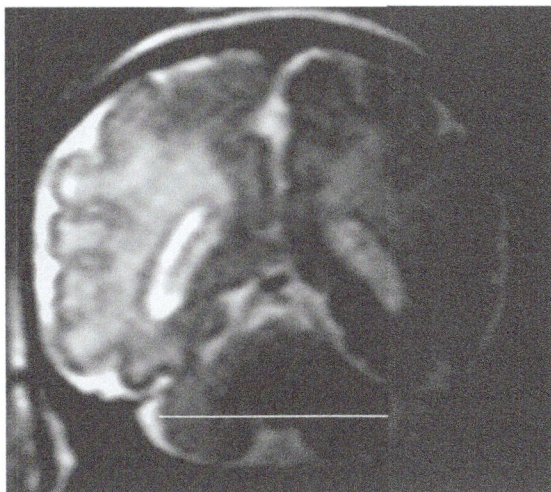

Fig. 34

Surface of the Vermis (Fig. 33)

Measurement of the surface of the vermis (SV) is made by manual computer planimetry on the midline sagittal slice (slice no. 1).

This surface was not at first measured in our study. It was hence taken in a limited number of examinations ($n = 133$) from 28 weeks of gestation. Measurement of the vermis's surface contributes to the estimation of its normality in the absence of reliable morphological criteria in antenatal period.

Transverse Cerebellar Diameter (Fig. 34)

The transverse cerebellar diameter (TCD) is measured on the posterior coronal slice at the level of the atria (slice no. 7). This measurement is superimposable to that obtained by antenatal ultrasonography, but it is more reliable in late stages.

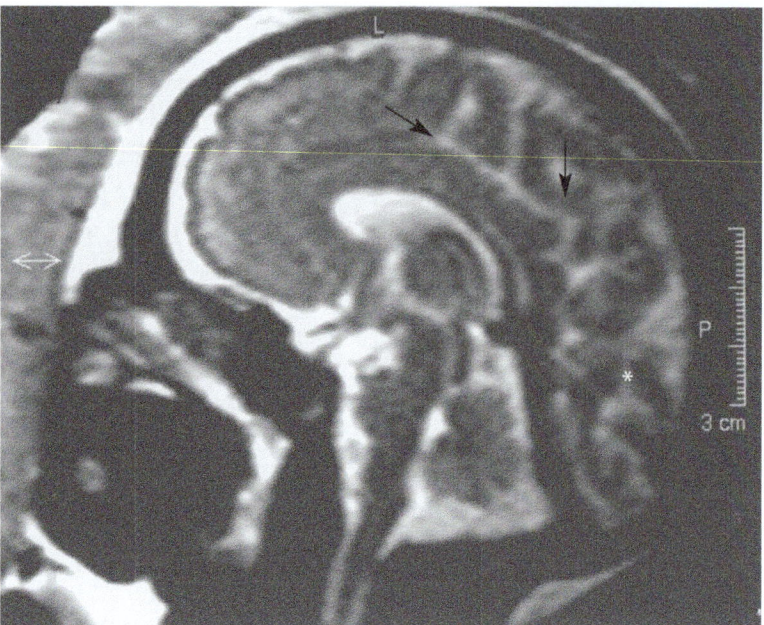

Fig. 35. Slice no. 1 at 35 weeks of gestation

Study of Gyration (Fig. 35–38)

The study of gyration was conducted on all slices except slices nos. 2 and 8. We considered a sulcus was identifiable when we could clearly see an indentation on the surface of the brain. A sulcus is labelled absent when it is identified in less than 25% of cases, detectable when it is visualized in between 25% and 75% of cases and present when it is visible in more than 75% of cases.

The reader is referred to the ten reference slices for the precise anatomy of sulci. The sulci on the internal face of the hemispheres (cingular sulcus, marginal sulcus, callosal sulcus, internal parieto-occipital fissure and calcarine fissure) are best studied on the midline sagittal slice (slice no. 1) and the coronal slices (slices nos. 4–7). These coronal slices also make it possible to study the sulci of the inferior face (hippocampal fissure, collateral sulcus and external occipitotemporal sulcus) and of the external face of the hemispheres (frontal and temporal superior and inferior sulci, intraparietal sulcus).

The sylvian fissure is studied on coronal slice no. 5 and axial slice no. 9. The very lateral parasagittal slice (slice no. 3) gives a morphological overall picture of opercularization.

The central, precentral and postcentral sulci are analysed on the axial slice at the level of the convexity (slice no. 10). These sulci may also be analysed on a parasagittal slice, less lateral than slice no. 3, which was not systematically made for examinations done on the 0.5-Tesla MRI unit (slice no. 2). Although this slice could not be analysed consistently for all the fetuses examined, it was included in this atlas since it can now be fairly easily done in single-shot mode. Using this slice is strongly recommended as an indispensable complement of axial slice no. 10 for the analysis of vertex gyration.

All the sulci whose localizations are given above are primary sulci, i. e. indentations that appear on the brain surface. We have also analysed some secondary sulci, which correspond to secondary ramifications of the primary sulci and appear at a later stage of development.

The cingular (arrows) and occipital (asterisk) secondary sulci are best studied on the midline sagittal slice (slice no. 1) (Fig. 35).

The insular sulci (arrows) appear as undulations on the edges of the sylvian fissure. They are best observed on the slices at the level of the latter (Figs. 36–38).

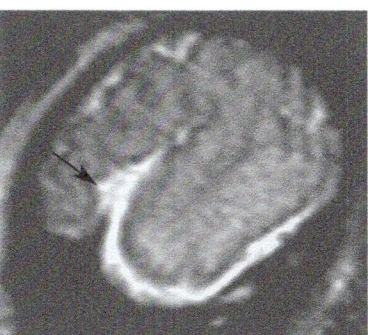

Fig. 36. Slice no. 3 at 33 weeks of gestation

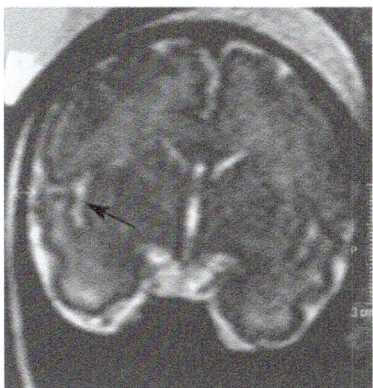

Fig. 37. Slice no. 5 at 35 weeks of gestation

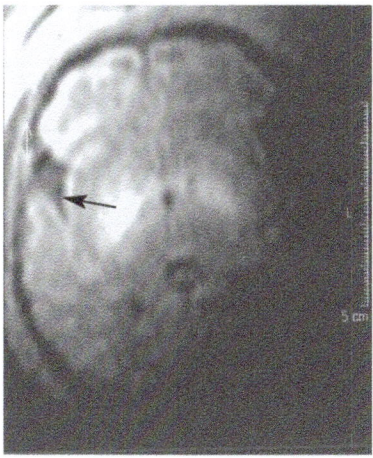

Fig. 38. Slice no. 9 at 34 weeks of gestation

Study of Myelination

Myelination was studied on a T1-weighted sequence of the axial slice at the level of the fourth ventricle (slice no. 8). On this slice, we noted the presence of a hypersignal at the level of the pons, particularly in the tegmentum area, in the vermis and in the middle cerebellar peduncles. The hypersignal is defined as being of an intensity equal to or less than that of the cortex, and greater than that of the white matter of the oval centre.

On axial slice no. 9, we noted the presence of a hypersignal at the level of the internal capsule and basal ganglia.

We have considered that myelination was present where the T1 hypersignal was detected in over 75 % of cases.

Results

We have chosen to present the results in two different manners corresponding to the two possible situations: either the precise stage is known, and one wants to know what morphological aspects one should expect to observe; or the stage is not known and one wants to try and date the pregnancy as precisely as possible based on fetal brain maturation.

Chronological Presentation of the Results by Week of Gestation: From 22–23 Weeks of Gestation to 37–38 Weeks of Gestation

Within each group of fetal MRIs that were made for a given week, we have selected ten slices corresponding to the ten reference slices of this atlas that seemed to be the most representative of that week. **Dr. Laurent Guibaud (Hôpital Debrousse, Lyons) kindly provided us with slices nos. 4–7 at 27 weeks of gestation. On the facing page of these ten slices, the results for each week are presented in a synthetic manner, as follows.

Biometrics

Only the measurements of the fronto-occipital diameter, bone and cerebral biparietal diameters, length of the corpus callosum, height of the vermis, anteroposterior diameter of the vermis, transverse cerebellar diameter and surface of the vermis are shown.

Biometric data for 35 and 36 weeks of gestation were grouped due to the small number of cases in the 36th-gestational-week cohort.

Indeed, we did not consider it useful to overload this voluntarily synthetic presentation, and all the biometric data can be found at the end of this chapter in the form of tables and graphs. The biometrical values given for each week only show the minimum and maximum values found.

The surface of the vermis was not measured on every fetus, and the results are only given for cases after 28 weeks of gestation.

Gyration

For each week, a table gives the list of the absent, detectable and present sulci.

The detectable sulci are presented in an order corresponding to their presence gradient, i.e. the percentage of visualization of these sulci, the most frequently visible sulcus appearing on top. Furthermore, we voluntarily show in bold characters the name of the sulci appearing for the first time in the "Present" column.

Following these results on gyration are a few comments corresponding to the events in gyration we thought should be highlighted.

Myelination and Cellular Migration

These steps of cerebral development manifest themselves in signal modifications in T1-weighted sequences. The main events that can be observed on slices nos. 8 and 9 are briefly overviewed.

22–23 Weeks of Gestation

Biometrics (in mm)

	FOD	Cerebral BPD	Bone BPD	LCC	HV	APDV	TCD
Min–max	60–73	45–55	50–63	28–34	10–12	8–9	22–34

Morphology

At this stage of fetal development, the vermis has finished its rotation and the posterior fossa takes its definitive morphological aspect. The pericerebral space shows a physiological broadening.

Gyration

Sulci present (≥75%)	Sulci detectable (25%–75%)	Sulci absent (<25%)
Interhemispheric fissure	Calcarine fissure	Collateral sulcus
Lateral sulcus[a]	Cingular sulcus	Central sulcus
Internal parieto-occipital fissure	Marginal sulcus	Precentral sulcus
Hippocampal fissure		Postcentral sulcus
Callosal sulcus[b]		Intraparietal sulcus
		Superior temporal sulcus
		Inferior temporal sulcus
		External occipitotemporal sulcus
		Superior frontal sulcus
		Inferior frontal sulcus
		Secondary cingular sulci
		Secondary occipital sulci
		Insular sulci

[a] The sylvian fissure is widely open at this stage.
[b] The callosal sulcus is hardly visible on the represented midline sagittal slice because of partial volume effect, but it is clearly visible on the coronal slice.
The convexity, temporal and frontal lobes and inferior faces of the hemispheres appear smooth.

Myelination

The hypersignal of myelin in T1 (see Appendix) is clearly detectable at the level of the tegmentum, and more uncertainly at the level of the vermis and the middle cerebellar peduncles.

No T1 hypersignal is observed at the level of the internal capsule at this stage.

Cellular Migration

Three distinct layers are visible: the germinal zone in the form of a preventricular strip in T1 hypersignal, wide at this stage, an intermediate area in hyposignal and the cortical ribbon, which appears in clear hypersignal (see Appendix).

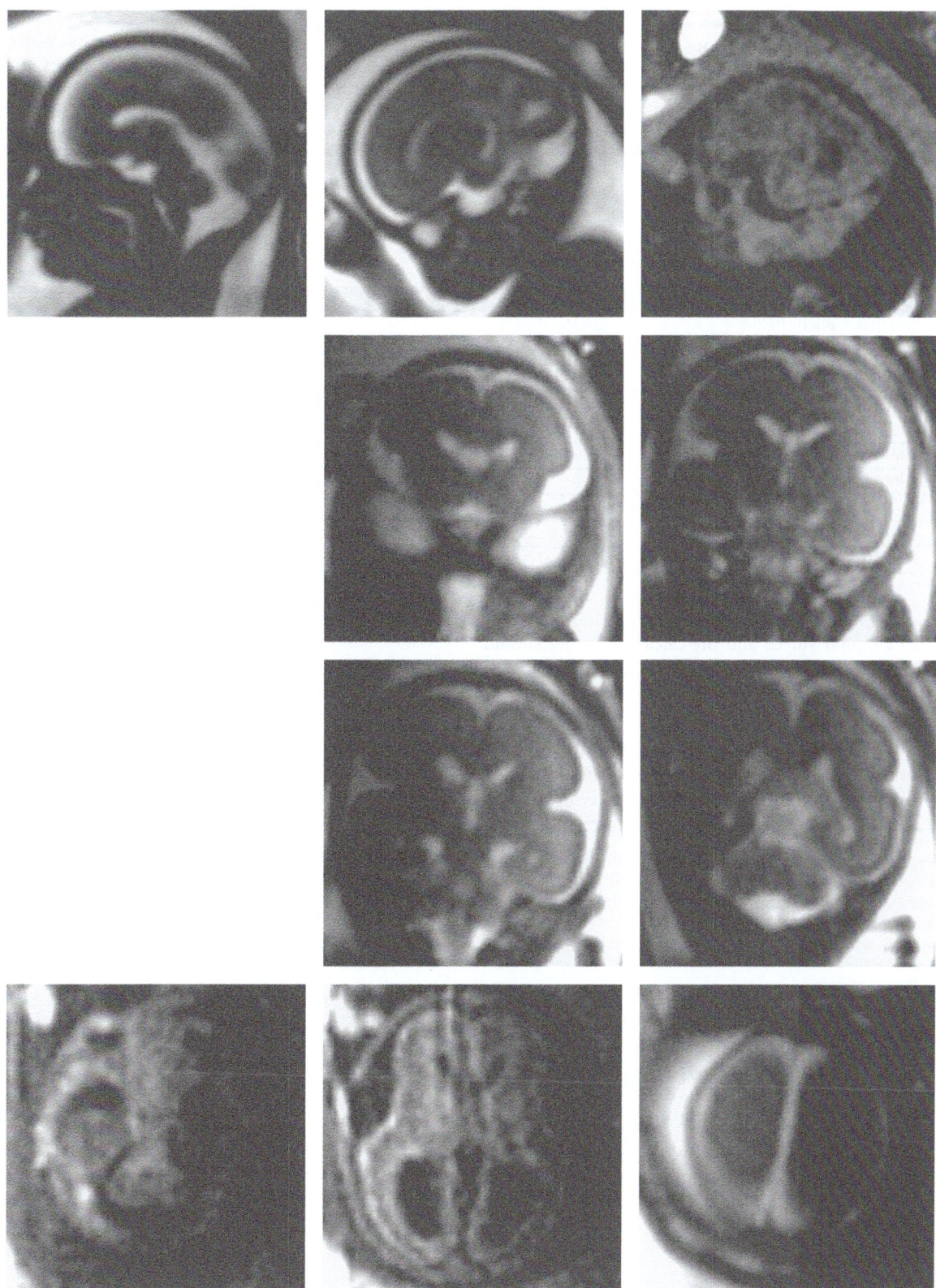

24–25 Weeks of Gestation

Biometrics (in mm)

	FOD	Cerebral BPD	Bone BPD	LCC	HV	APDV	TCD
Min–max	60–81	44–58	53–68	27–36	10–15	6—10	24—30

Gyration

Sulci present (≥75%)	Sulci detectable (25%–75%)	Sulci absent (<25%)
Interhemispheric fissure	Collateral sulcus	Superior temporal sulcus
Lateral sulcus	Superior frontal sulcus	Inferior temporal sulcus
Internal parieto-occipital fissure	Central sulcus	External occipitotemporal sulcus
Hippocampal fissure	Marginal sulcus	Intraparietal sulcus
Callosal sulcus		Precentral sulcus
Calcarine fissure		Postcentral sulcus
Cingular sulcus		Inferior frontal sulcus
		Secondary cingular sulci
		Secondary occipital sulci
		Insular sulci

The cingular sulcus and the calcarine fissure should be visible. The calcarine fissure is at right angles to the internal parieto-occipital sulcus.

Some sulci become detectable (the collateral sulcus, and less consistently and less distinctly the superior frontal, central and marginal sulci) in the form of a discrete cortical depression. The posterior opercularization of the sylvian fissure has clearly started.

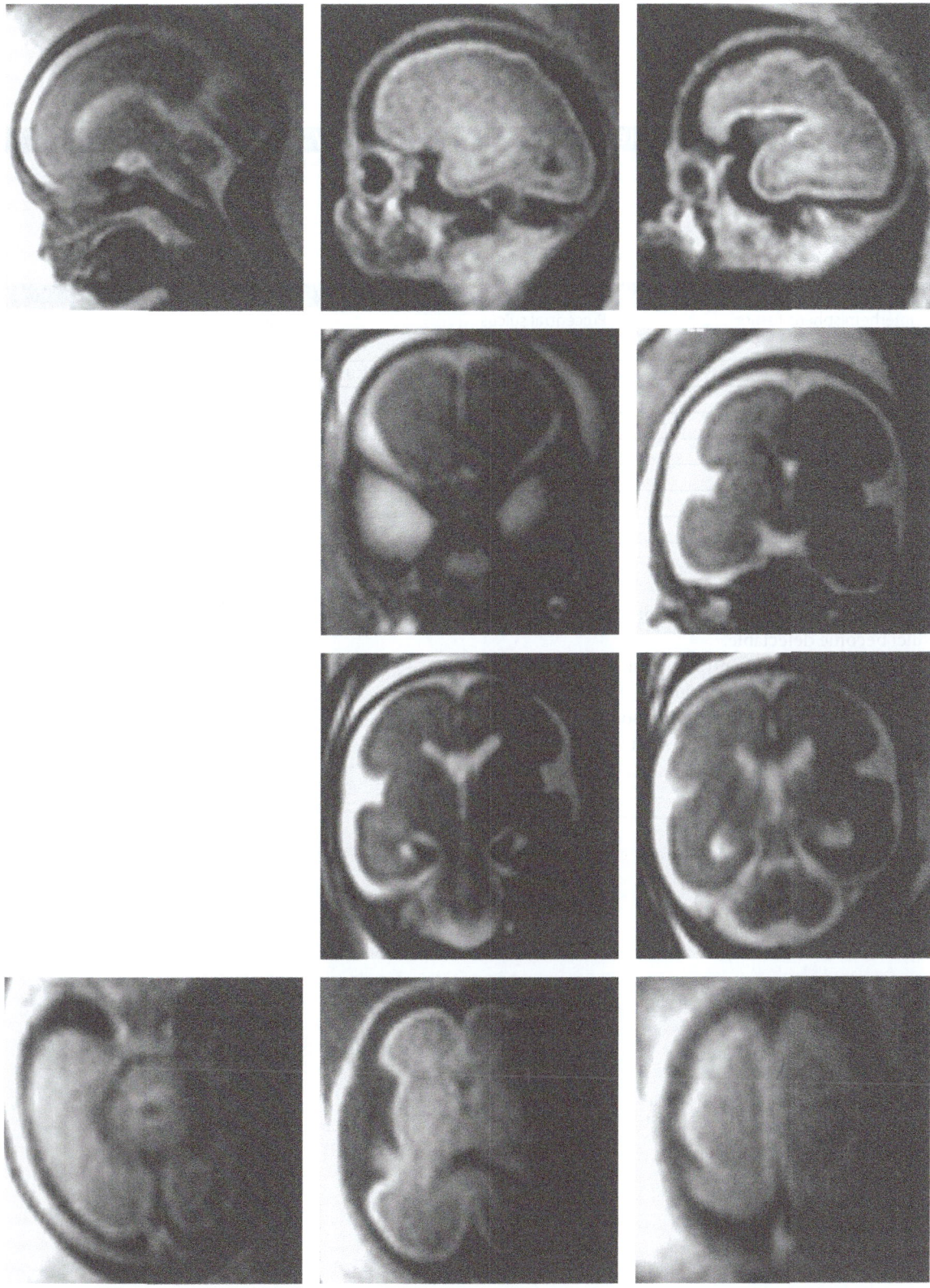

26 Weeks of Gestation

Biometrics (in mm)

	FOD	Cerebral BPD	Bone BPD	LCC	HV	APDV	TCD
Min–max	71–90	52–63	60–73	30–37	13–15	9–10	26–35

Gyration

Sulci present (≥75%)	Sulci detectable (25%–75%)	Sulci absent (<25%)
Interhemispheric fissure	Precentral sulcus	Superior (anterior) temporal sulcus
Lateral sulcus	Marginal sulcus	Inferior temporal sulcus
Internal parieto-occipital fissure	Superior (posterior) temporal sulcus	External occipitotemporal sulcus
Hippocampal fissure	Intraparietal sulcus	Secondary cingular sulci
Callosal sulcus	Postcentral sulcus	Secondary occipital sulci
Calcarine fissure	Superior frontal sulcus	Inferior frontal sulcus
Cingular sulcus		Insular sulci
Central sulcus		
Collateral sulcus		

The intraparietal sulcus and the pre- and postcentral sulci become detectable.

The collateral and central sulci should be visible.

In half the cases, a posterior temporal cortical depression is visible, which corresponds to an early form of the superior temporal sulcus.

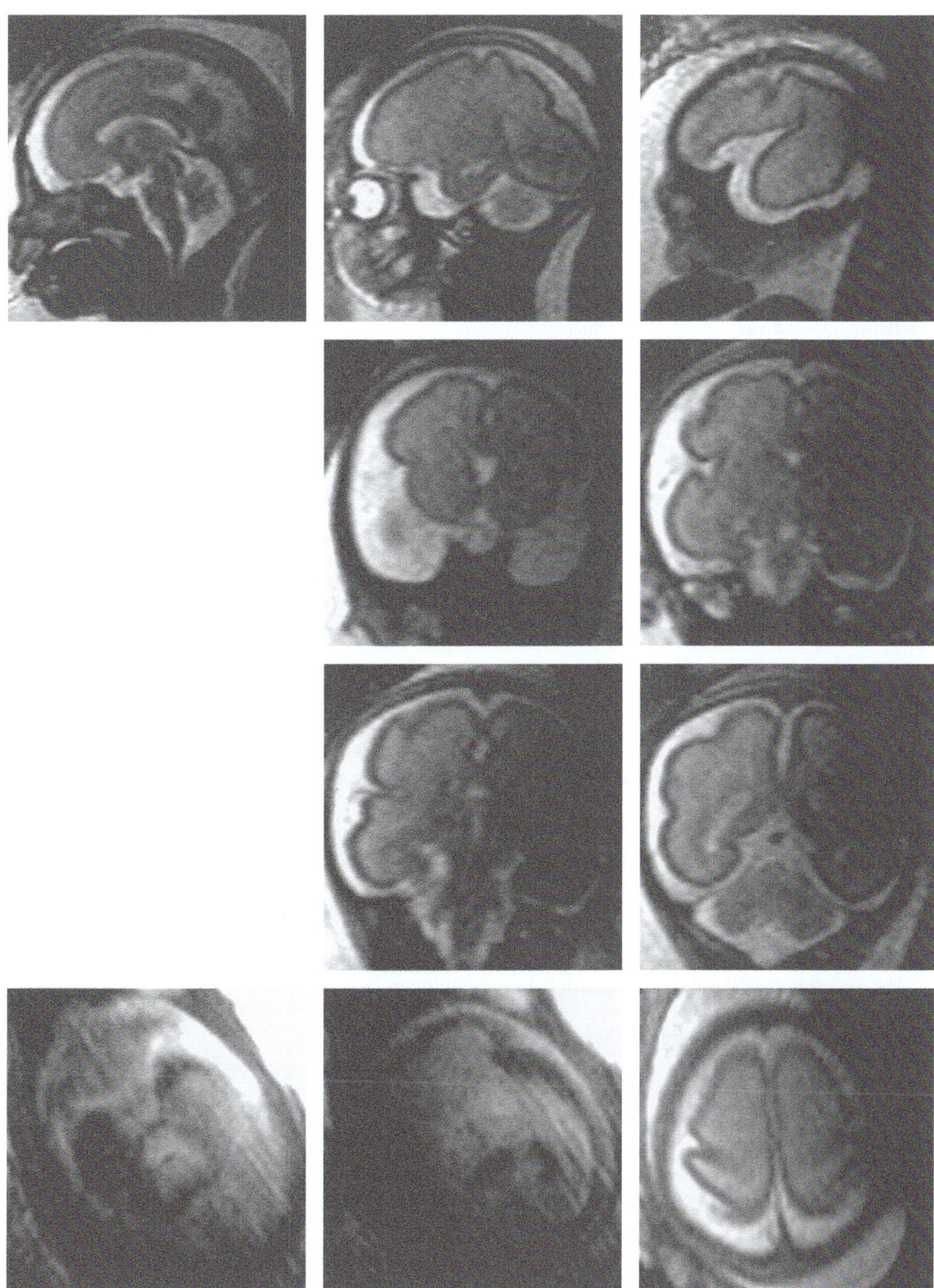

27 Weeks of Gestation

Biometrics (in mm)

	FOD	Cerebral BPD	Bone BPD	LCC	HV	APDV	TCD
Min–max	73–90	55–63	60–70	28–41	12–18	7–13	26–40

Gyration

Sulci present (≥75%)	Sulci detectable (25%–75%)	Sulci absent (<25%)
Interhemispheric fissure	Intraparietal sulcus	Superior (anterior) temporal sulcus
Lateral sulcus	Superior frontal sulcus	Inferior temporal sulcus
Internal parieto-occipital fissure	Inferior frontal sulcus	External occipitotemporal sulcus
Hippocampal fissure	Postcentral sulcus	Secondary cingular sulci
Callosal sulcus		Secondary occipital sulci
Calcarine fissure		Insular sulci
Cingular sulcus		
Marginal sulcus		
Central sulcus		
Precentral sulcus		
Collateral sulcus		
Superior (posterior) temporal sulcus		

The cingular sulcus should be visible in its various parts (the marginal posterior part is also visible).

The central sulcus is present in 100 % of cases.

The precentral sulcus and the collateral sulcus are normally visible.

Only the posterior part of the superior temporal sulcus is visible. This sulcus develops from back to front, and its anterior part will therefore be visible at a later stage.

The postcentral sulcus and the inferior frontal sulcus are detectable.

The superior frontal sulcus is distinctly deeper than in the previous weeks.

Opercularization is in progress at the back and appears at the front.

Myelination

No significant modification is noted. The myelin is more visible at the level of the vermis and the middle cerebellar peduncles.

The central basal ganglia are visible in a more moderate hypersignal, while the internal capsule appears in hyposignal. This aspect is probably explained by a hypercellularity of the basal ganglia, and not by the presence of myelin (see Appendix).

The germinal zone is visible and seems a little thinner.

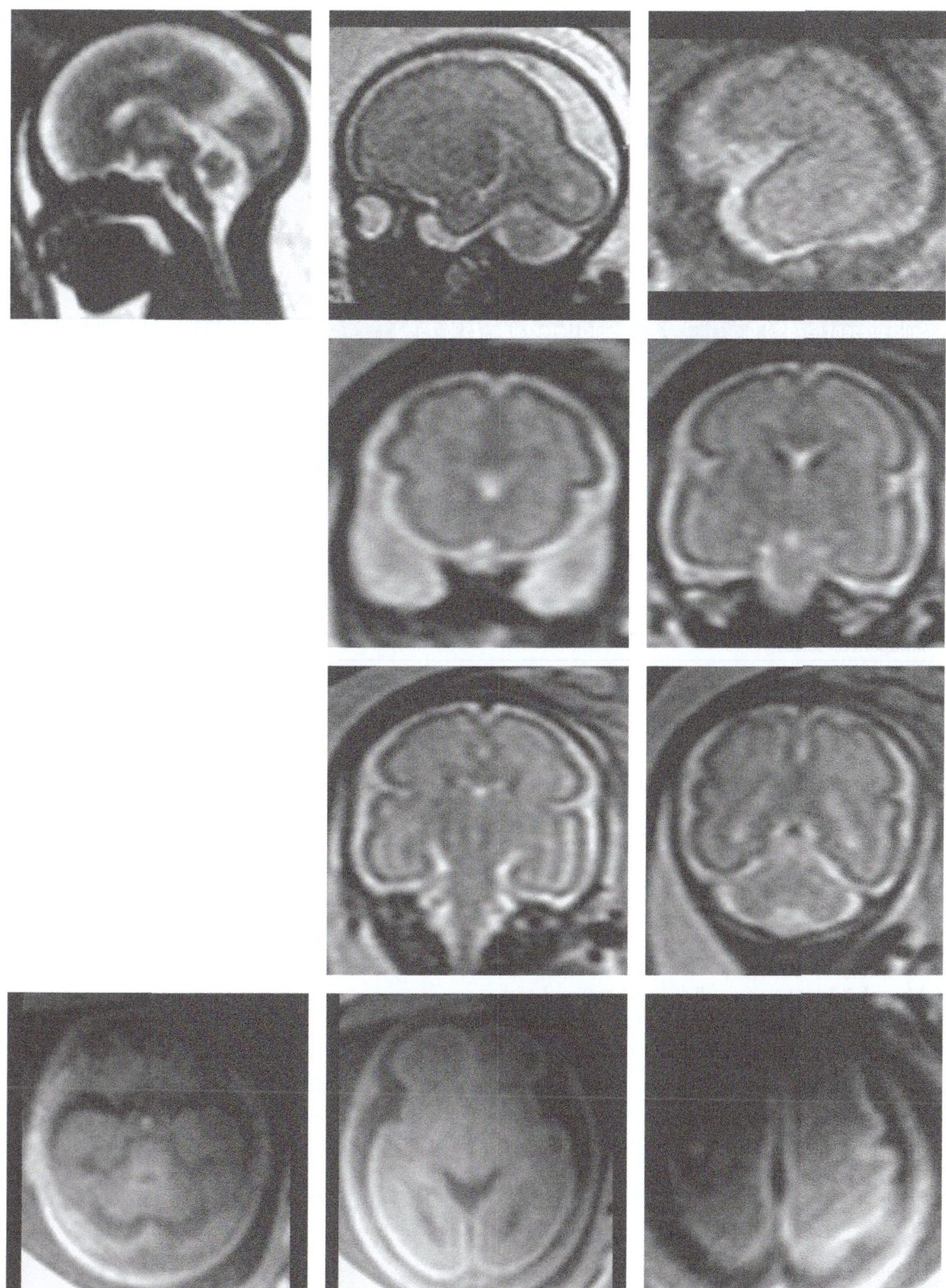

28 Weeks of Gestation

Biometrics (in mm)

	FOD	Cerebral BPD	Bone BPD	LCC	HV	APDV	TCD
Min–max	70–90	52–69	55–80	32–40	13–18	8–11	29–36

Surface of the vermis (mm^2): 146–229 (min–max).

Gyration

Sulci present (≥75%)	Sulci detectable (25%–75%)	Sulci absent (<25%)
Interhemispheric fissure	Superior frontal sulcus	Superior (anterior) temporal sulcus
Lateral sulcus	Inferior frontal sulcus	Inferior temporal sulcus
Internal parieto-occipital fissure		External occipitotemporal sulcus
Hippocampal fissure		Secondary cingular sulci
Callosal sulcus		Secondary occipital sulci
Calcarine fissure		Insular sulci
Cingular sulcus		
Marginal sulcus		
Central sulcus		
Precentral sulcus		
Postcentral sulcus		
Intraparietal sulcus		
Collateral sulcus		
Superior (posterior) temporal sulcus		

The postcentral sulcus and the intraparietal sulcus should be visible.

The cingular sulcus looks more tortuous.

Myelination

The myelin should be visible at the level of the vermis (although it is not seen on slice no. 8 here) and of the middle cerebellar peduncles.

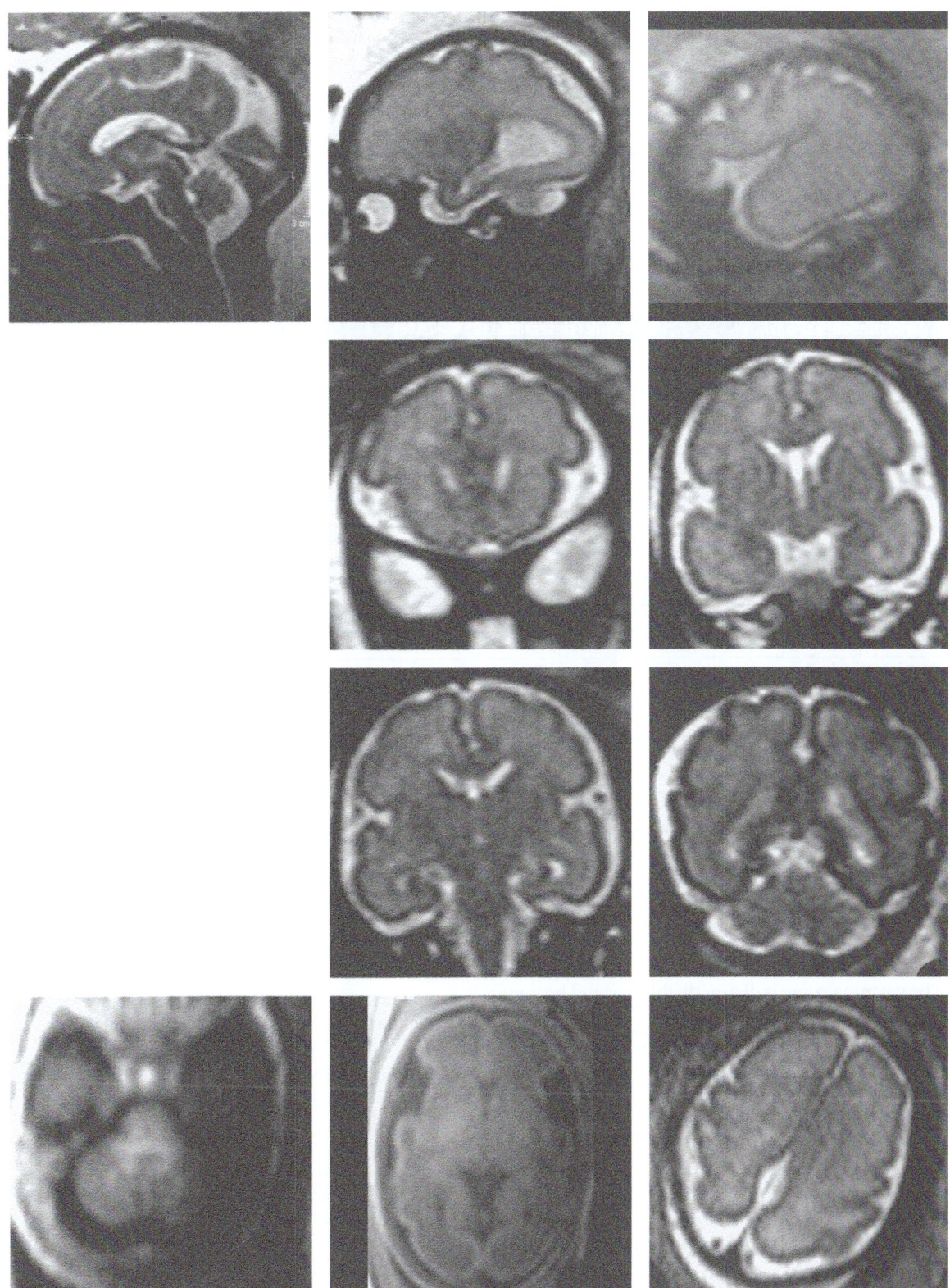

29 Weeks of Gestation

Biometrics (in mm)

	FOD	Cerebral BPD	Bone BPD	LCC	HV	APDV	TCD
Min–max	75–95	57–72	61–82	28–42	14–18	8–13	31–42

Surface of the vermis (mm^2): 151–231 (min–max).

Gyration

Sulci present (≥75%)	Sulci detectable (25%–75%)	Sulci absent (<25%)
Interhemispheric fissure		Superior (anterior) temporal sulcus
Lateral sulcus		Inferior temporal sulcus
Internal parieto-occipital fissure		Secondary cingular sulci
Hippocampal fissure		Secondary occipital sulci
Callosal sulcus		Insular sulci
Calcarine fissure		External occipitotemporal sulcus
Cingular sulcus		
Marginal sulcus		
Central sulcus		
Precentral sulcus		
Postcentral sulcus		
Intraparietal sulcus		
Collateral sulcus		
Superior (posterior) temporal sulcus		
Superior frontal sulcus		
Inferior frontal sulcus		

The frontal sulci (superior and inferior) should be present.

Cellular Migration

The germinal zone is distinctly thinner, and becomes only just visible.

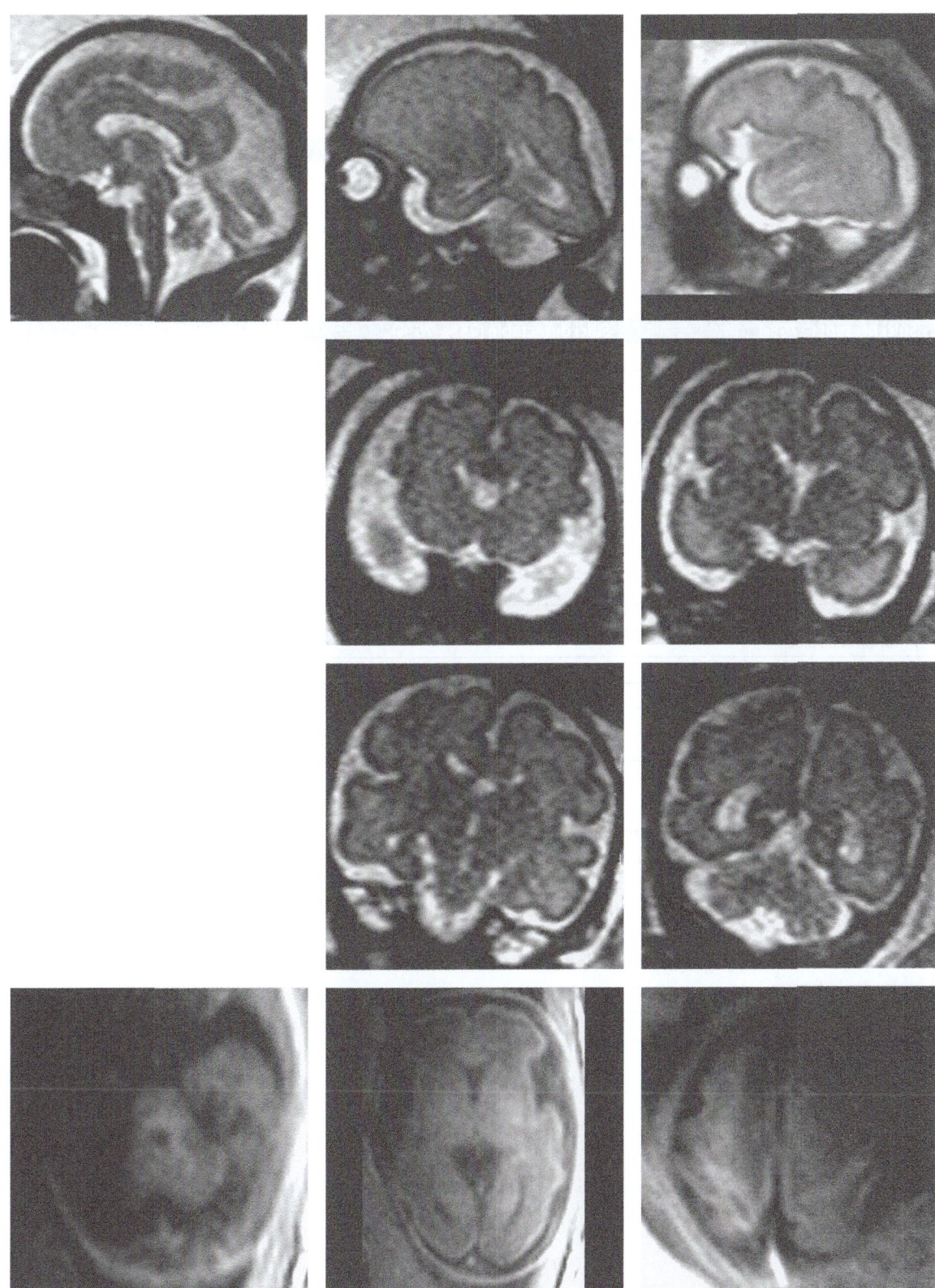

30 Weeks of Gestation

Biometrics (in mm)

	FOD	Cerebral BPD	Bone BPD	LCC	HV	APDV	TCD
Min–max	77–108	62–82	66–88	33–46	13–20	9–15	32–45

Surface of the vermis (mm^2): 159–274 (min–max).

Gyration

Sulci present (≥75%)	Sulci detectable (25%–75%)	Sulci absent (<25%)
Interhemispheric fissure	Inferior temporal sulcus	Secondary cingular sulci
Lateral sulcus	External occipitotemporal sulcus	Secondary occipital sulci
Internal parieto-occipital fissure		Insular sulci
Hippocampal fissure		Superior (anterior) temporal sulcus
Callosal sulcus		
Calcarine fissure		
Cingular sulcus		
Marginal sulcus		
Central sulcus		
Precentral sulcus		
Postcentral sulcus		
Intraparietal sulcus		
Collateral sulcus		
Superior (posterior) temporal sulcus		
Superior frontal sulcus		
Inferior frontal sulcus		

The cingular sulcus is even more tortuous.

The inferior temporal sulcus appears in the shape of a discrete cortical depression.

The external occipitotemporal sulcus is detectable, it appears on slice no. 6 here.

The central sulcus progresses towards the interhemispheric fissure.

Opercularization is in progress; it appears very advanced at the back.

Myelination

A hypersignal is visible at the level of the lateral part of the posterior limb of the internal capsule.

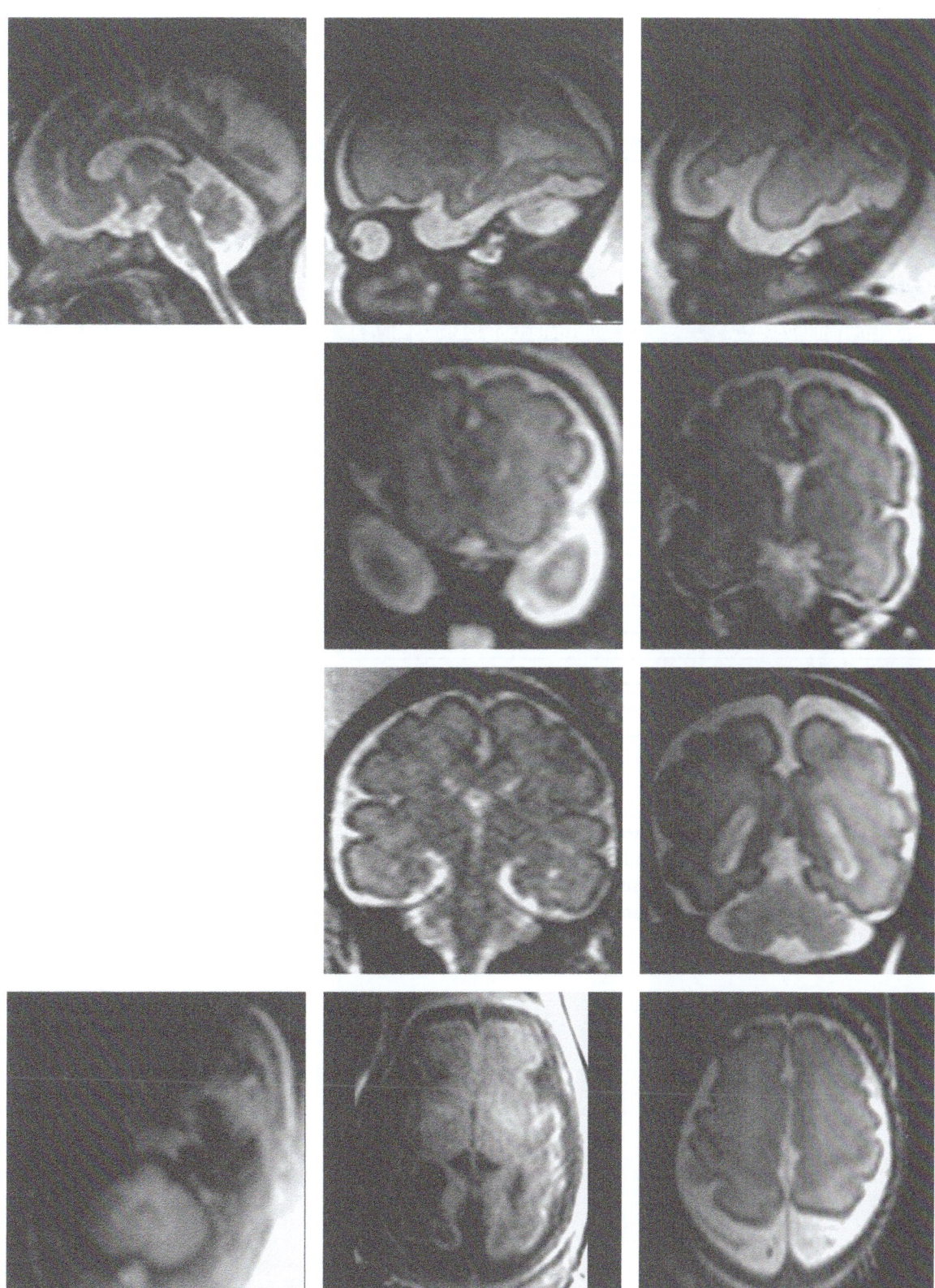

31 Weeks of Gestation

Biometrics (in mm)

	FOD	Cerebral BPD	Bone BPD	LCC	HV	APDV	TCD
Min–max	82–97	60–80	66–85	32–44	15–20	10–16	35–43

Surface of the vermis (mm²): 168–282 (min–max).

Gyration

Sulci present (≥75%)	Sulci detectable (25%–75%)	Sulci absent (<25%)
Interhemispheric fissure	Inferior temporal sulcus	Secondary occipital sulci
Lateral sulcus	External occipitotemporal sulcus	Insular sulci
Internal parieto-occipital fissure	Superior (anterior) temporal sulcus	
Hippocampal fissure	Secondary cingular sulci	
Callosal sulcus		
Calcarine fissure		
Cingular sulcus		
Marginal sulcus		
Central sulcus		
Precentral sulcus		
Postcentral sulcus		
Intraparietal sulcus		
Collateral sulcus		
Superior (posterior) temporal sulcus		
Superior frontal sulcus		
Inferior frontal sulcus		

At this stage, most primary sulci are present, except for the temporal sulcus (inferior and superior, anterior part) and the occipitotemporal sulcus.

The secondary cingular sulci are detectable (although they do not appear on slice no. 1 here).

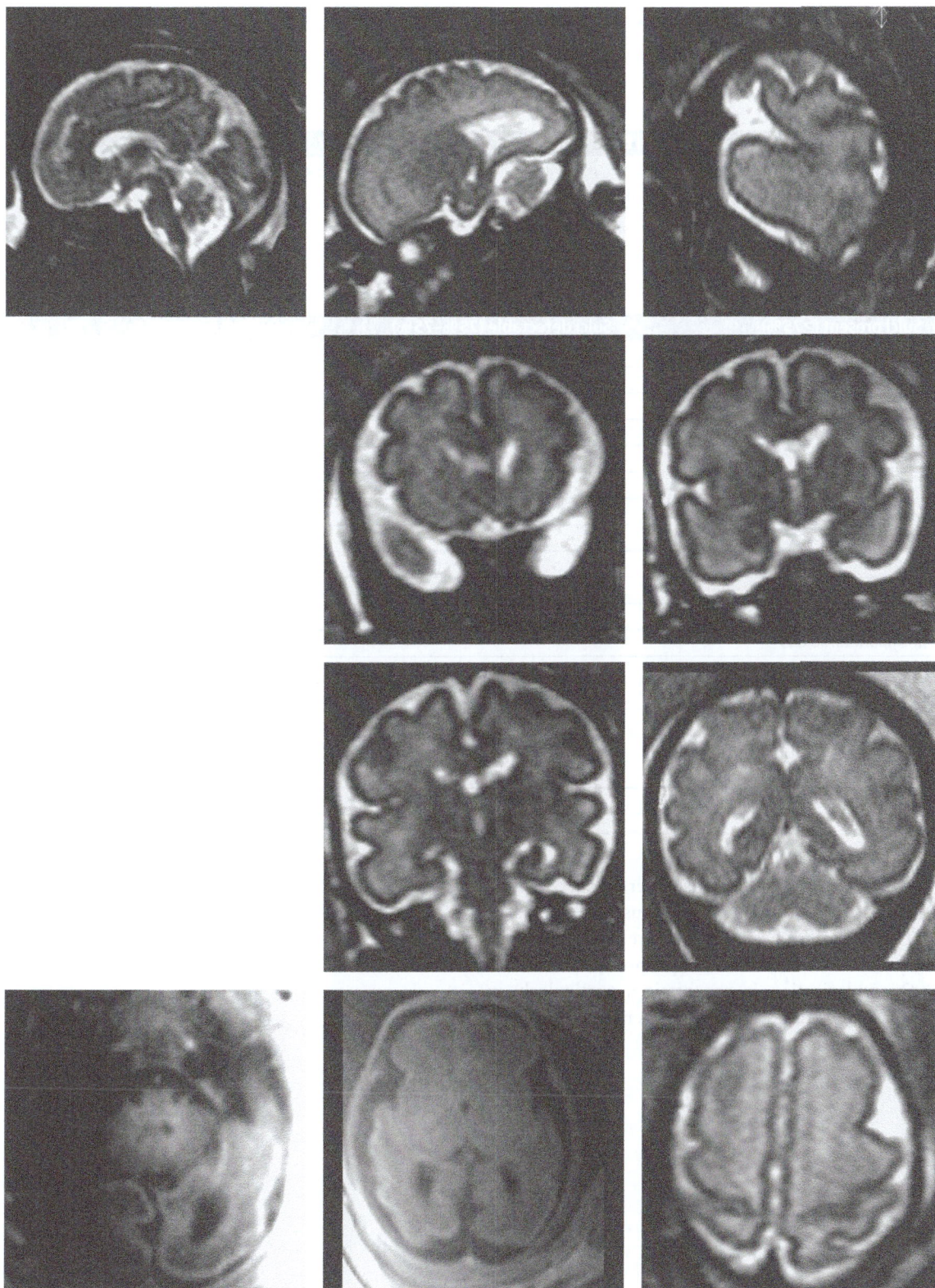

32 Weeks of Gestation

Biometrics (in mm)

	FOD	Cerebral BPD	Bone BPD	LCC	HV	APDV	TCD
Min–max	82–106	63–86	70–91	33–46	15–22	8–17	34–43

Surface of the vermis (mm^2): 165–287 (min–max).

Gyration

Sulci present (≥75%)	Sulci detectable (25%–75%)	Sulci absent (<25%)
Interhemispheric fissure	External occipitotemporal sulcus	
Lateral sulcus	Secondary cingular sulci	
Internal parieto-occipital fissure	Insular sulci	
Hippocampal fissure	Secondary occipital sulci	
Callosal sulcus		
Calcarine fissure		
Cingular sulcus		
Marginal sulcus		
Central sulcus		
Precentral sulcus		
Postcentral sulcus		
Intraparietal sulcus		
Collateral sulcus		
Superior (posterior) temporal sulcus		
Superior (anterior) temporal sulcus		
Inferior temporal sulcus		
Superior frontal sulcus		
Inferior frontal sulcus		

The superior temporal sulcus, anterior part, is present, as is the inferior temporal sulcus.

The secondary occipital sulci are now detectable. They are not seen on the example presented here.

Opercularization is progressing, particularly in the back (the craniocaudal interopercular distance is almost nonexistent).

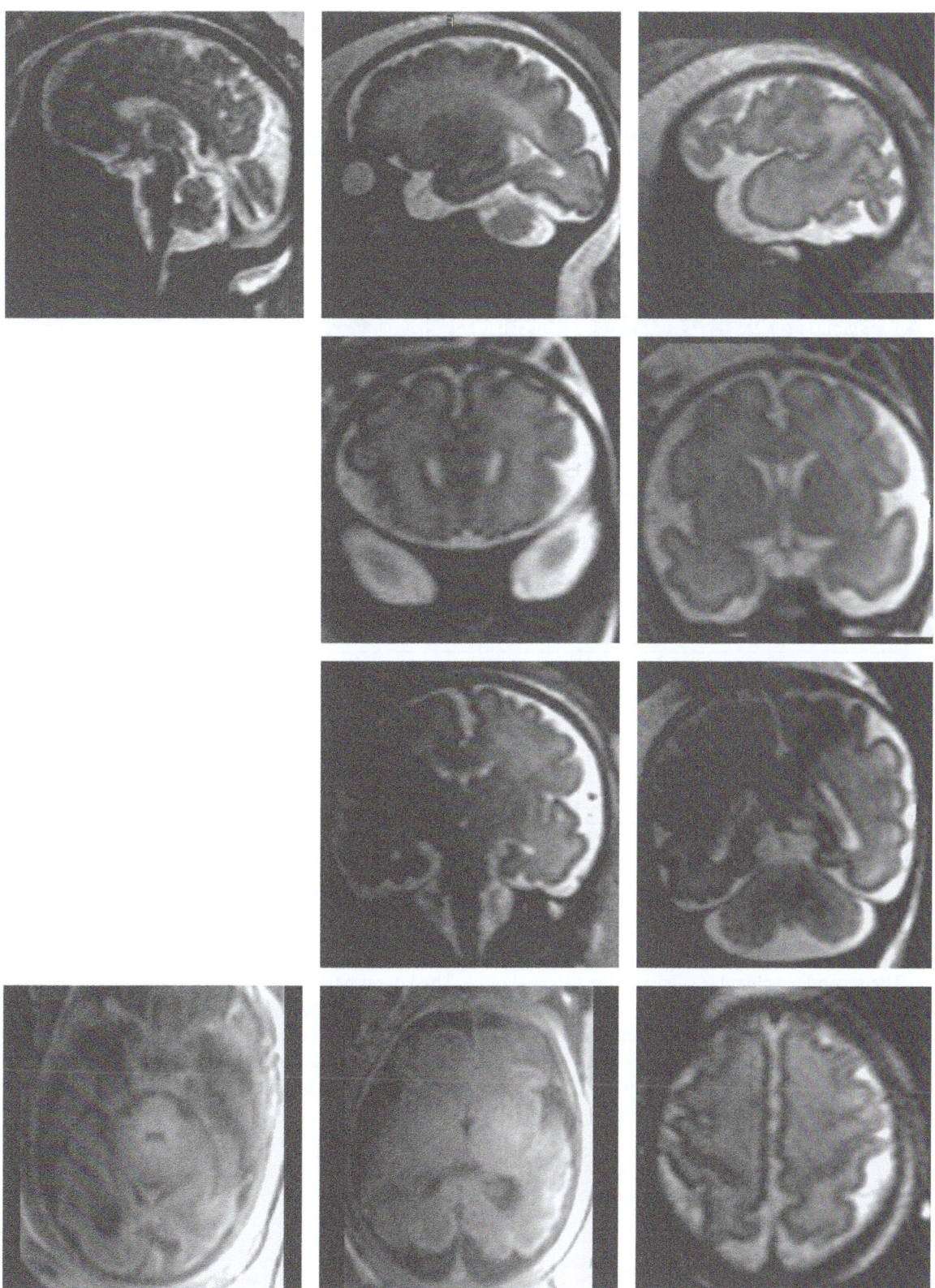

33 Weeks of Gestation

Biometrics (in mm)

	FOD	Cerebral BPD	Bone BPD	LCC	HV	APDV	TCD
Min–max	90–105	68–83	74–89	36–49	15–22	10–20	37–46

Surface of the vermis (mm^2): 174–336 (min–max).

Gyration

Sulci present (≥75%)	Sulci detectable (25%–75%)
Interhemispheric fissure	Insular sulci
Lateral sulcus	Secondary occipital sulci
Internal parieto-occipital fissure	
Hippocampal fissure	
Callosal sulcus	
Calcarine fissure	
Cingular sulcus	
Marginal sulcus	
Central sulcus	
Precentral sulcus	
Postcentral sulcus	
Intraparietal sulcus	
Collateral sulcus	
Superior (posterior) temporal sulcus	
Superior (anterior) temporal sulcus	
Inferior temporal sulcus	
External occipitotemporal sulcus	
Superior frontal sulcus	
Inferior frontal sulcus	
Secondary cingular sulci	

All primary sulci are present at this stage, the inferior temporal sulcus included.

The secondary cingular sulci and the external occipitotemporal sulcus are present.

On the slices exploring the vertex, the central sulcus reaches the interhemispheric fissure.

Opercularization is further progressing in its posterior and median parts.

Myelination

The lateral part of the posterior limb of the internal capsule should be myelinated, while the presence of a hypersignal in its medial part is less systematic, and hence merely detectable in a number of cases (it is only just visible on the example presented).

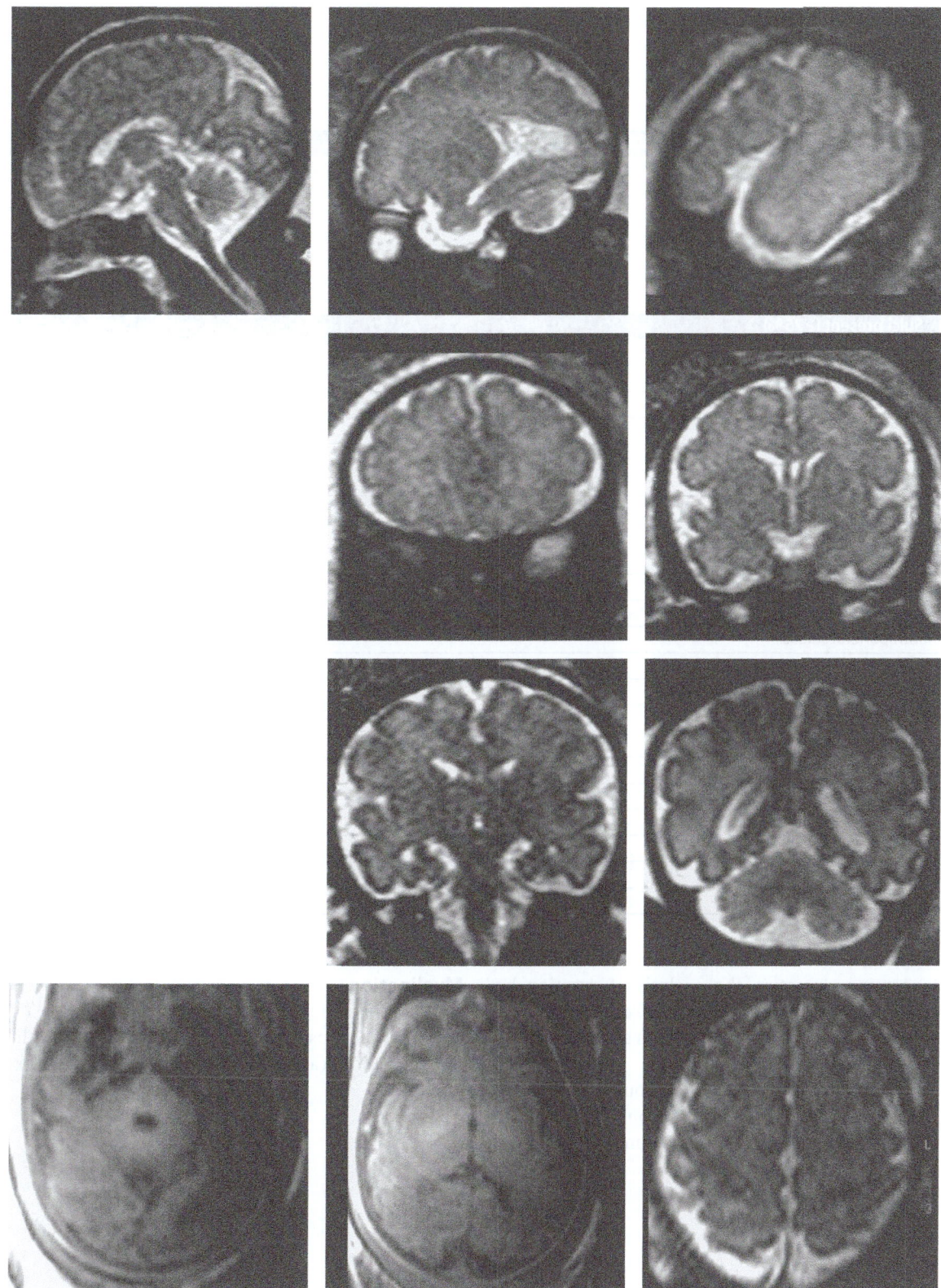

34 Weeks of Gestation

Biometrics (in mm)

	FOD	Cerebral BPD	Bone BPD	LCC	HV	APDV	TCD
Min–max	90–114	64–85	69–92	30–43	16–26	11–20	38–50

Surface of the vermis (mm^2): 215–303 (min–max).

Gyration

Sulci present (≥75%)
Interhemispheric fissure
Lateral sulcus
Internal parieto-occipital fissure
Hippocampal fissure
Callosal sulcus
Calcarine fissure
Cingular sulcus
Marginal sulcus
Central sulcus
Precentral sulcus
Postcentral sulcus
Intraparietal sulcus
Collateral sulcus
Superior (posterior) temporal sulcus
Superior (anterior) temporal sulcus
Inferior temporal sulcus
External occipitotemporal sulcus
Superior frontal sulcus
Inferior frontal sulcus
Secondary cingular sulci
Insular sulci
Secondary occipital sulci

In common practice, the analysis of gyration becomes more difficult at this stage, even though the sulci are clearly visible on the slices shown.

The insular sulci are present.

The secondary occipital sulci should be visible (although they do not appear clearly on the sagittal slice shown here because of partial volume effect).

Myelination

The internal capsule hypersignal may extend to the globus pallidus (although only just visible on this example).

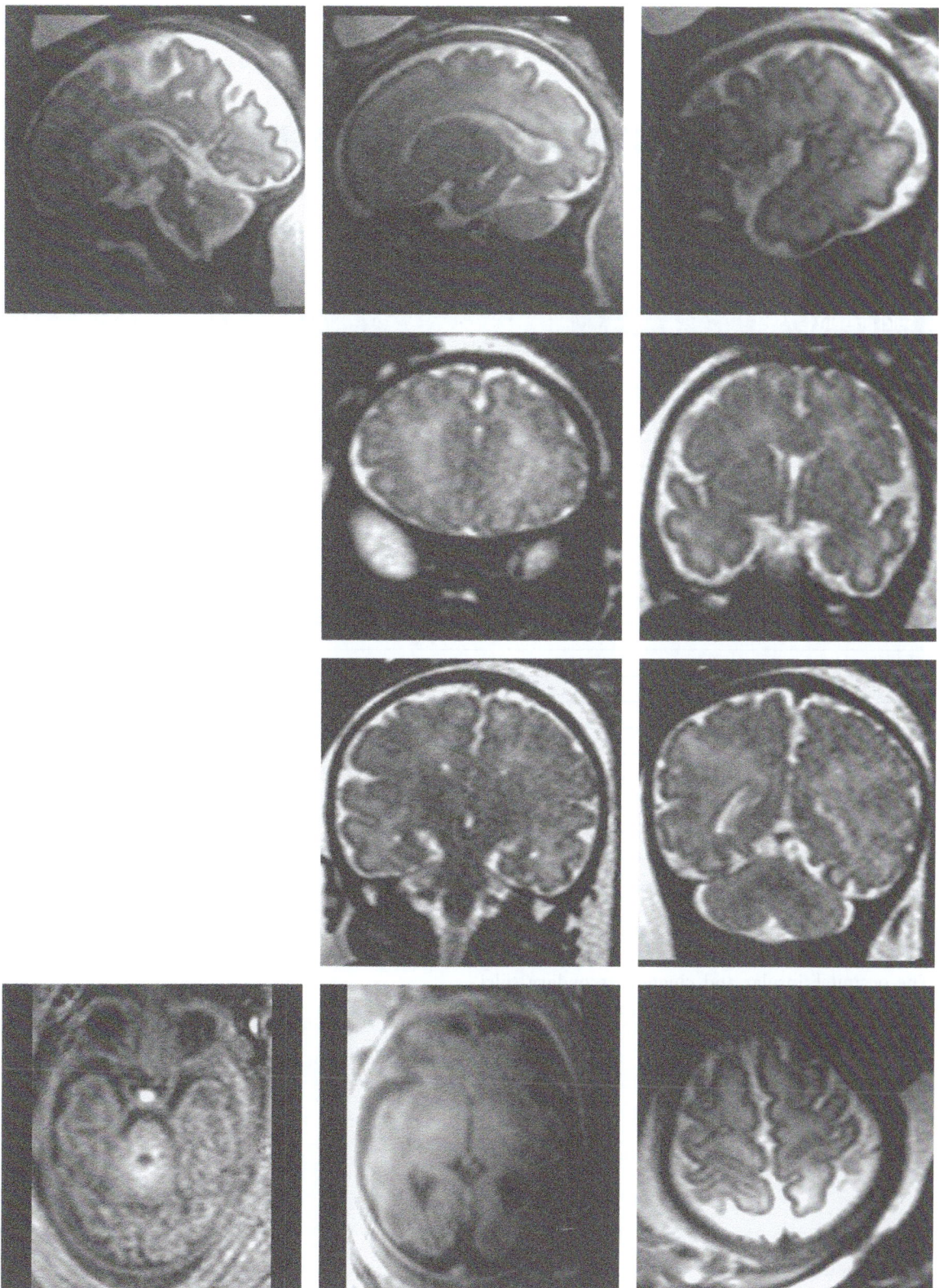

35 Weeks of Gestation

Biometrics (in mm)

	FOD	Cerebral BPD	Bone BPD	LCC	HV	APDV	TCD
Min–max	97–113	70–87	78–93	33–49	18–25	10–18	43–53

Surface of the vermis (mm²): 240–456 (min–max).

Gyration

Sulci present (≥ 75 %)
Interhemispheric fissure
Lateral sulcus
Internal parieto-occipital fissure
Hippocampal fissure
Callosal sulcus
Calcarine fissure
Cingular sulcus
Marginal sulcus
Central sulcus
Precentral sulcus
Postcentral sulcus
Intraparietal sulcus
Collateral sulcus
Superior (posterior) temporal sulcus
Superior (anterior) temporal sulcus
Inferior temporal sulcus
External occipitotemporal sulcus
Superior frontal sulcus
Inferior frontal sulcus
Secondary cingular sulci
Insular sulci
Secondary occipital sulci

The occipital, insular and cingular secondary sulci are very distinctly seen on this example.

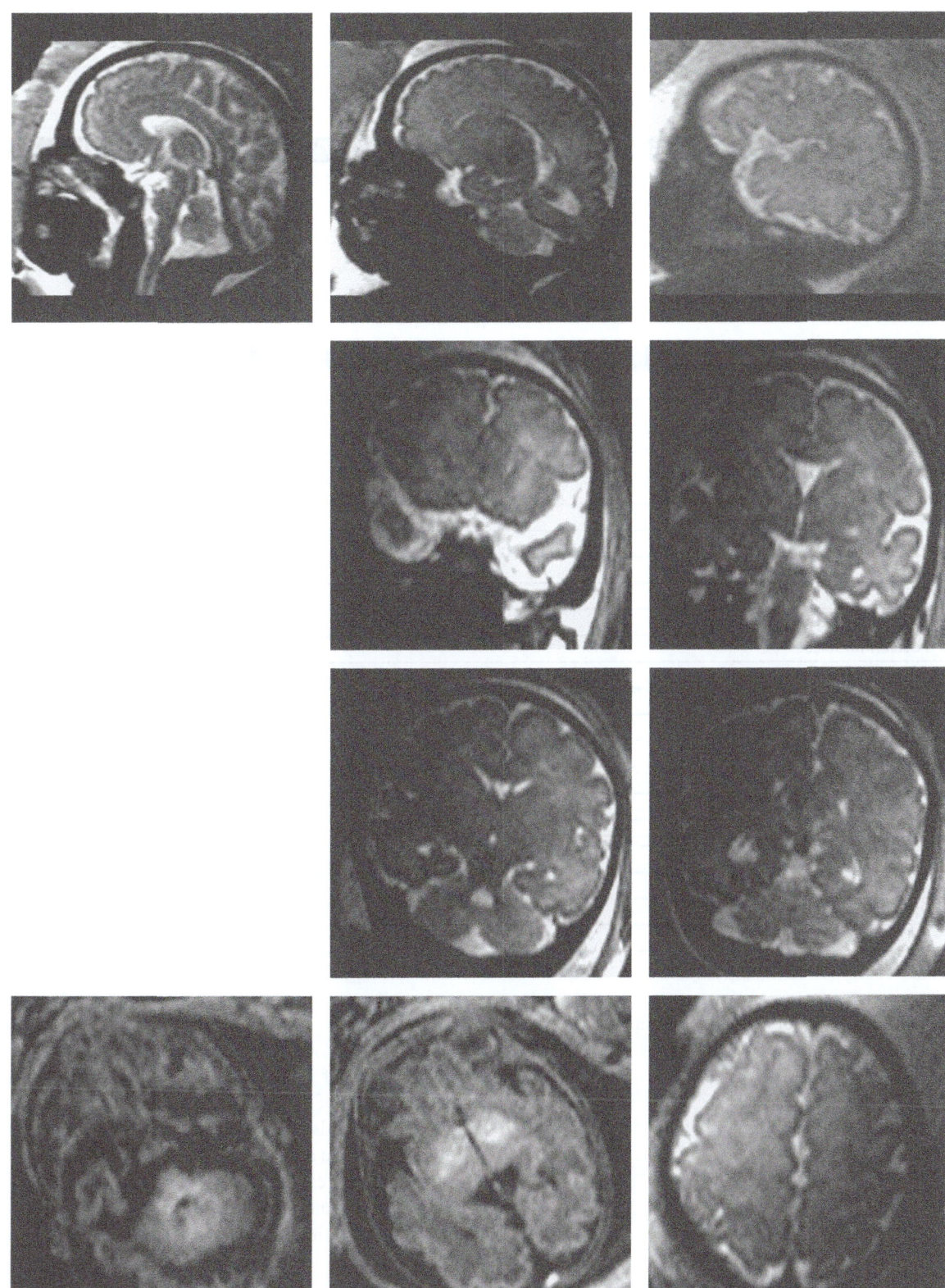

36 Weeks of Gestation

Biometrics (in mm)

	FOD	Cerebral BPD	Bone BPD	LCC	HV	APDV	TCD
Min–max	97–113	70–87	78–93	33–49	18–25	10–18	43–53

Surface of the vermis (mm²): 240–456 (min–max).

Gyration

Sulci present (≥75%)
Interhemispheric fissure
Lateral sulcus
Internal parieto-occipital fissure
Hippocampal fissure
Callosal sulcus
Calcarine fissure
Cingular sulcus
Marginal sulcus
Central sulcus
Precentral sulcus
Postcentral sulcus
Intraparietal sulcus
Collateral sulcus
Superior (posterior) temporal sulcus
Superior (anterior) temporal sulcus
Inferior temporal sulcus
External occipitotemporal sulcus
Superior frontal sulcus
Inferior frontal sulcus
Secondary cingular sulci
Insular sulci
Secondary occipital sulci

Opercularization of the sylvian fissure is complete in its median and posterior parts.

Myelination

The presence of myelin should be observed in the posterior limb of the internal capsule, not only in its lateral part but also in its medial part. The globus pallidus should also appear in T1 hypersignal.

In some rare cases, we can see an aspect of myelination of the pons in its most anterior part, with a start of myelination of the pyramidal tract.

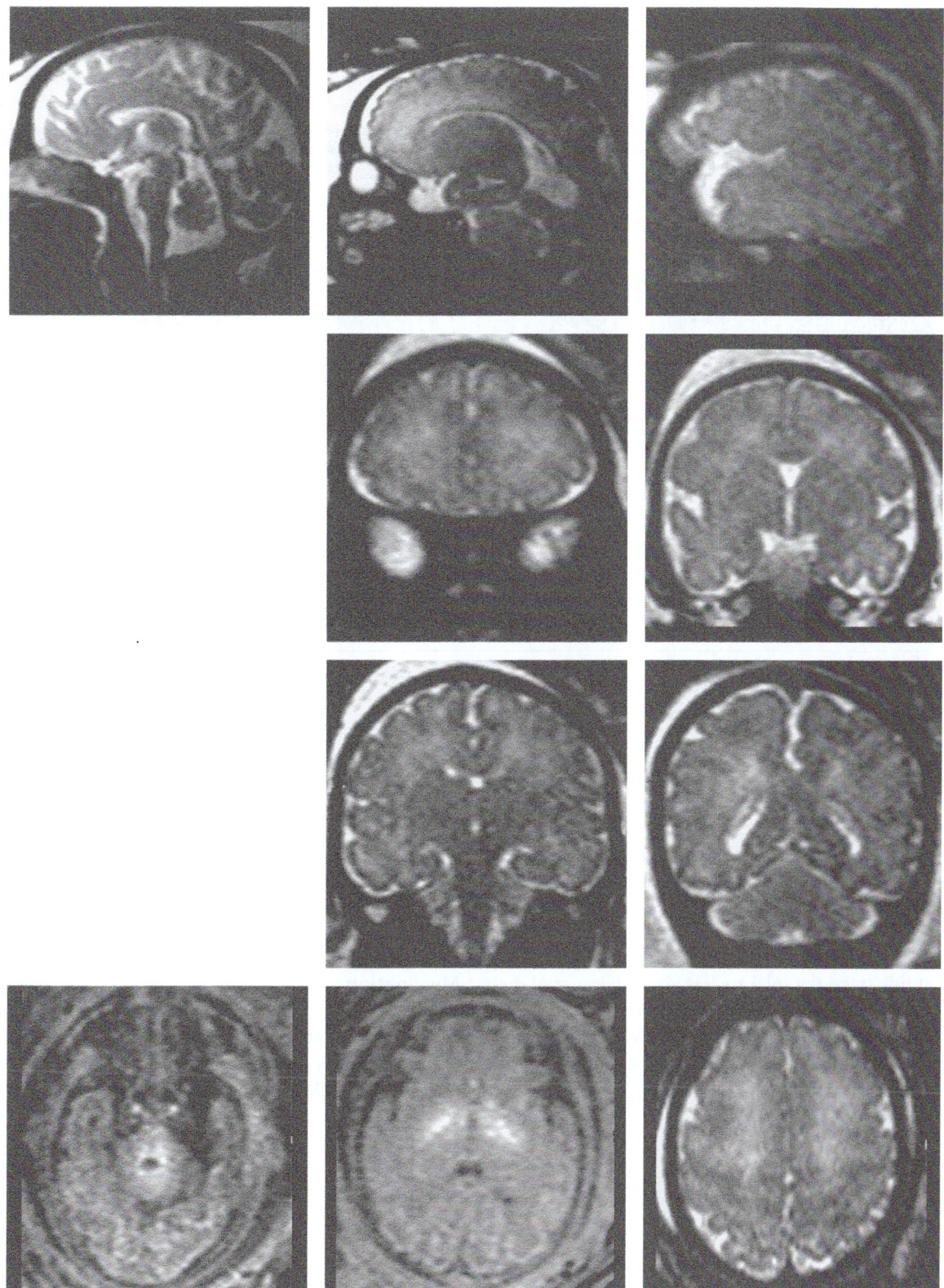

37–38 Weeks of Gestation

Biometrics (in mm)

	FOD	Cerebral BPD	Bone BPD	LCC	HV	APDV	TCD
Min–max	90–112	74–91	77–100	32–55	16–29	10–20	42–55

Surface of the vermis (mm^2): 274–470 (min–max).

Gyration

Sulci present (≥75%)
Interhemispheric fissure
Lateral sulcus
Internal parieto-occipital fissure
Hippocampal fissure
Callosal sulcus
Calcarine fissure
Cingular sulcus
Marginal sulcus
Central sulcus
Precentral sulcus
Postcentral sulcus
Intraparietal sulcus
Collateral sulcus
Superior (posterior) temporal sulcus
Superior (anterior) temporal sulcus
Inferior temporal sulcus
External occipitotemporal sulcus
Superior frontal sulcus
Inferior frontal sulcus
Secondary cingular sulci
Insular sulci
Secondary occipital sulci

At this stage, the sulci are less visible because of their narrowness and the small size of pericerebral spaces. This is seen rather distinctly on the anterior coronal slice. MRI is therefore less effective at this stage for the study of gyration.

Myelination

In a nonsignificant number of cases (less than 25%), we discerned the presence of a hypersignal at the level of the ventral lateral nucleus of the thalamus.

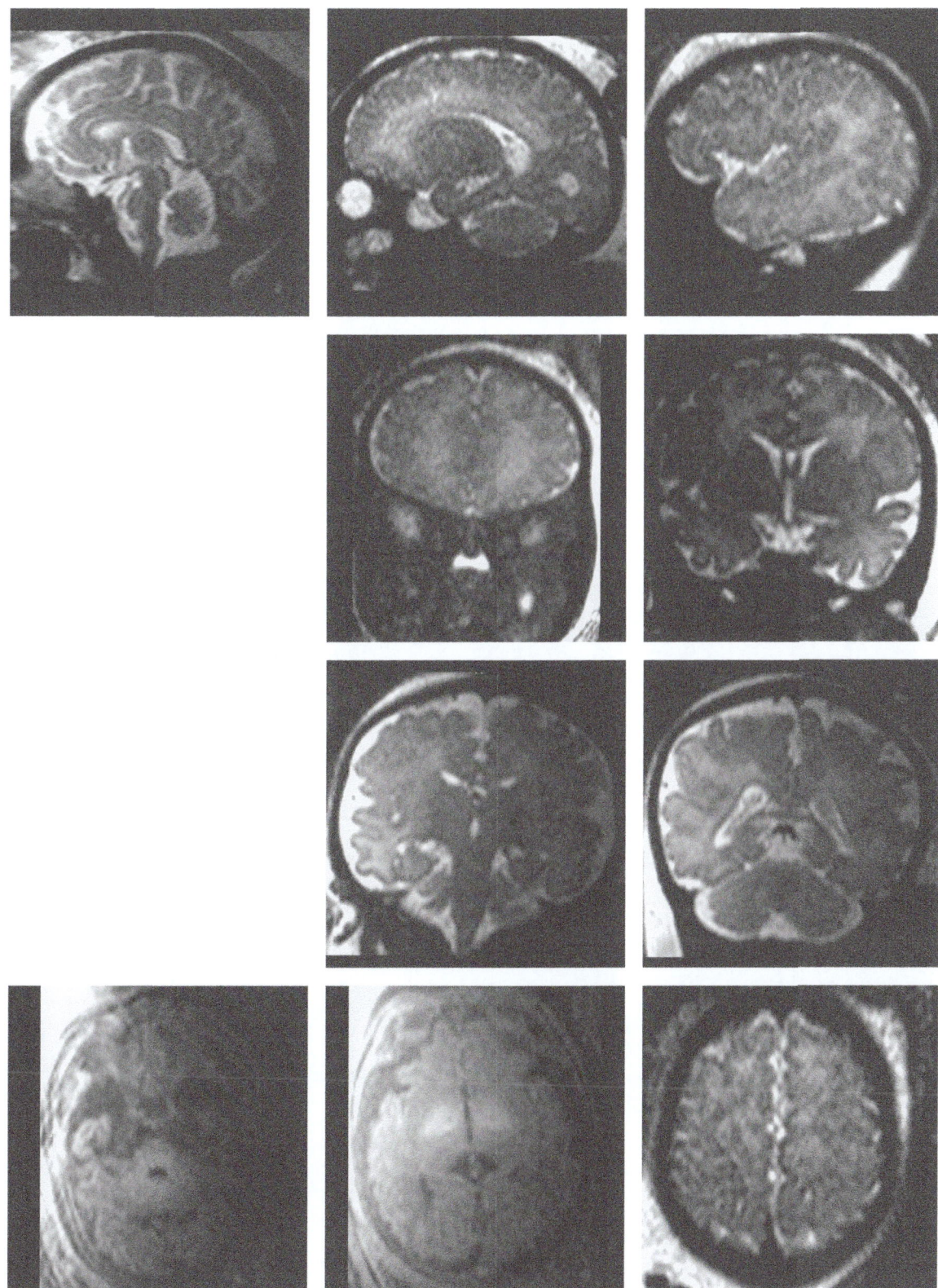

Chronological Presentation of the Results by Slice

We thought it useful to provide the reader with a vision of the changes on each one of the ten reference slices between 22 and 38 weeks of gestation. Indeed, precisely situating any given slice chronologically in the pregnancy can prove quite difficult. In this respect, it is interesting to compare it to the same slice in the preceding and following weeks, and to proceed in a manner similar to that of an estimation of bone age. Moreover, it is often useful to regroup the sulci of the different aspects of the brain in the gyration analysis.

The sulci on the internal faces of the hemispheres (cingular sulcus, marginal sulcus, callosal sulcus, internal parieto-occipital fissure and calcarine fissure) are analysed on slices nos. 1, 4, 5, 6 and 7. These sulci are among the earliest to appear during the gyration of the fetal brain. Between 22 and 38 weeks of gestation, the internal face is subjected to profound and extensive modifications. Easily visible at 22 weeks of gestation, the sulci are progressively hidden by the development of cingular and occipital secondary sulci from 32 weeks of gestation.

The callosal sulcus is very thin, and often best seen on coronal slices because of partial volume effect, which precludes satisfactory observation on a midline sagittal slice.

The posterior coronal slices (nos. 6 and 7) provide a good analysis of the gyration on the hemispheres' inferior faces (hippocampal fissure, collateral sulcus and external occipitotemporal sulcus). For neurofetopathologists, the orbital sulci are an excellent index of fetal maturation in the last weeks of pregnancy. Their visualization by MRI requires very anterior coronal slices. The same applies to olfactory sulci (see Appendix).

The sulci on the external face of the hemispheres (frontal, temporal and intraparietal sulci) are studied on the coronal slices. The development of the frontal sulci is best seen on the two most anterior coronal slices between 22 and 38 weeks of gestation. The middle frontal sulcus is not constant. On the more posterior coronal slices, the temporal sulci appear progressively, starting with the superior and continuing with the inferior, from back to front.

The axial slice at the level of the vertex (no. 10) and the parasagittal slice provide a good view of the progressive development between 22 and 38 weeks of gestation of the convexity sulci (central, pre- and postcentral sulci). These sulci initially appear at the convexity of the brain and progressively deepen towards the interhemispheric fissure.

The opercularization of the sylvian fissure is one of the major events of the fetal brain gyration. It is observed in the three planes: sagittal (no. 3), coronal (no. 5) and axial (no. 9). The sylvian fissure, still wide open at 22 weeks of gestation, progressively closes from back to front between 22 and 38 weeks of gestation. The opercularization of the sylvian fissure is complete at 40 weeks of gestation.

Slices 1–10

Slice 1

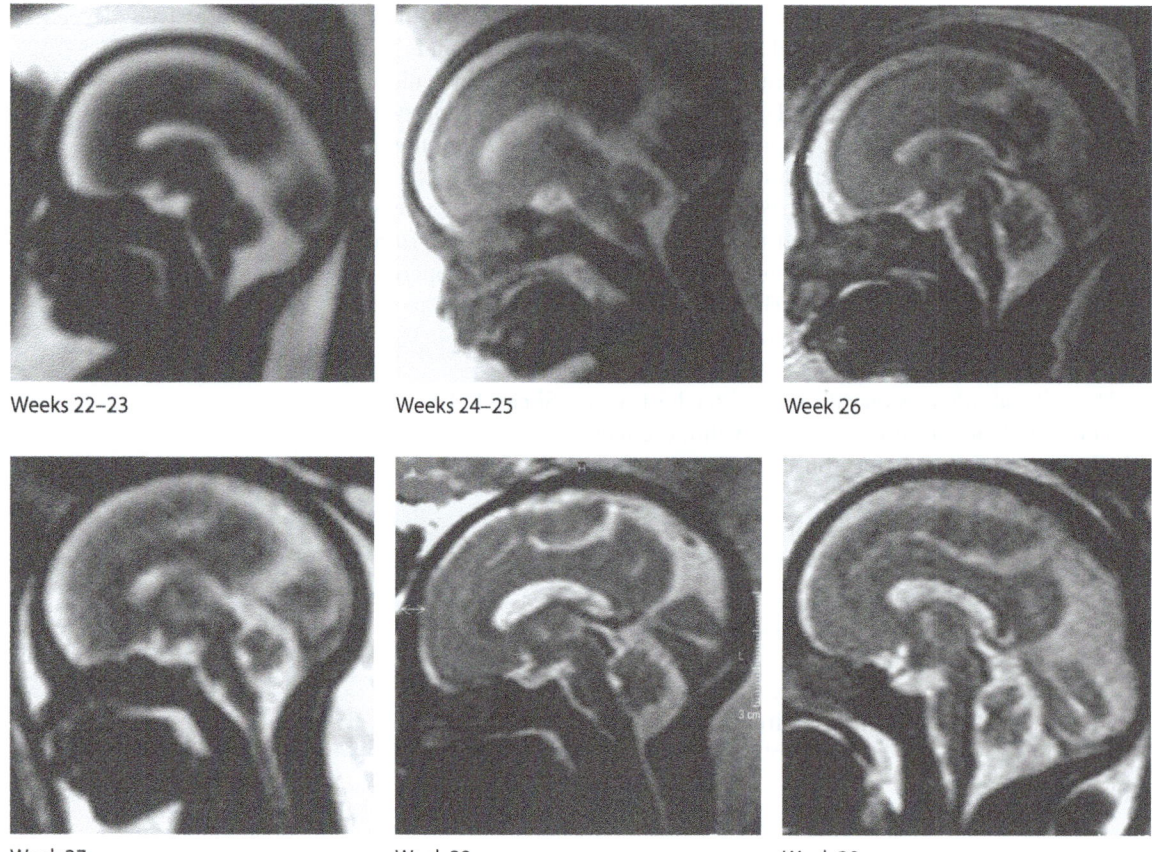

Weeks 22–23   Weeks 24–25   Week 26

Week 27   Week 28   Week 29

Slice 1

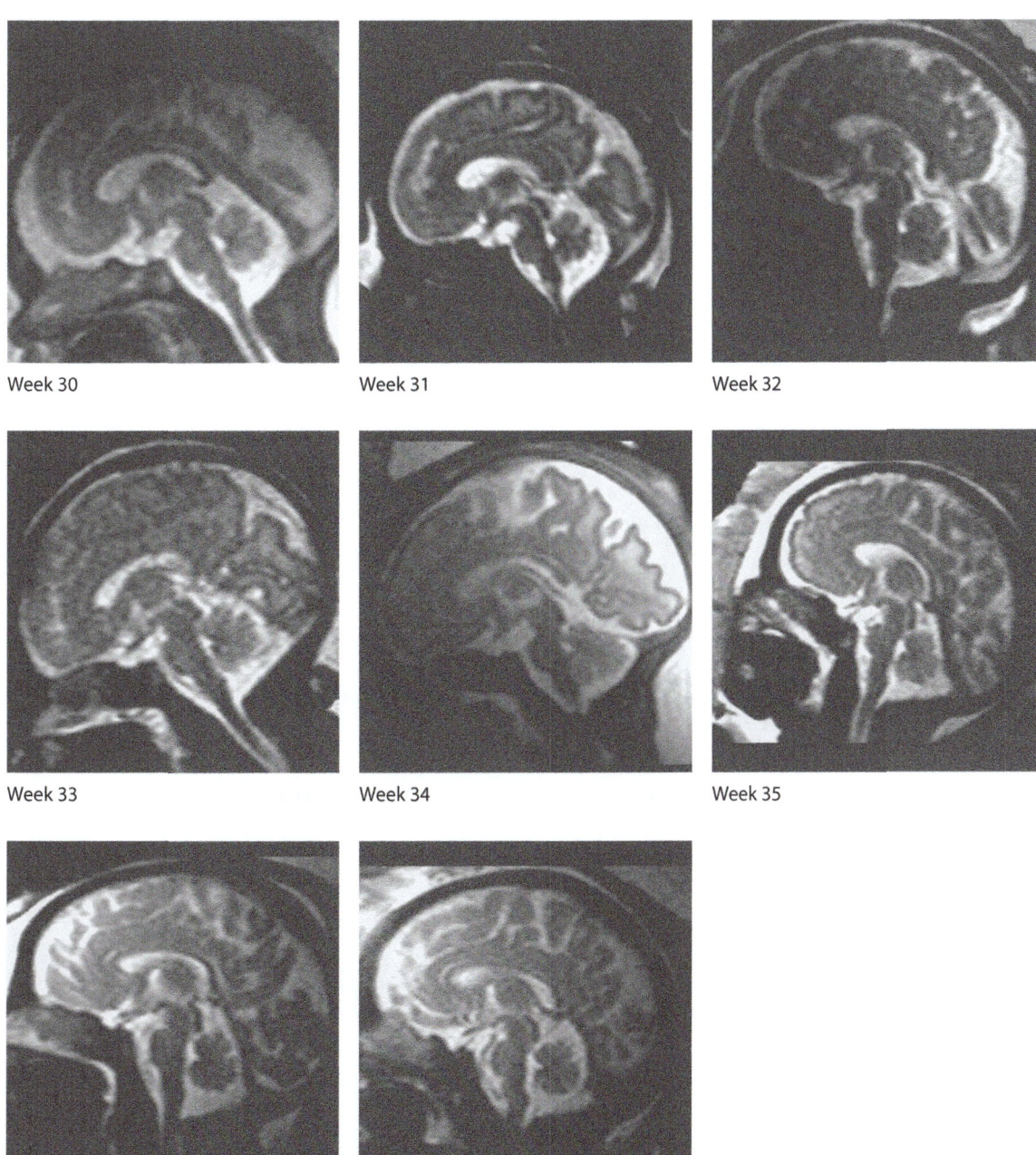

Week 30

Week 31

Week 32

Week 33

Week 34

Week 35

Week 36

Weeks 37–38

Slice 2

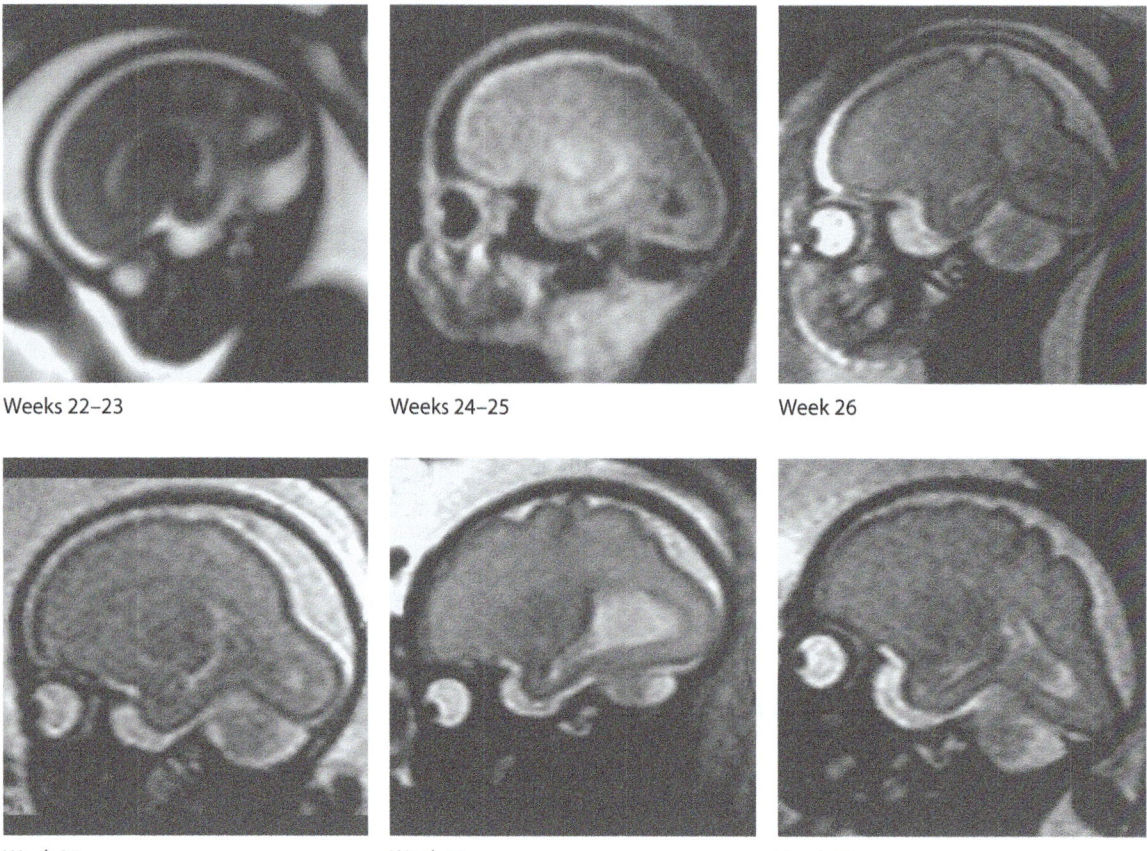

Weeks 22–23   Weeks 24–25   Week 26

Week 27   Week 28   Week 29

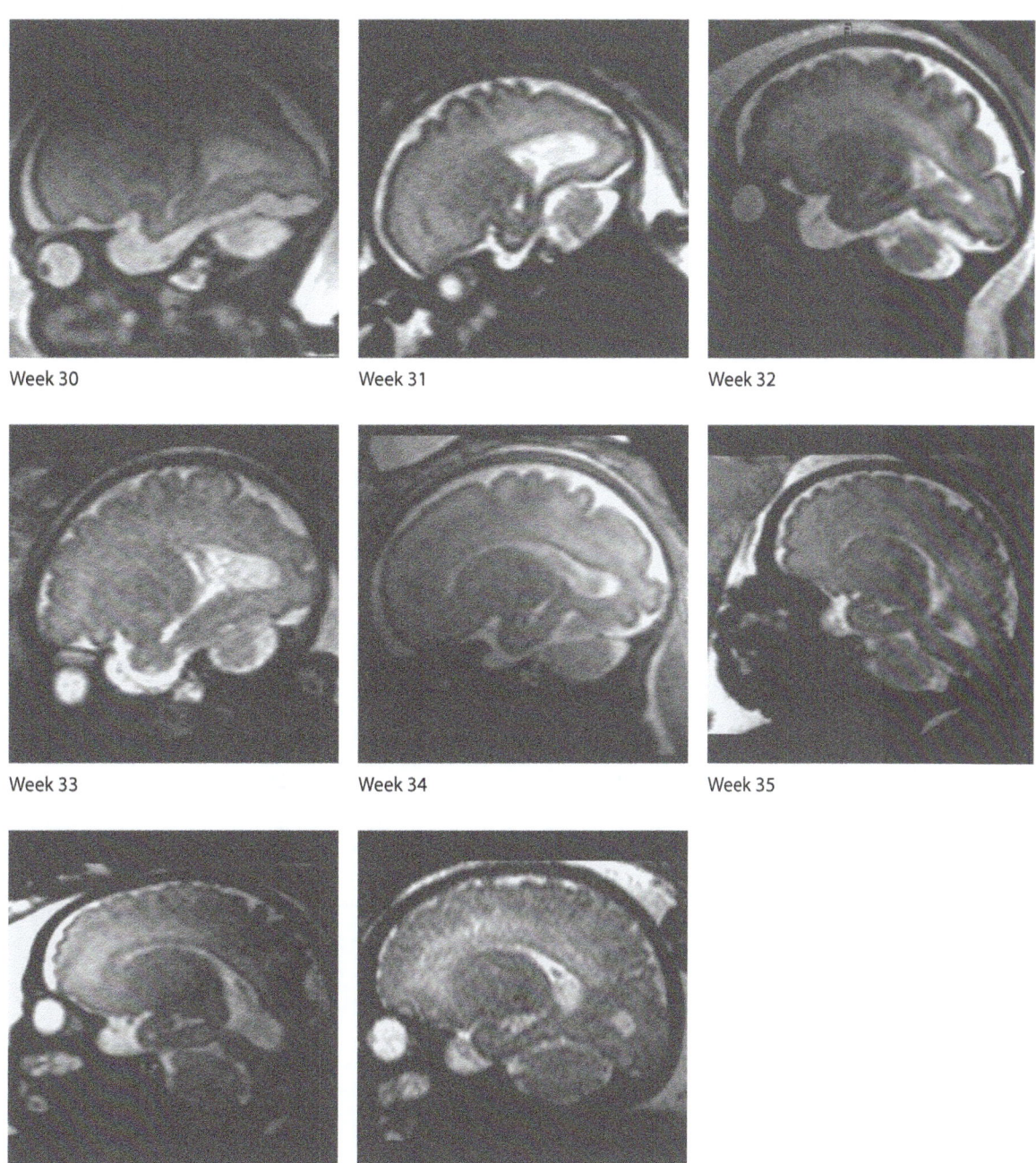

Week 30

Week 31

Week 32

Week 33

Week 34

Week 35

Week 36

Weeks 37–38

Slice 3

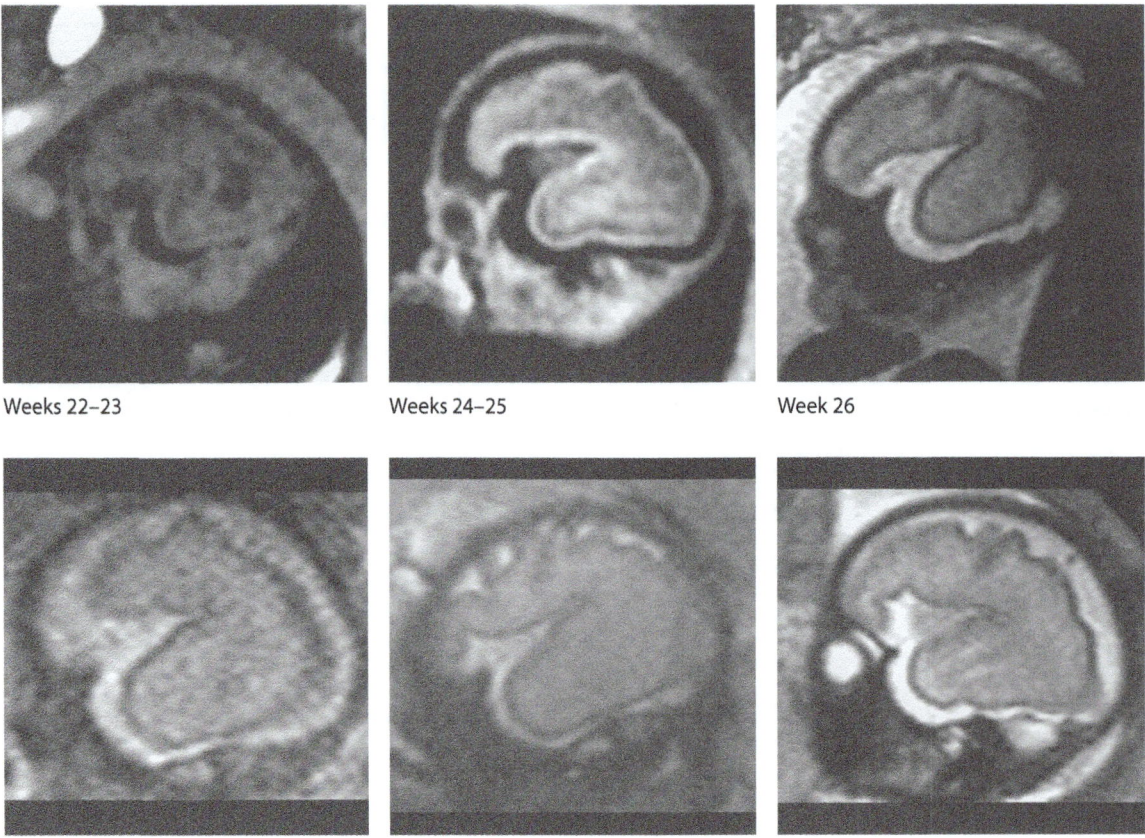

Weeks 22–23   Weeks 24–25   Week 26

Week 27   Week 28   Week 29

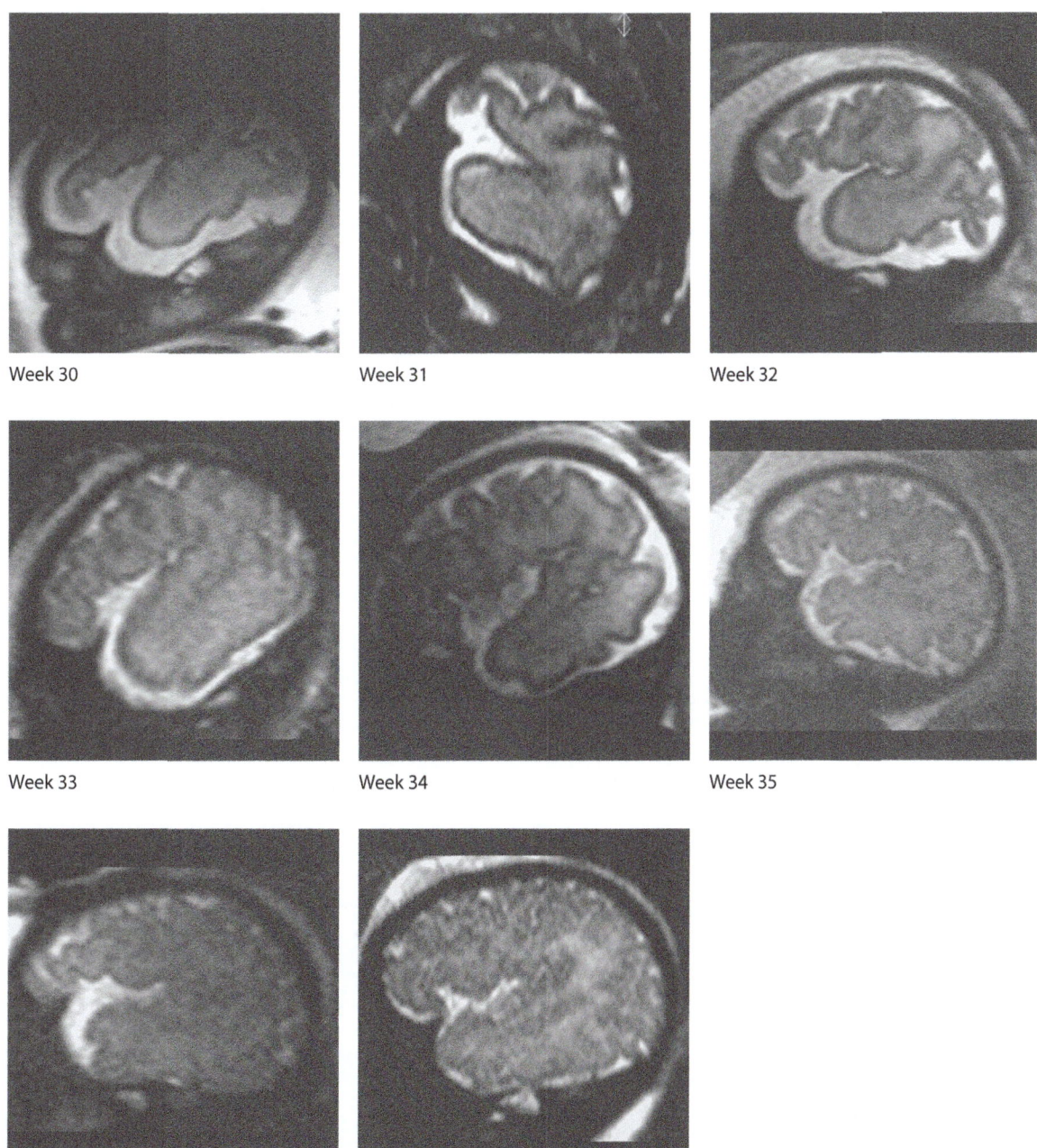

Week 30

Week 31

Week 32

Week 33

Week 34

Week 35

Week 36

Weeks 37–38

Slice 4

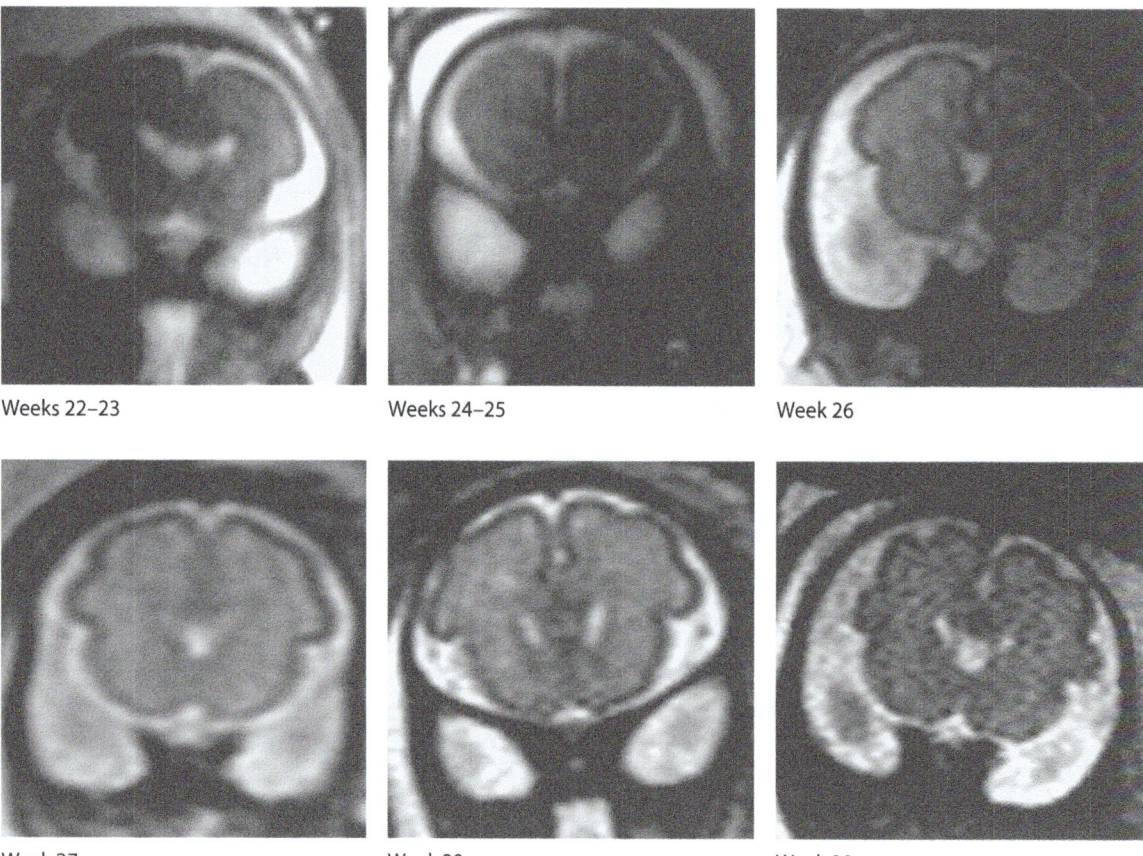

Weeks 22–23

Weeks 24–25

Week 26

Week 27

Week 28

Week 29

Slice 4

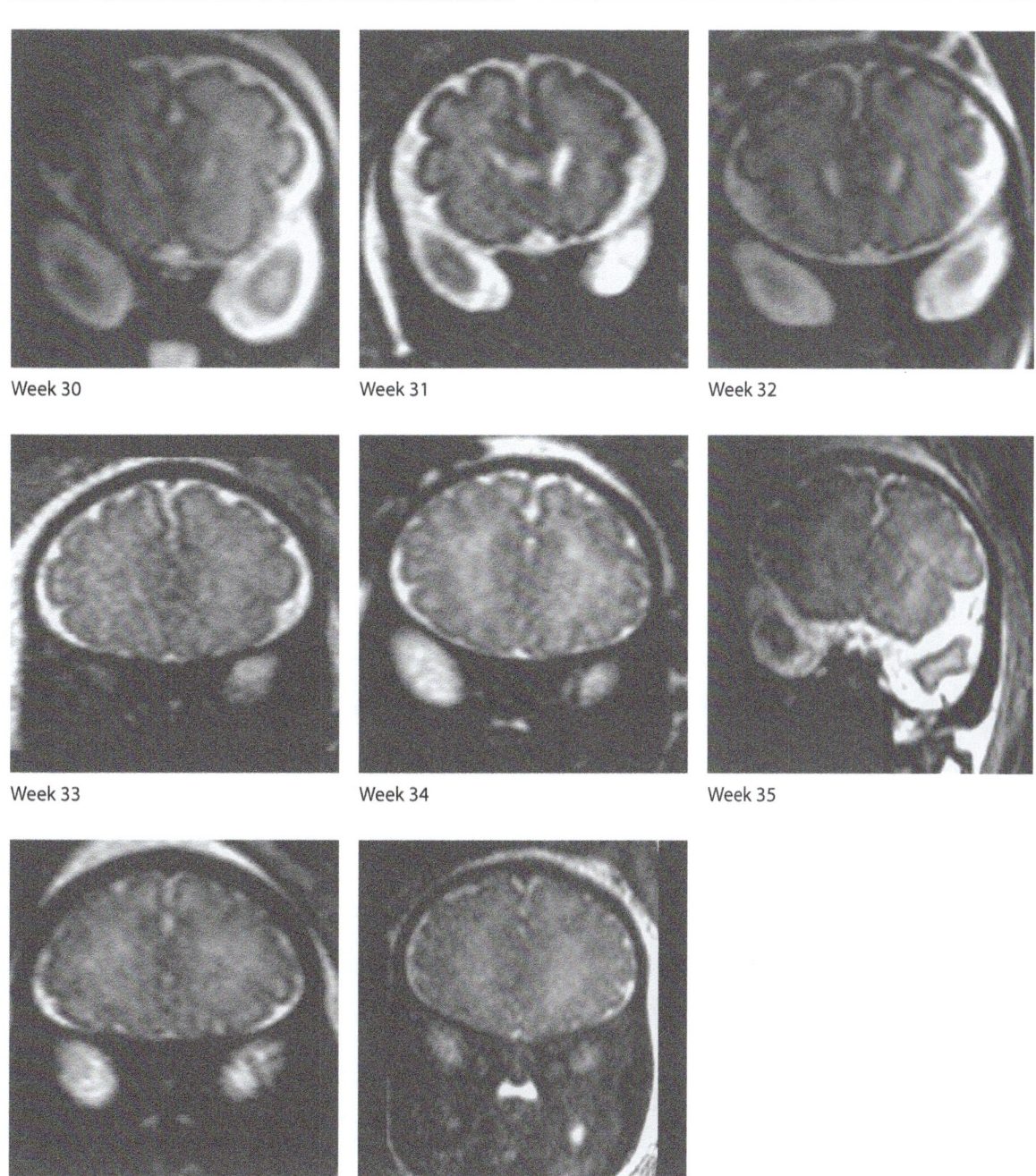

Week 30

Week 31

Week 32

Week 33

Week 34

Week 35

Week 36

Weeks 37–38

Slice 5

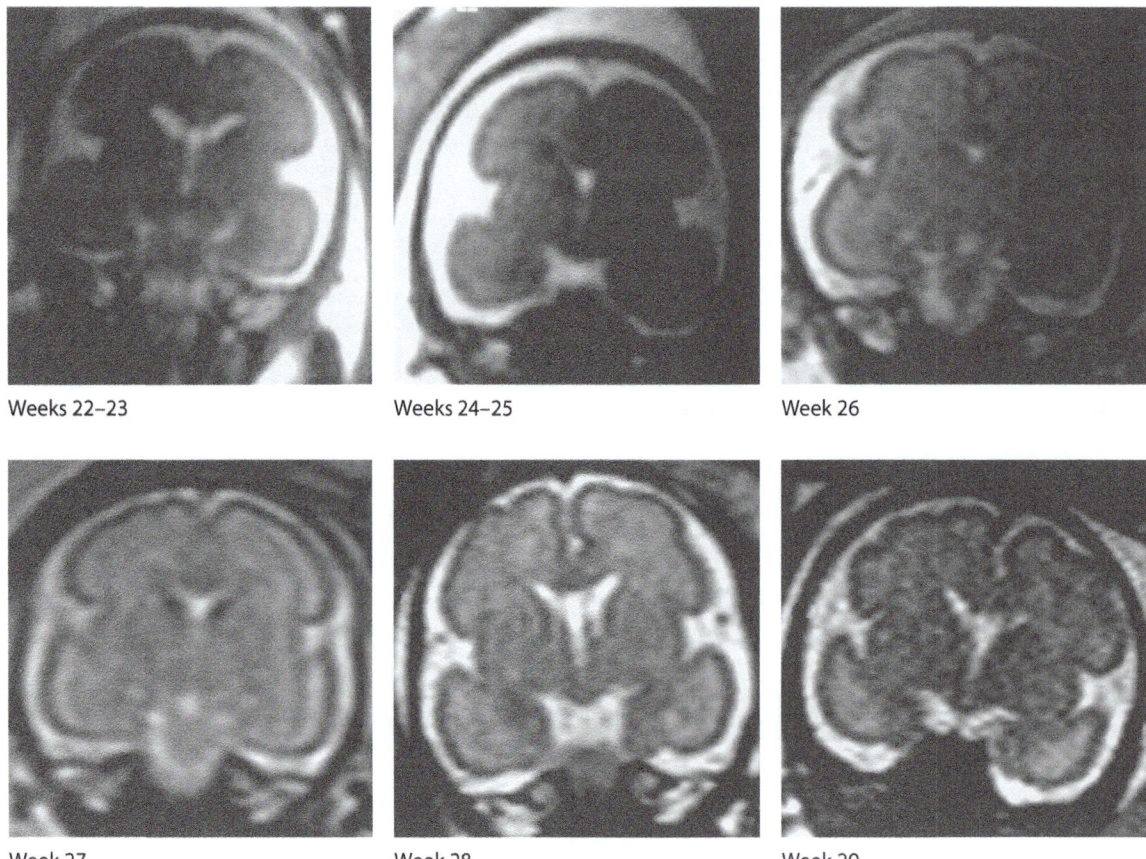

Weeks 22–23   Weeks 24–25   Week 26

Week 27   Week 28   Week 29

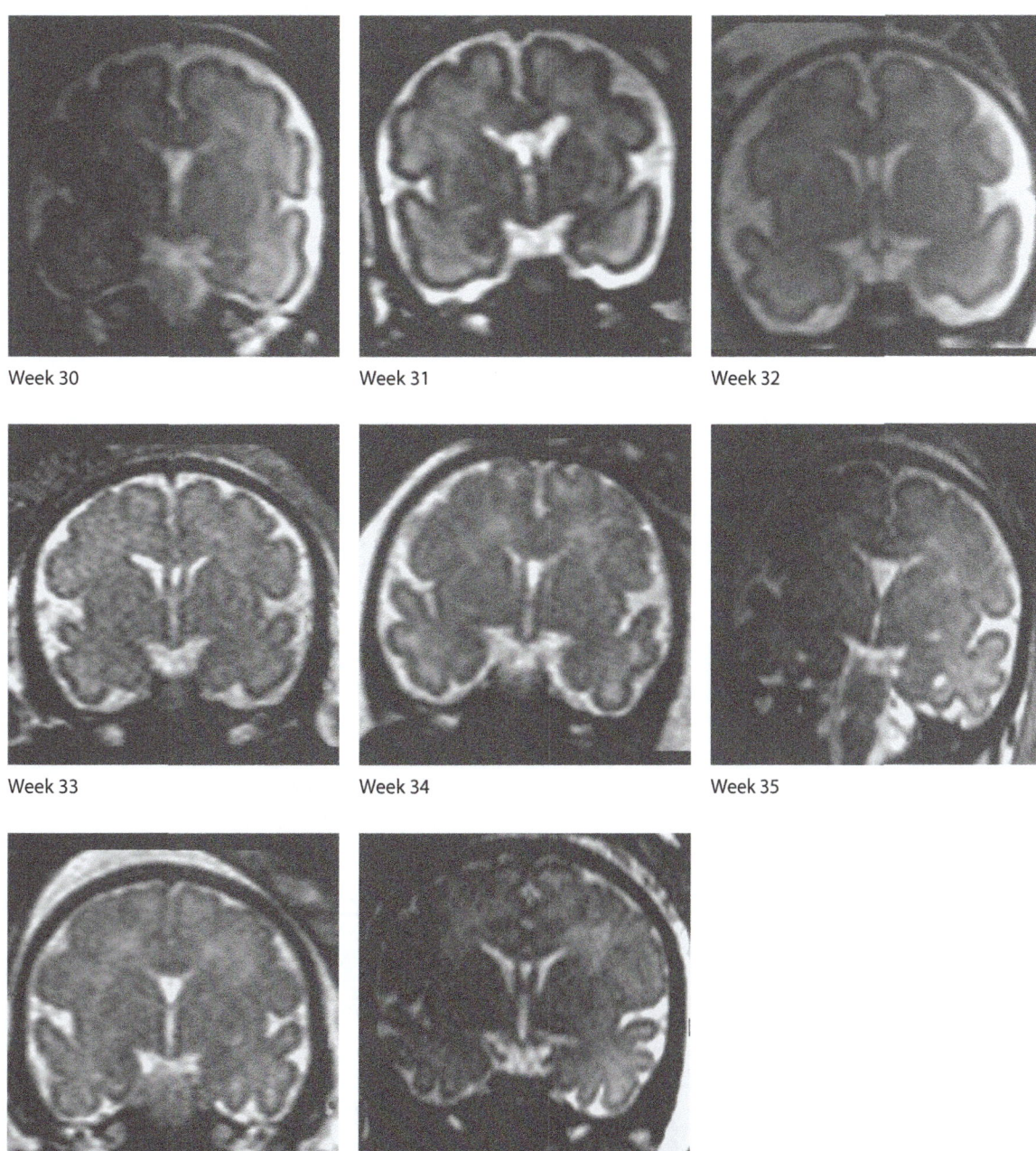

Week 30

Week 31

Week 32

Week 33

Week 34

Week 35

Week 36

Weeks 37–38

Slice 6

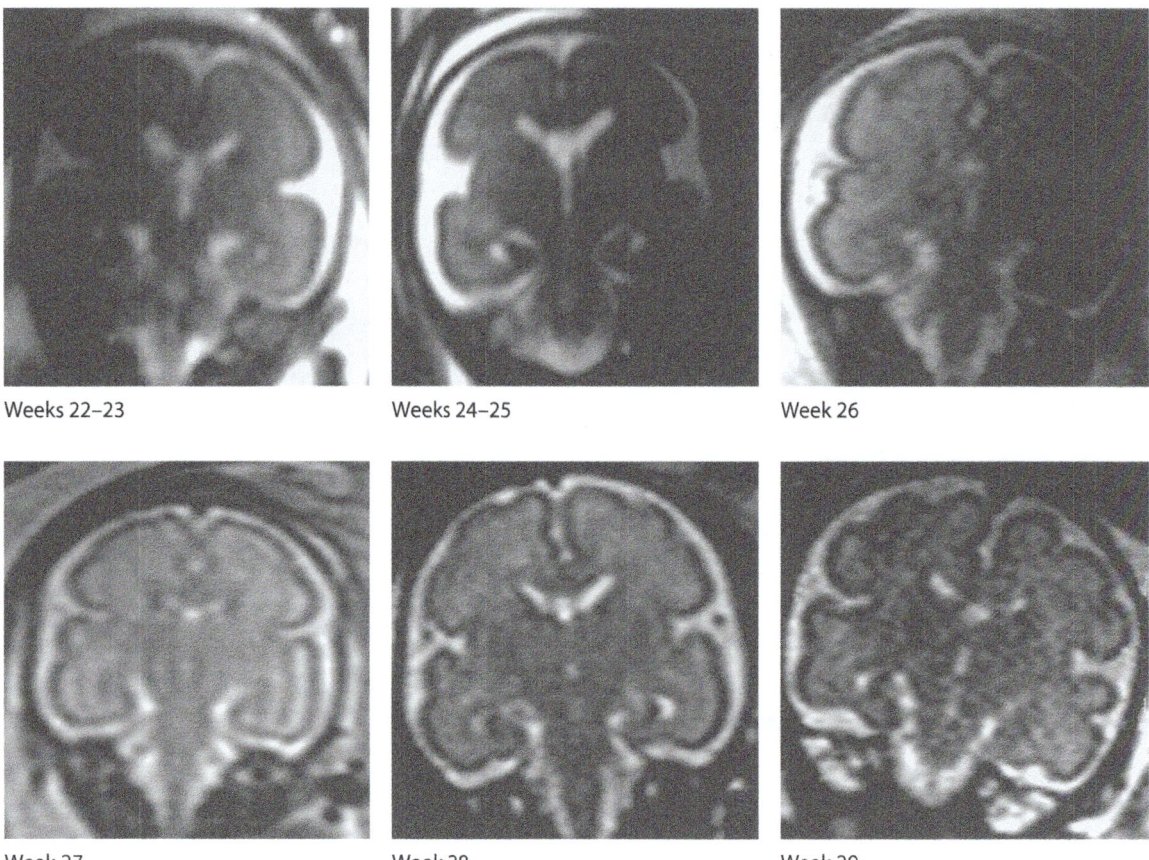

Weeks 22–23   Weeks 24–25   Week 26

Week 27   Week 28   Week 29

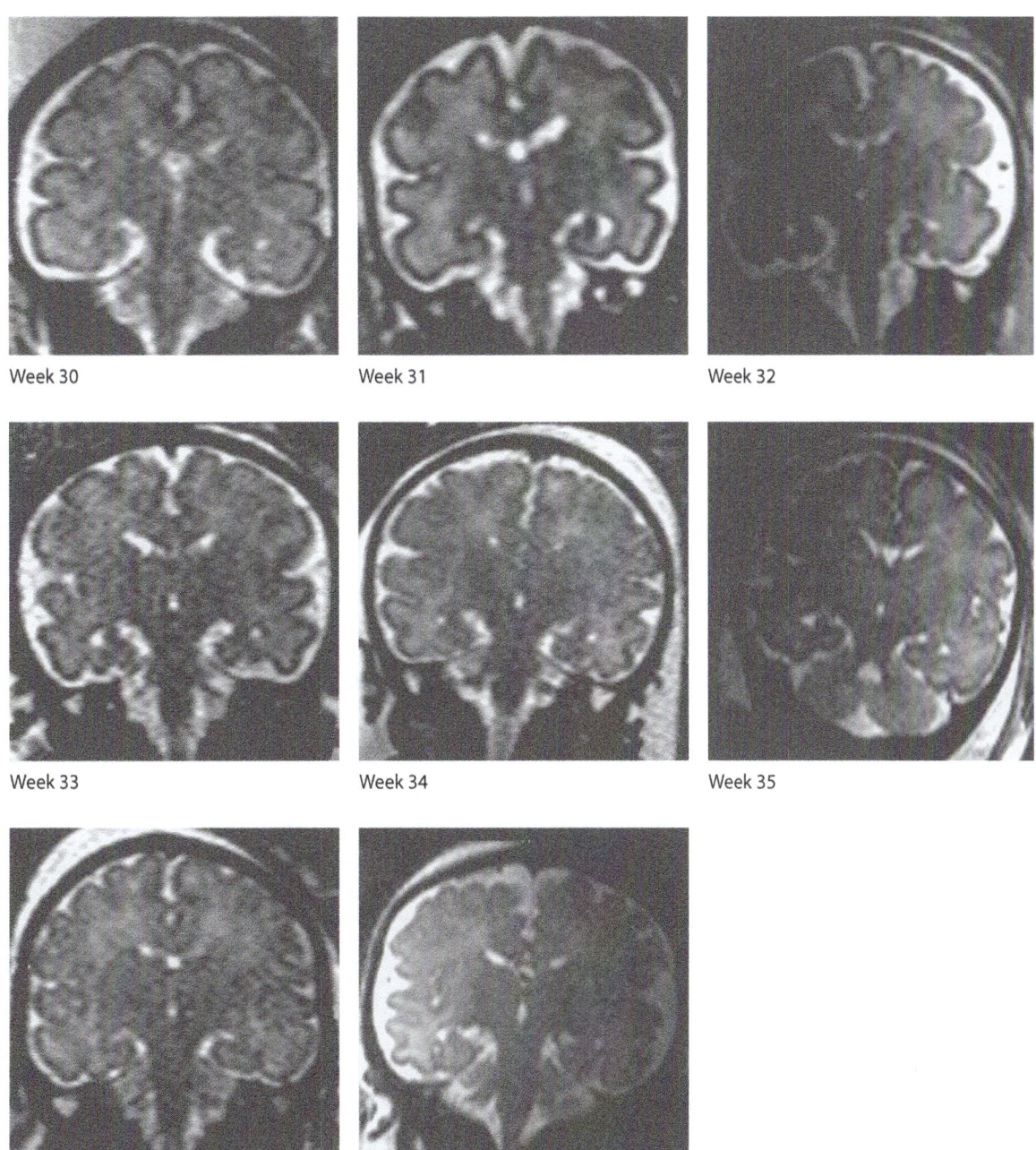

Week 30

Week 31

Week 32

Week 33

Week 34

Week 35

Week 36

Weeks 37–38

Slice 7

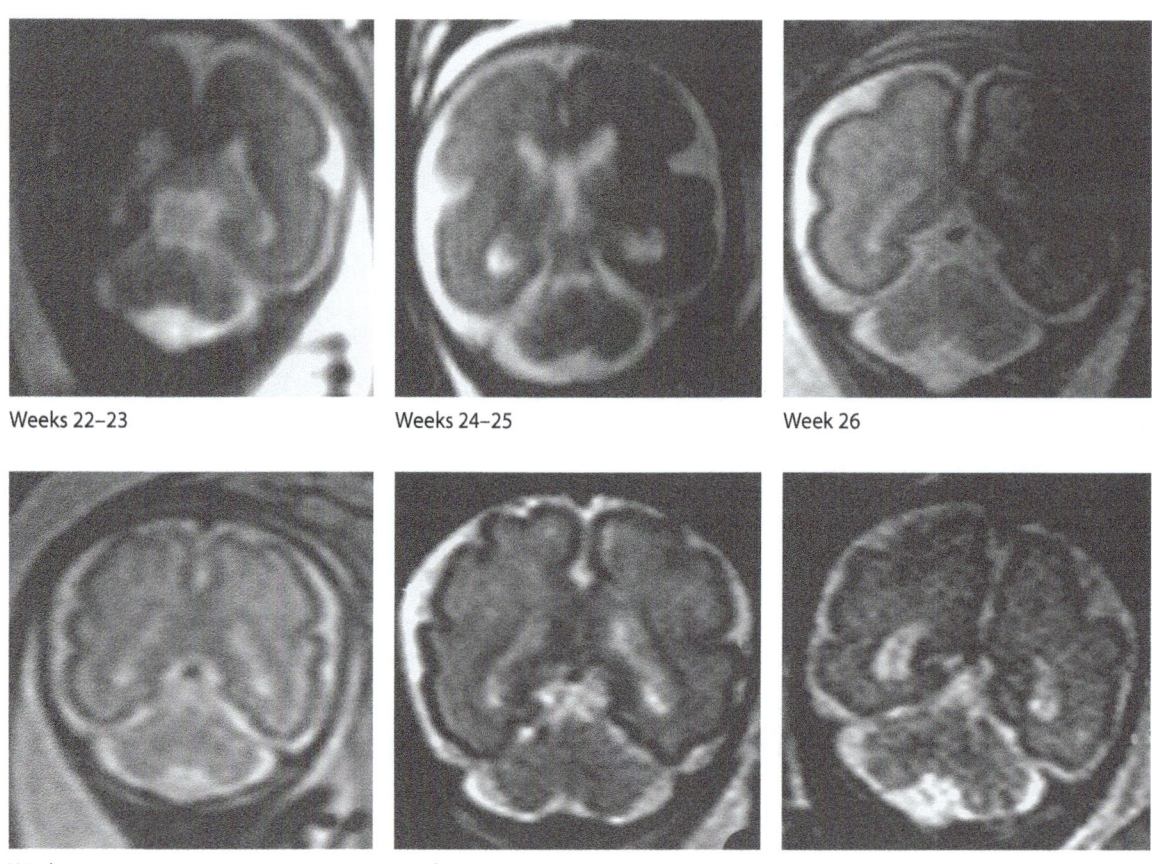

Weeks 22–23

Weeks 24–25

Week 26

Week 27

Week 28

Week 29

Slice 7

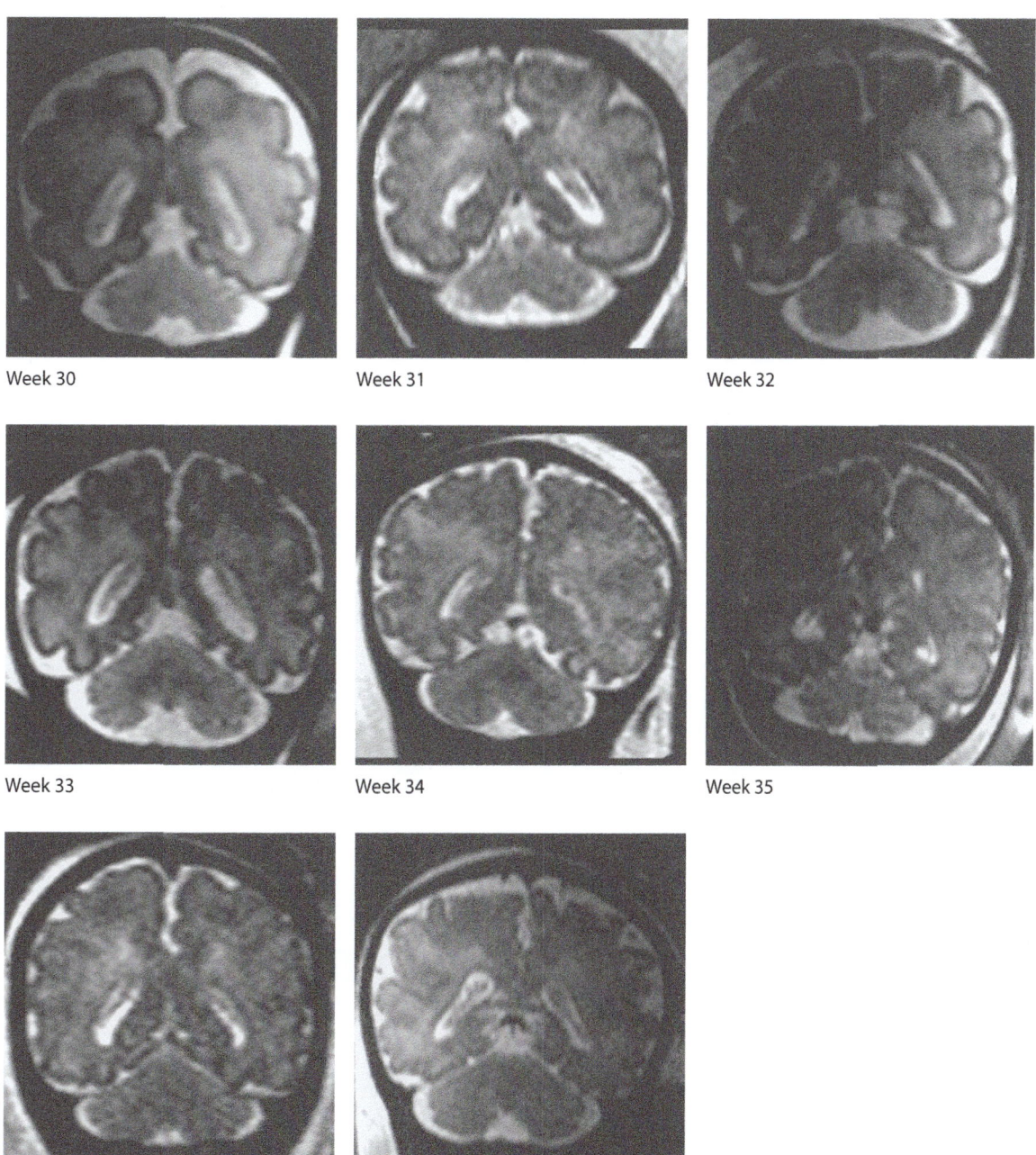

Week 30   Week 31   Week 32

Week 33   Week 34   Week 35

Week 36   Weeks 37–38

Slice 8

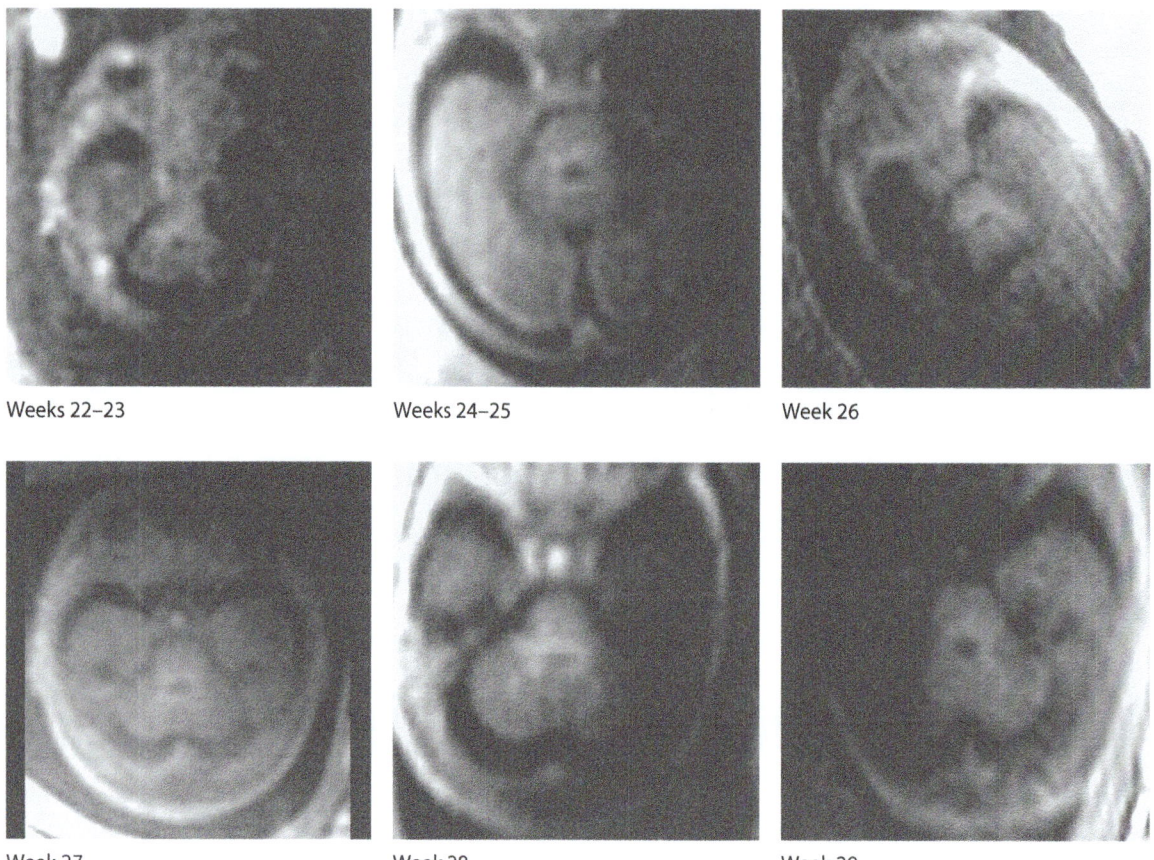

Weeks 22–23   Weeks 24–25   Week 26

Week 27   Week 28   Week 29

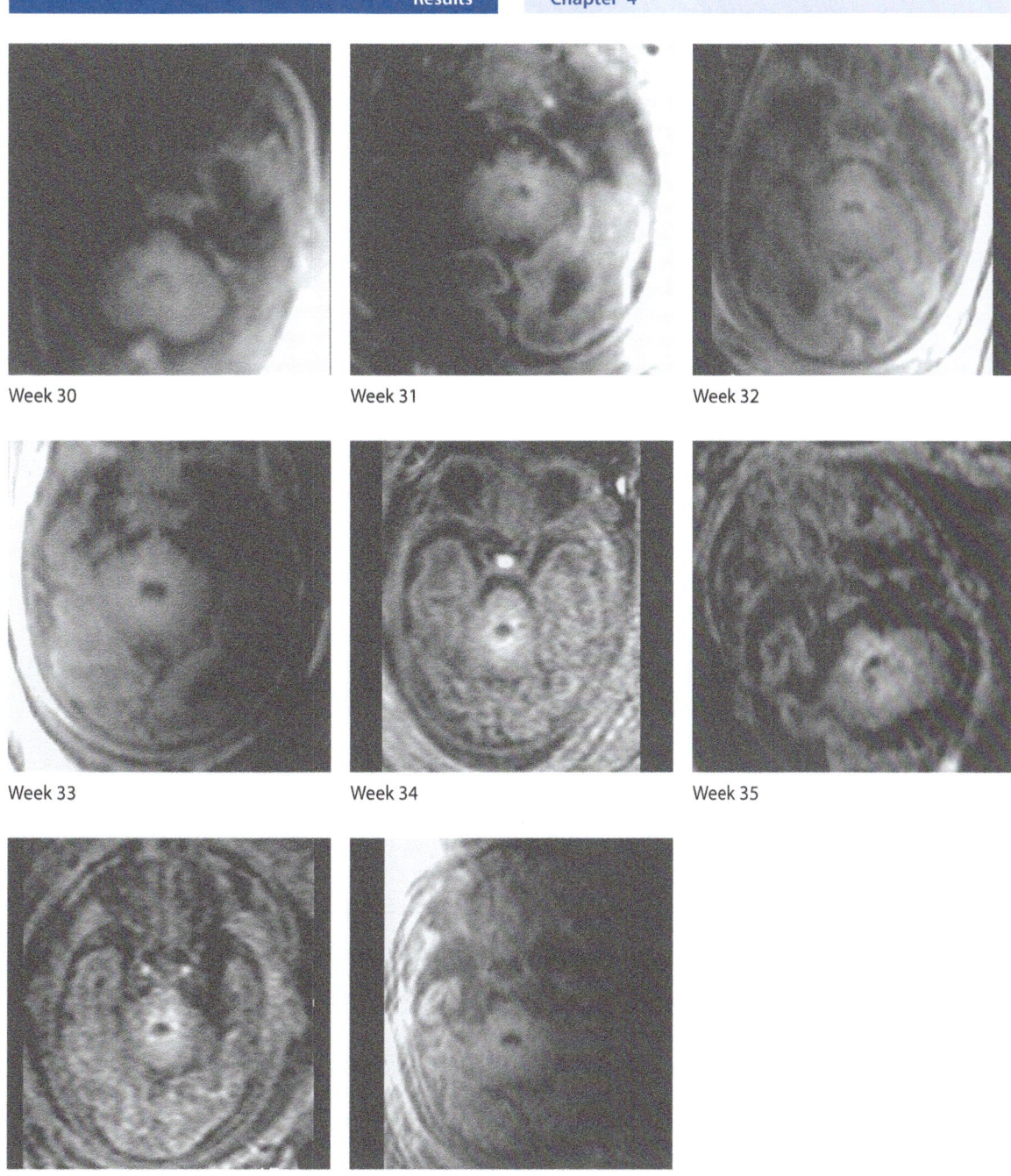

Week 30

Week 31

Week 32

Week 33

Week 34

Week 35

Week 36

Weeks 37–38

Slice 9

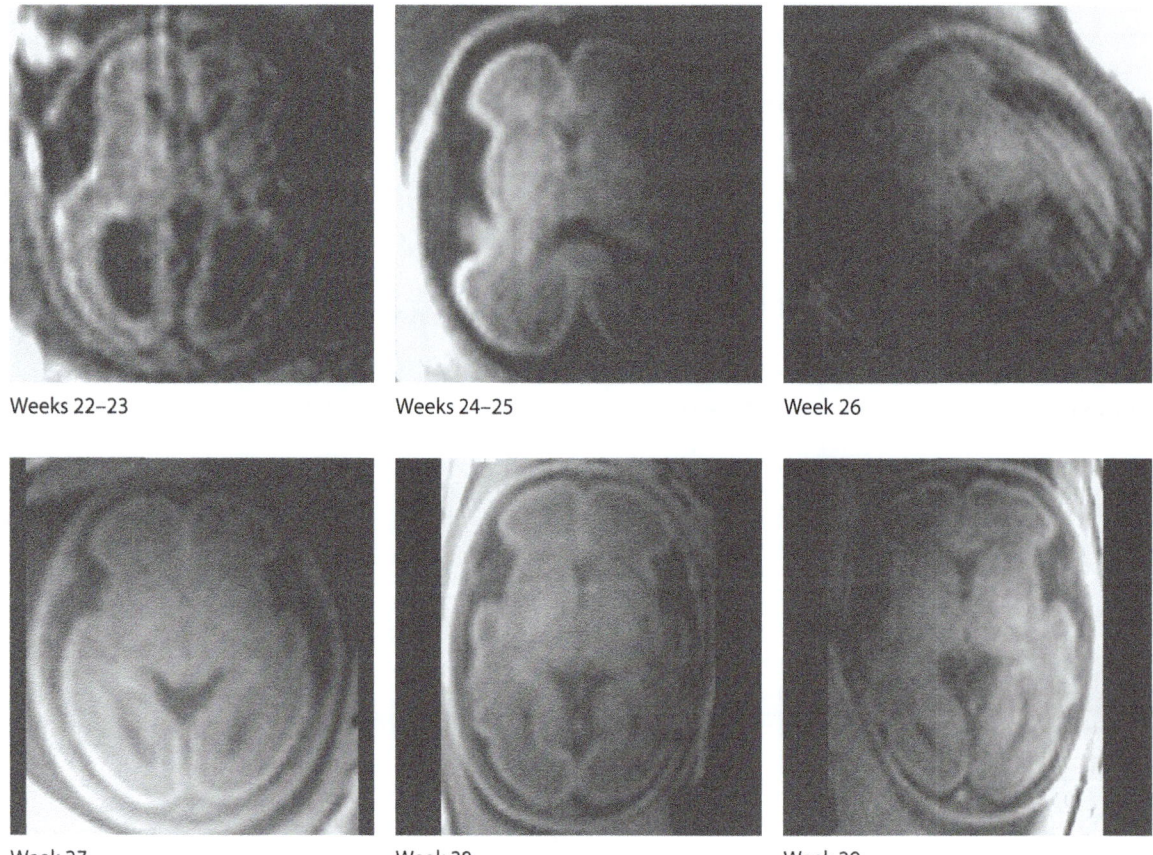

Weeks 22–23   Weeks 24–25   Week 26

Week 27   Week 28   Week 29

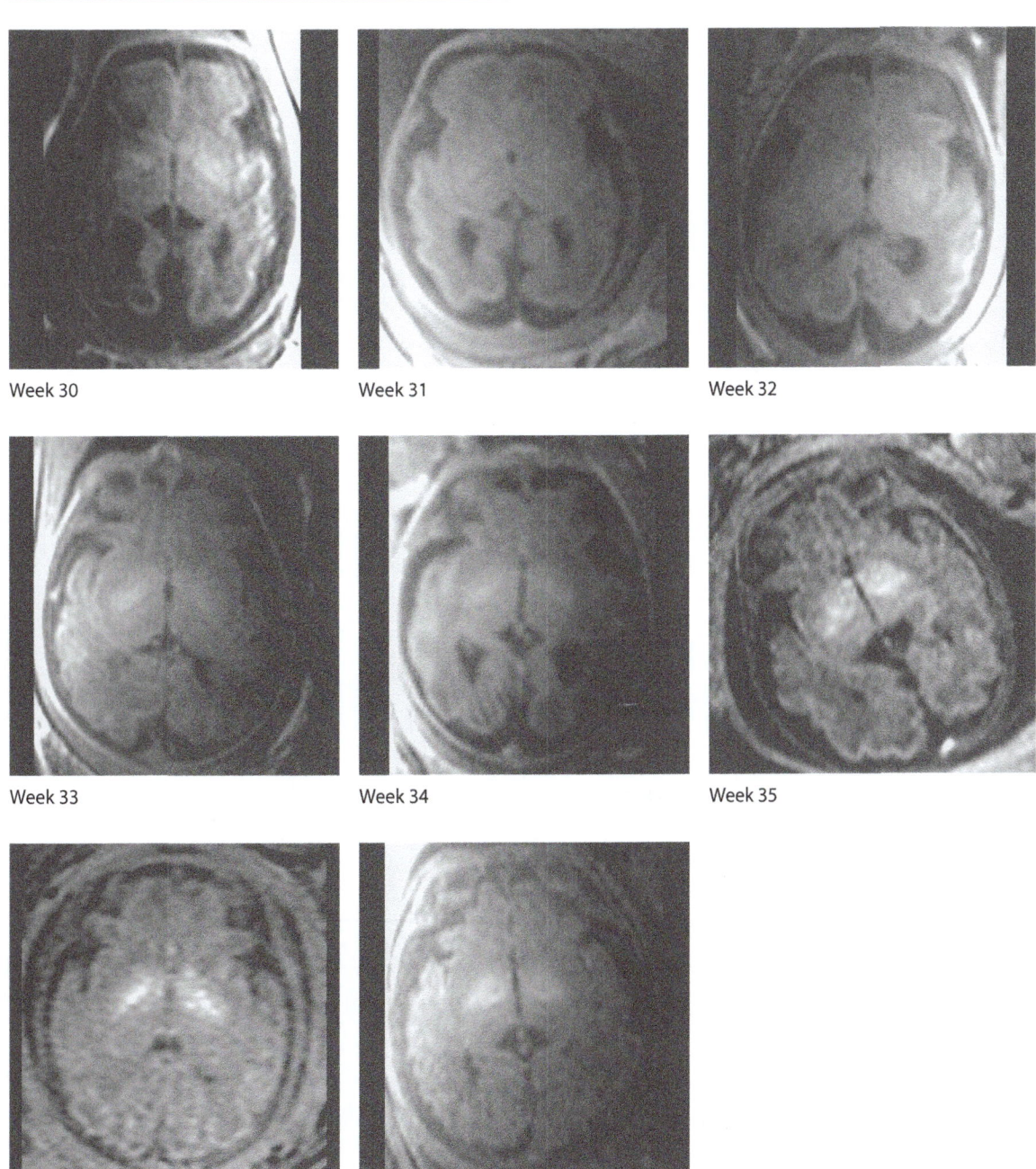

Week 30

Week 31

Week 32

Week 33

Week 34

Week 35

Week 36

Weeks 37–38

Slice 10

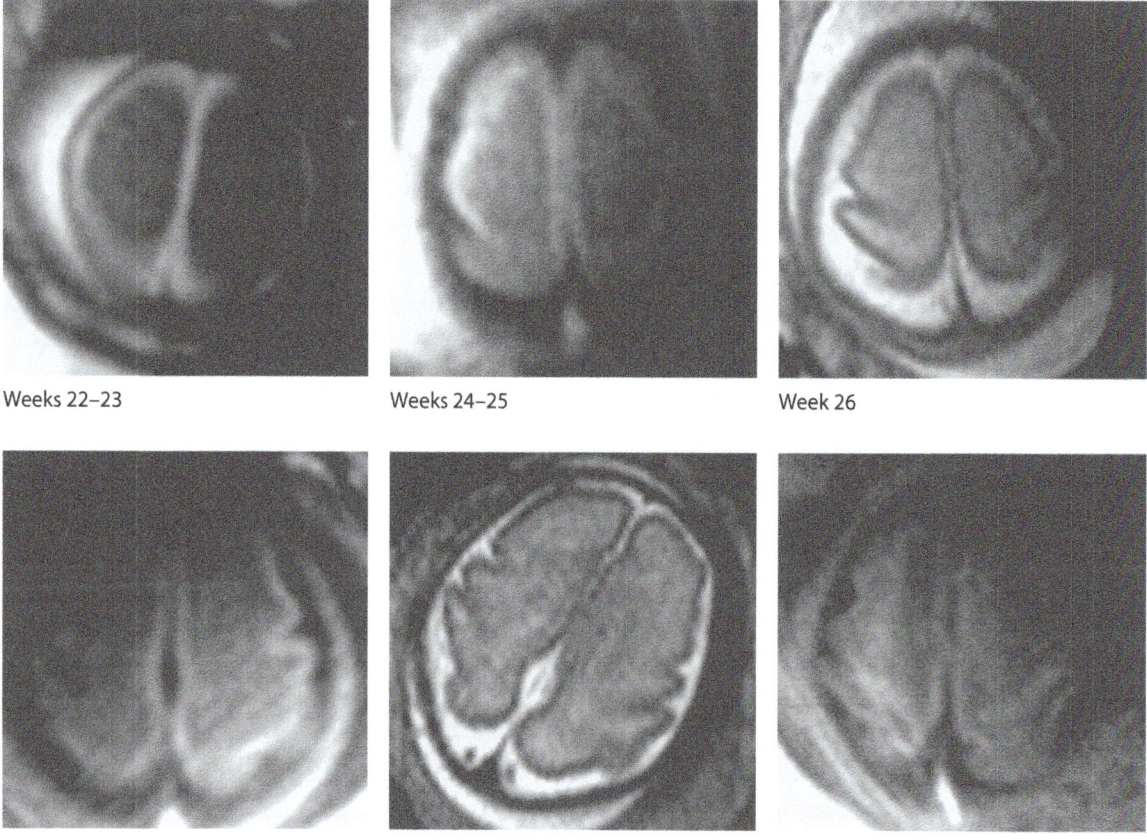

Weeks 22–23   Weeks 24–25   Week 26

Week 27   Week 28   Week 29

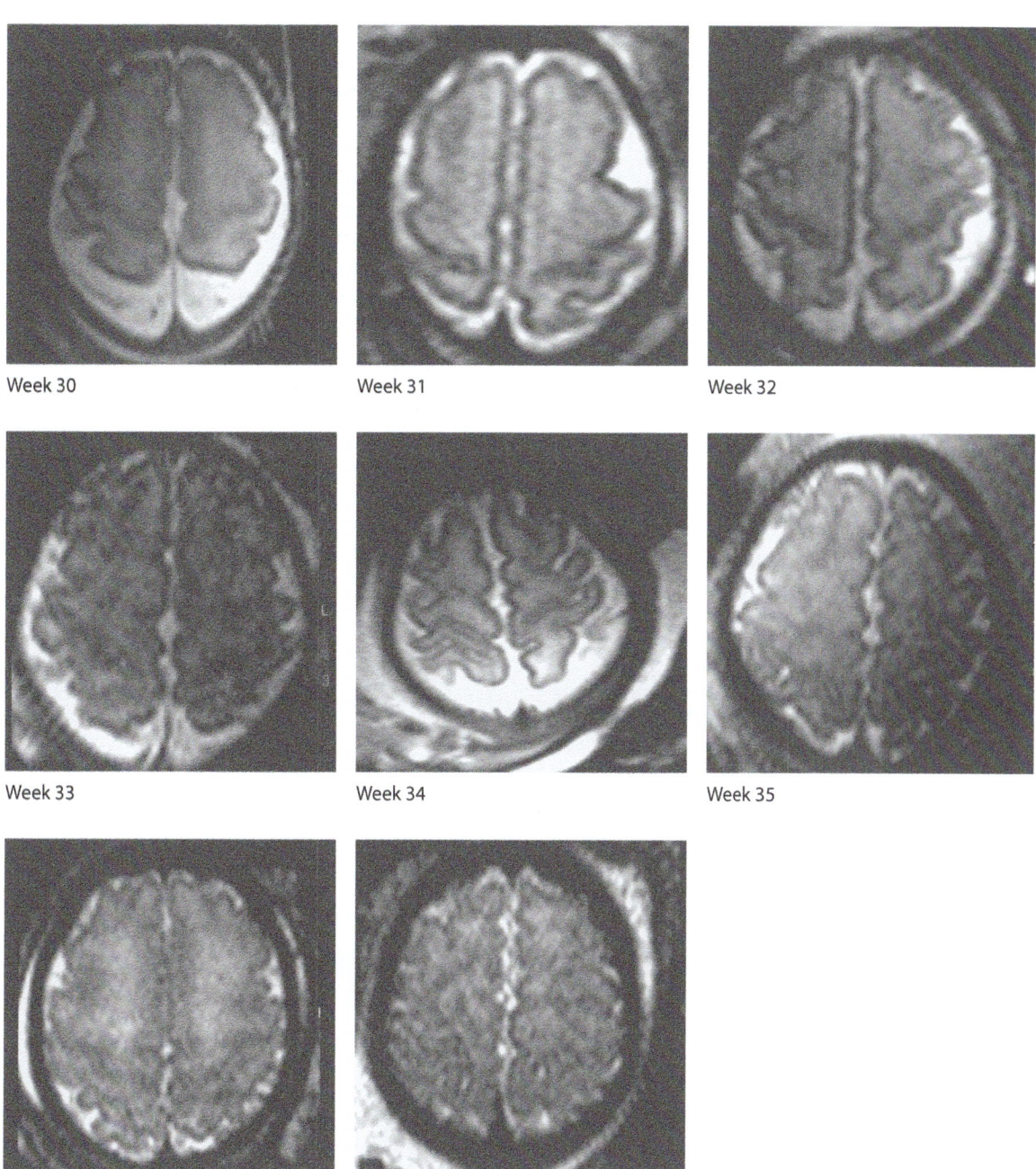

Week 30

Week 31

Week 32

Week 33

Week 34

Week 35

Week 36

Weeks 37–38

Detailed Results of Biometry for Each Parameter Studied

As mentioned in Chap. 3, the results are presented in their raw state, without any smoothing of the imperfections related to the small study population. These results give an order of magnitude rather than exact values for each parameter. They cannot be as precise as the biometrical values established in much larger-scale fetal sonographic studies. Hence, the reader should always refer to the results for the preceding and following weeks. Aberrant results (e.g. 10th percentile for a value lower than that of the preceding week, or a higher value for a given percentile than in the following 2 or 3 weeks) appear in bold characters in order to encourage the reader's critical thinking.

Fronto-occipital Diameter

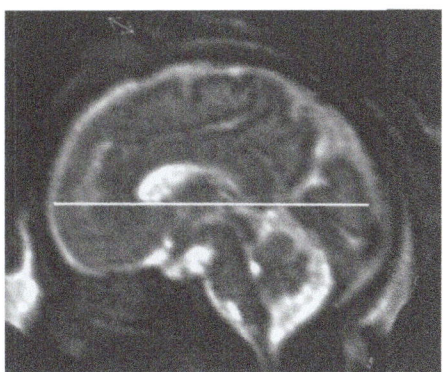

WG	Cohort	Average	SD	10th perc.	25th perc.	50th perc.	75th perc.	90th perc.	Min.	Max.
22–23	8	67.5	3.1	60	65	67	71	72	60	73
24–25	7	69.7	8.12	63	66	71	74	79	60	81
26	5	76.8	7.91	71	71	74	78	85	71	90
27	16	81.3	4.68	78	78	80	86	88	73	90
28	11	81.5	4.15	77	79	81	82	88	70	90
29	18	85.3	5.84	79	81	86	90	91	75	95
30	23	89.2	5.94	83	86	89	91	95	77	108
31	21	91	3.85	86	90	91	94	96	82	97
32	25	93.4	5.43	88	90	92	96	99	82	106
33	20	97	4.48	92	94	96	100	103	90	105
34	24	99	5.28	**94**	96	98	101	104	90	114
35–36	28	102.2	3.92	98	99	101	104	106	97	113
37–38	17	103	5.78	98	100	103	108	110	90	112

The values in bold characters correspond to aberrant results. Please refer to the comment at the beginning of „Detailed Results of Biometry for Each Parameter Studied", p. 86.

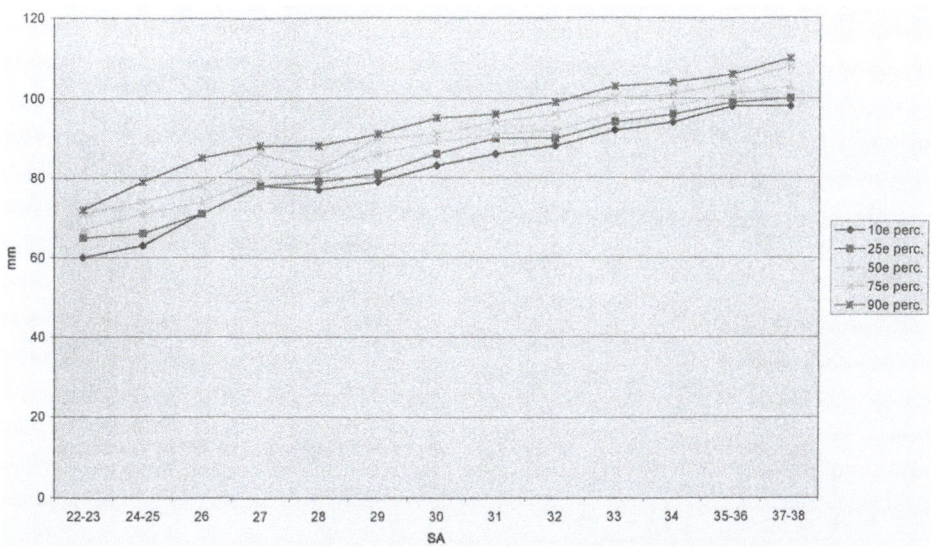

Cerebral Biparietal Diameter

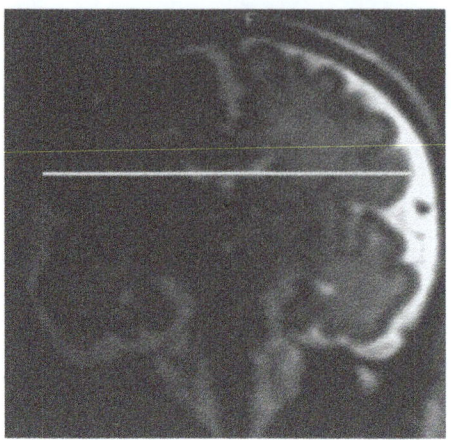

WG	Cohort	Average	SD	10th perc.	25th perc.	50th perc.	75th perc.	90th perc.	Min.	Max.
22–23	7	49	4.24	46	46	49	53	54	45	55
24–25	7	51.8	5.76	47	50	52	55	57	44	58
26	5	57.8	4.14	54	56	58	60	62	52	63
27	16	59.4	3.65	55	58	59	60	62	55	63
28	9	61.3	4.73	57	59	62	64	65	52	69
29	16	65.7	3.71	62	64	66	67	70	57	72
30	23	69	4.55	65	66	68	70	74	62	82
31	21	70.5	4.42	65	68	70	73	76	60	80
32	21	72.4	5.85	**64**	69	72	77	78	63	86
33	20	77.7	3.89	70	74	76	79	80	63	83
34	20	**76.7**	4.81	72	75	77	79	81	64	85
35–36	27	81.2	3.72	76	80	82	84	85	70	87
37–38	18	83.6	5.63	77	80	83	86	89	74	91

The values in bold characters correspond to aberrant results. Please refer to the comment at the beginning of „Detailed Results of Biometry for Each Parameter Studied", p. 86.

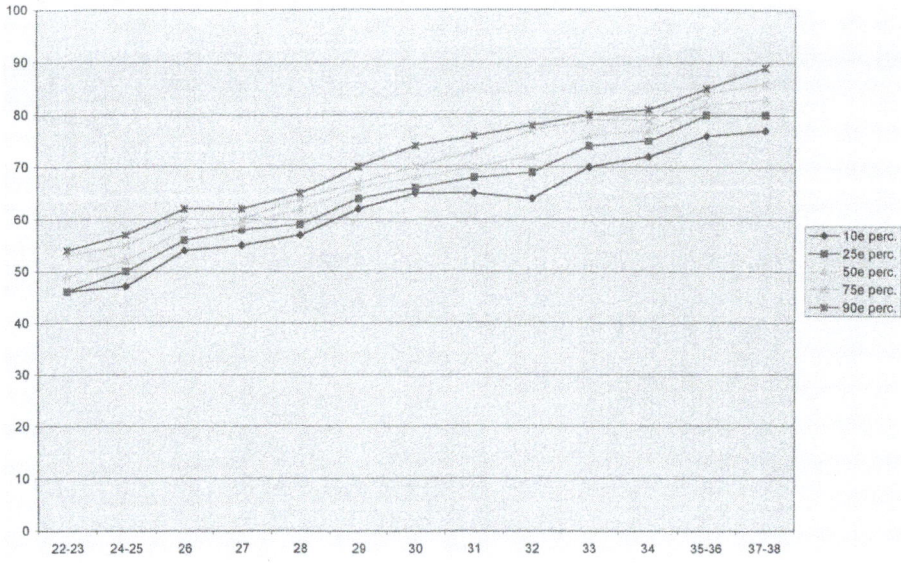

Bone Biparietal Diameter

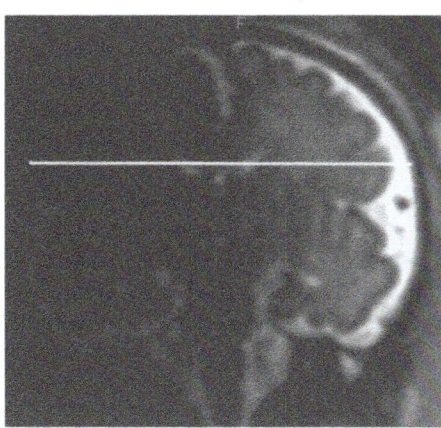

WG	Cohort	Average	SD	10th perc.	25th perc.	50th perc.	75th perc.	90th perc.	Min.	Max.
22–23	7	55.5	5.07	51	52	55	58	61	50	63
24–25	7	60	6.78	54	56	63	66	67	53	68
26	5	65.2	4.86	61	63	64	66	70	60	73
27	16	66.8	3.86	62	66	67	69	**69**	60	70
28	9	67.8	6.93	**61**	**65**	68	70	74	55	80
29	16	71.8	4.73	67	71	72	73	76	61	82
30	23	75.7	5.36	70	73	75	77	83	66	88
31	21	76.7	4.99	70	72	77	79	**81**	66	85
32	21	78.9	6.51	70	74	78	84	86	70	91
33	20	81.5	4.74	74	80	81	86	87	74	89
34	20	**81.1**	5.68	74	**79**	81	**84**	88	69	92
35–36	27	86.4	4.08	81	83	87	89	91	78	93
37–38	18	87.6	5.89	**80**	83	88	91	93	77	100

The values in bold characters correspond to aberrant results. Please refer to the comment at the beginning of „Detailed Results of Biometry for Each Parameter Studied", p. 86.

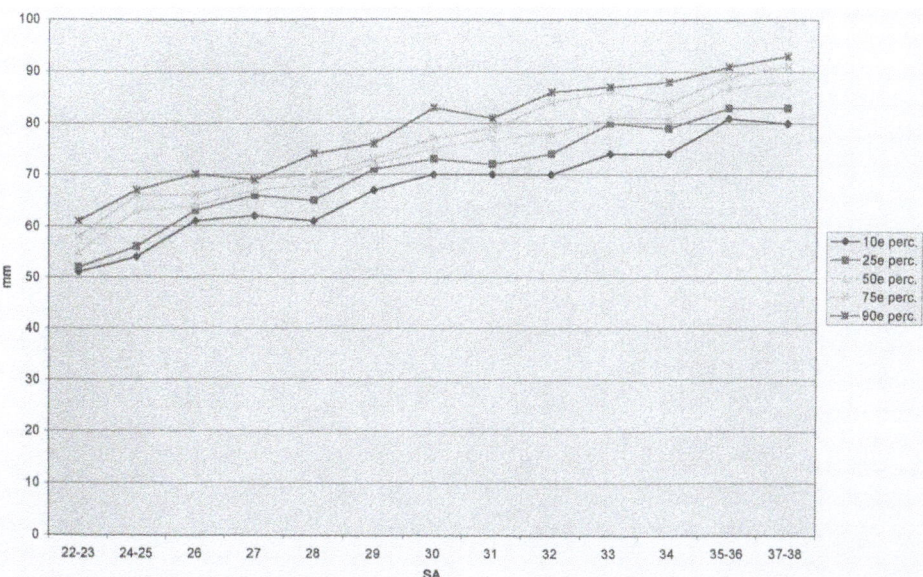

Craniocerebral Index (Bone BPD – Cerebral BPD/Bone BPD)

WG	Average bone BPD	Average cerebral BPD	Bone BPD–Cerebral BPD	Ratio (%)
22–23	55.5	49	**6.5**	11.7
24–25	60	51.8	8.2	13.6
26	65.2	57.8	7.4	11.3
27	66.8	59.4	7.4	11
28	67.8	61.3	6.5	9.5
29	71.8	65.7	6.1	8.5
30	75.7	69	6.7	8.8
31	76.7	70.5	6.2	8
32	78.9	72.4	6.5	8.2
33	81.5	77.7	3.8	**4.7**
34	81.1	76.7	4.4	5.4
35–36	86.4	81.2	5.2	6
37–38	87.6	83.6	4	4.5

The values in bold characters correspond to aberrant results. Please refer to the comment at the beginning of „Detailed Results of Biometry for Each Parameter Studied", p. 86.

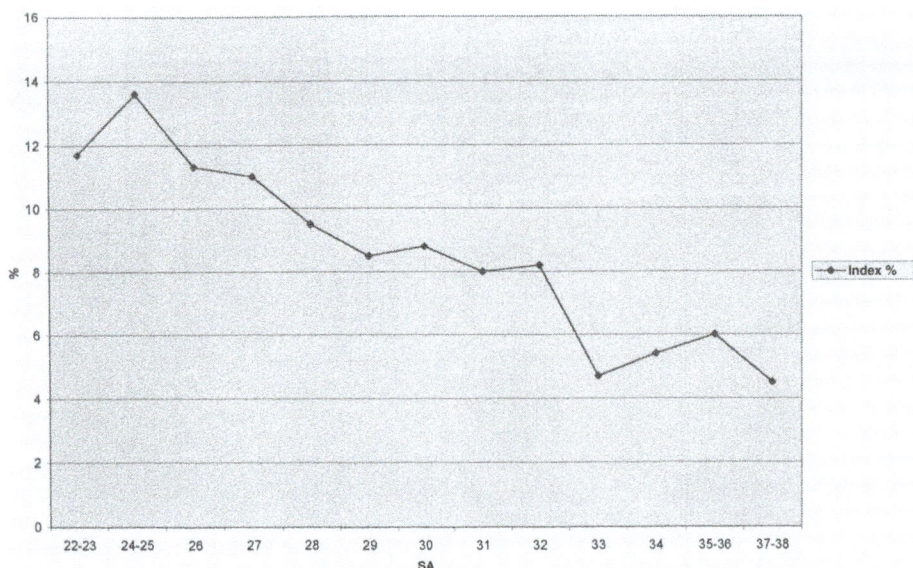

Interhemispheric Distance

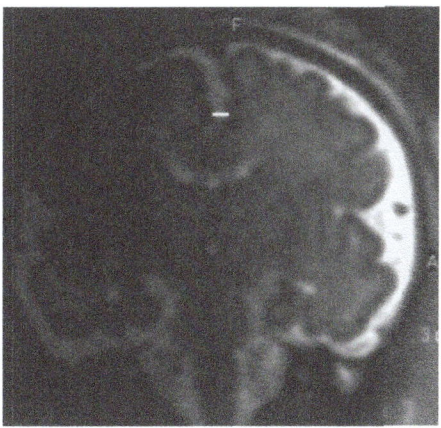

WG	Cohort	Average	SD	10th perc.	25th perc.	50th perc.	75th perc.	90th perc.	Min.	Max.
22–23	4	2.5	0.65	2	2	2.5	3	3	2	3
24–25	7	2.2	0.9	1.5	2	2	2	2.5	1.5	2.5
26	4	3	0.81	2	3	3	3	4	2	4
27	16	3	0.5	1.5	2	3	3	3.5	1.5	4
28	10	2.1	0.81	1.5	1.5	2	2	3	1.5	4
29	16	2.23	0.67	1.5	2	2	3	3	1	3
30	21	2.49	0.8	2	2	2.5	2.5	3.5	1	5
31	16	2.64	0.81	2	2	2.5	3	4	1.5	4
32	19	2.53	0.74	2	2	2.5	3	3	1.5	3.5
33	18	2.58	1.23	2	2	2	3	4	0.5	6
34	20	2.25	0.83	1.5	2	2	3	3	1	4.5
35–36	26	2.15	0.78	1	7.5	2	3	3	1	4
37–38	17	2.07	0.79	1	1.5	2	2.5	3	1	4

This measurement is not very precise, as it concerns a very small structure. However, despite some fluctuations the values are relatively constant throughout the pregnancy. The IHD/cerebral BPD index indicates that this structure becomes smaller and smaller in proportion to the fetal brain.

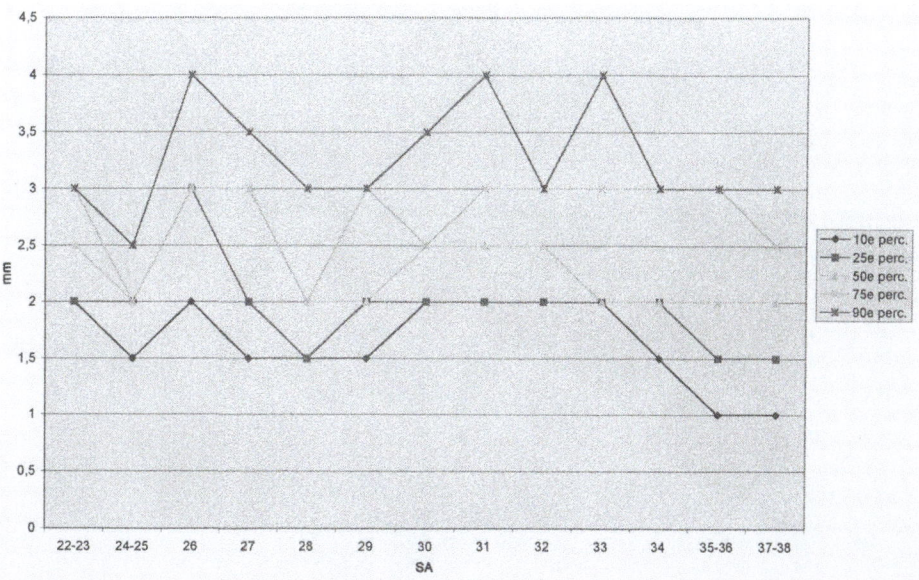

Interhemispheric Distance/Cerebral BPD Index

WG	Average cerebral BPD	Average IHD	Ratio (%)
22–23	49	2.5	5.1
24–25	51.8	2.2	4.2
26	57.8	3	5.2
27	59.4	3	5
28	61.3	2.1	3.4
29	65.7	2.23	3.4
30	69	2.49	3.6
31	70.5	2.64	3.7
32	72.4	2.53	3.5
33	77.7	2.58	3.3
34	76.7	2.25	2.9
35–36	81.2	2.15	2.6
37–38	83.6	2.07	2.4

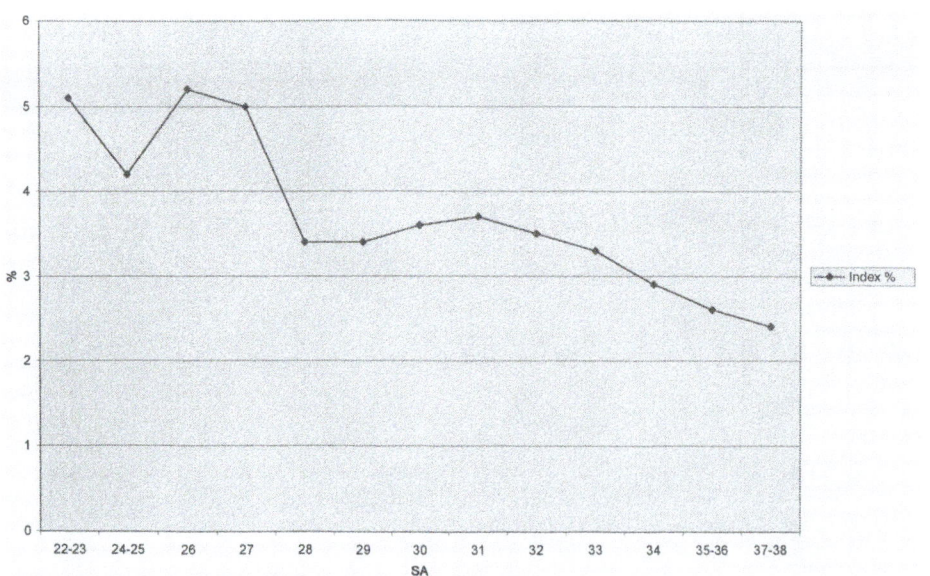

Length of the Corpus Callosum

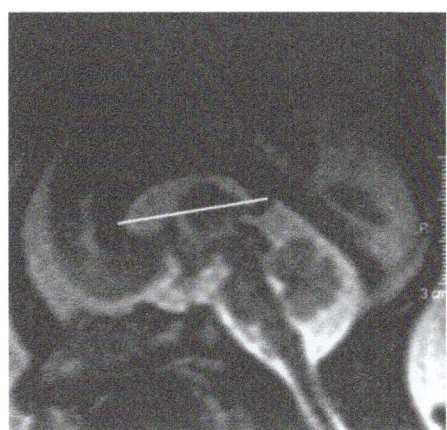

WG	Cohort	Average	SD	10th perc.	25th perc.	50th perc.	75th perc.	90th perc.	Min.	Max.
22–23	8	30.12	1.84	29	29	30	31	32	28	34
24–25	7	30.96	3.3	27	**28**	30	34	35	27	36
26	5	33.4	2.6	31	32	34	34	36	30	37
27	16	35.06	4.34	**30**	32	36	**39**	39	28	41
28	11	36.2	2.57	32	35	37	38	39	32	40
29	16	**35.62**	3.55	32	**33**	**35**	38	39	28	42
30	23	37.06	3.05	33	35	37	38	40	33	46
31	20	37.51	3.1	33	36	37	40	41	32	44
32	22	38.63	3.6	34	37	38	41	44	33	46
33	20	40.97	3.37	37	**40**	40	42	**46**	36	49
34	21	**38.89**	3.09	**36**	38	**39**	**41**	42	30	43
35–36	27	40.9	3.54	37	39	40	43	45	33	49
37–38	17	43.12	5.87	38	40	42	47	50	32	55

The values in bold characters correspond to aberrant results. Please refer to the comment at the beginning of „Detailed Results of Biometry for Each Parameter Studied", p. 86.

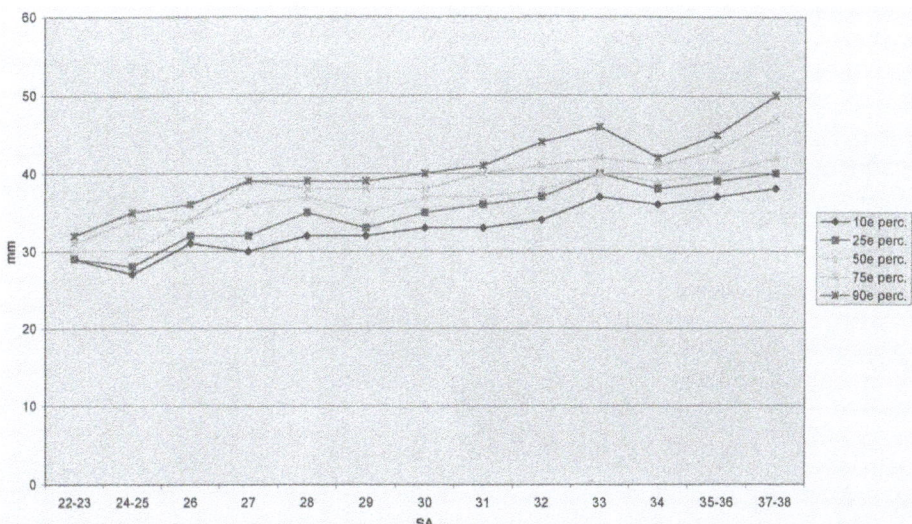

LCC/FOD Index

WG	Average FOD	Average LCC	Ratio (%)
22–23	67.5	30.12	44.6
24–25	69.7	30.96	44.4
26	76.8	33.4	43.5
27	81.3	35.06	43.1
28	81.5	36.2	44.4
29	85.3	35.62	41.7
30	89.2	37.06	41.5
31	91	37.51	41.2
32	93.4	38.63	41.3
33	97	40.97	42.2
34	99	38.89	39.3
35–36	102.2	40.9	40
37–38	103	43.12	41.8

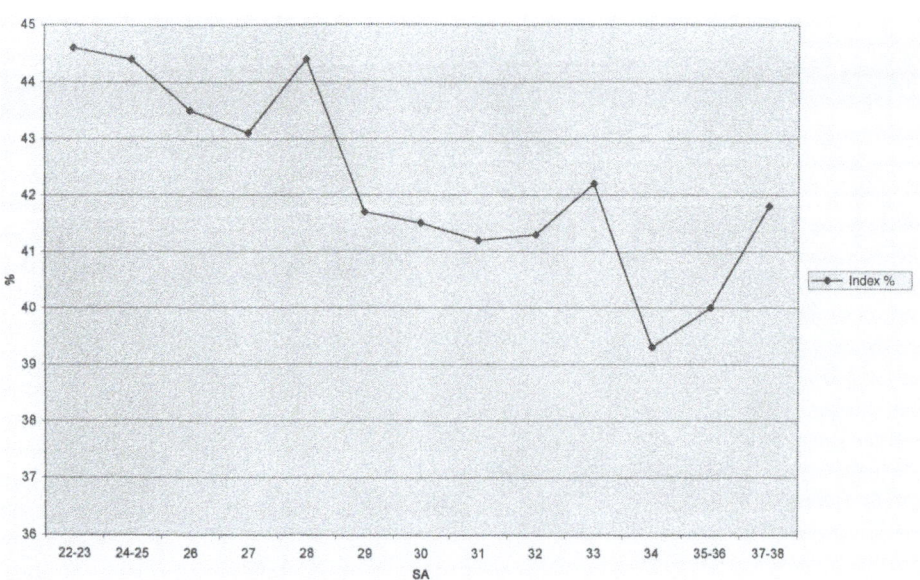

Height of the Vermis

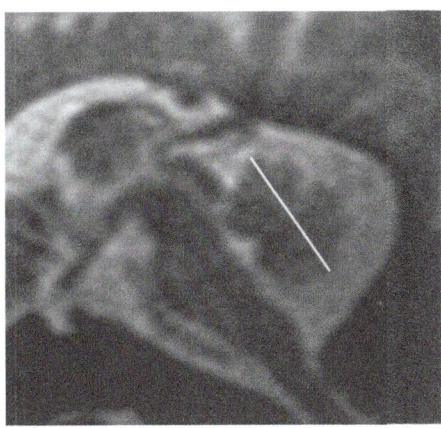

WG	Cohort	Average	SD	10th perc.	25th perc.	50th perc.	75th perc.	90th perc.	Min.	Max.
22–23	6	11.5	1	10	11	11	12	12	10	12
24–25	5	12.8	2.12	11	13	14	14	14	10	15
26	4	14	0.81	13	14	14	14	15	13	15
27	12	15.2	2.24	13	14	16	16	17	12	18
28	10	15.4	1.91	13	14	16	17	18	13	18
29	16	16	1.07	15	15	16	17	**17**	14	18
30	24	17.1	2.14	15	16	17	19	20	13	20
31	20	17.1	1.37	16	16	17	**18**	**19**	15	20
32	21	18.3	2.01	16	17	18	20	21	15	22
33	20	19.2	1.78	17	19	20	20	21	15	22
34	23	20.1	2.15	18	19	20	21	23	16	26
35–36	27	20.9	1.83	19	19	20	22	23	18	25
37–38	18	21.1	2.79	19	20	20	22	24	16	29

The values in bold characters correspond to aberrant results. Please refer to the comment at the beginning of „Detailed Results of Biometry for Each Parameter Studied", p. 86.

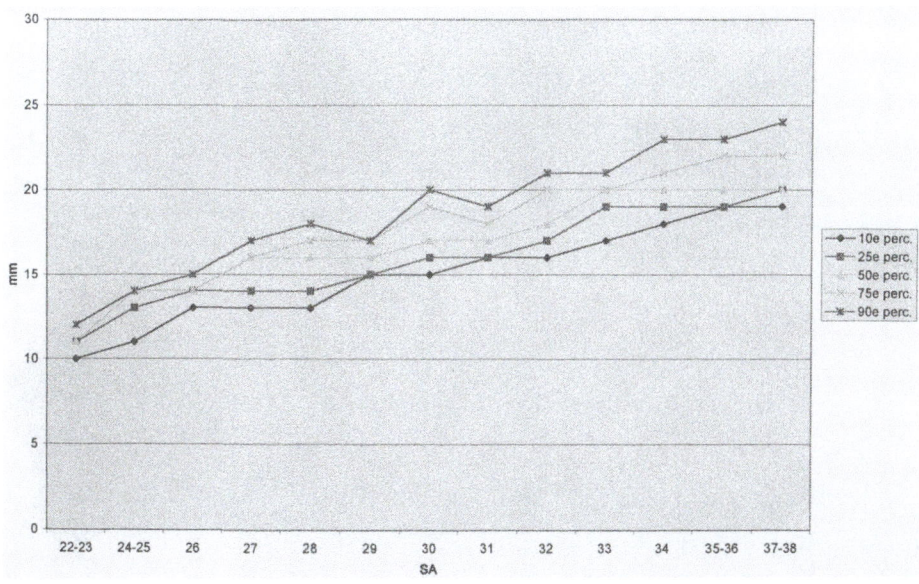

Anteroposterior Diameter of the Vermis

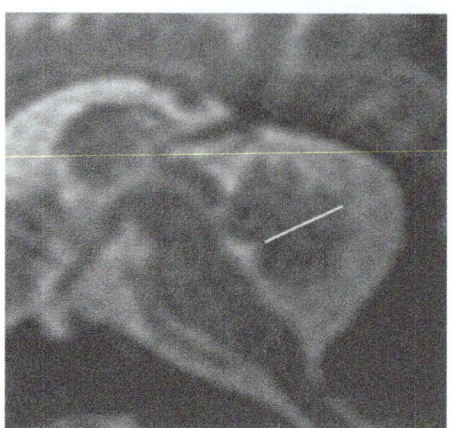

WG	Cohort	Average	SD	10th perc.	25th perc.	50th perc.	75th perc.	90th perc.	Min.	Max.
22–23	6	8.5	0.76	8	8	8	9	9	8	9
24–25	5	8.6	1.67	8	9	9	9	10	6	10
26	4	9.37	0.47	9	9	9	10	10	9	10
27	12	10.46	2.29	8	9	10	11	12	7	13
28	10	**9.85**	0.67	9	10	10	**10**	**10**	8	11
29	16	10.6	1.23	10	10	10	11	12	8	13
30	22	11.81	1.99	10	10	11	14	14	9	15
31	20	12.23	1.53	10	12	12	**12**	14	10	16
32	20	12.99	2.22	11	**11**	13	15	15	8	17
33	20	13.74	2.29	11	12	14	15	16	10	20
34	21	14.95	2.41	**13**	13	14	16	18	11	20
35–36	27	**14.8**	1.95	12	14	15	16	18	10	18
37–38	18	15.28	2.66	12	14	15	17	19	10	20

The values in bold characters correspond to aberrant results. Please refer to the comment at the beginning of „Detailed Results of Biometry for Each Parameter Studied", p. 86.

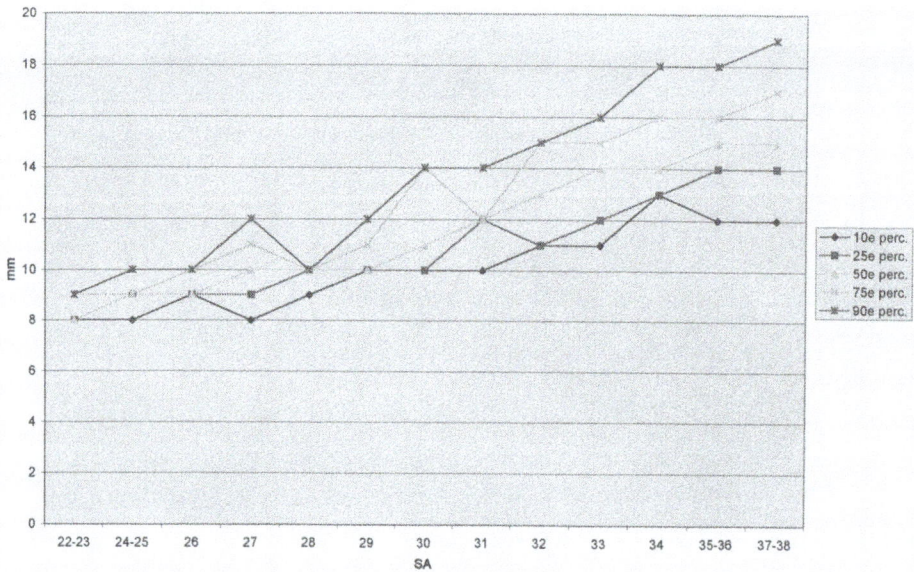

Transverse Cerebral Diameter

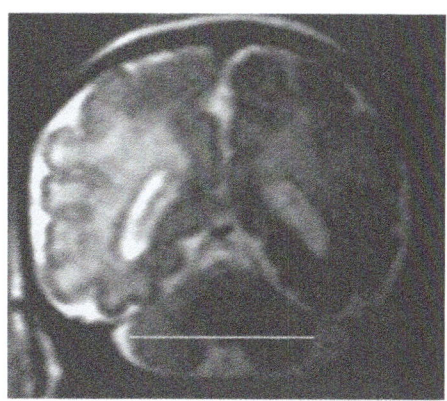

WG	Cohort	Average	SD	10th perc.	25th perc.	50th perc.	75th perc.	90th perc.	Min.	Max.
22–23	7	25.9	3.09	23	23	25	26	27	22	34
24–25	7	26.7	1.86	26	26	26	28	29	24	30
26	4	28.7	4.27	26	26	27	30	33	26	35
27	16	32.1	3.11	29	31	31	33	35	26	40
28	10	32.4	1.96	30	32	32	33	**34**	29	36
29	16	35.4	2.59	33	34	35	36	38	31	42
30	24	36.6	3.25	33	34	37	37	40	32	45
31	21	38.9	2.04	36	38	39	40	41	35	43
32	24	39.9	2.27	38	39	40	41	43	34	43
33	20	41.6	2.22	40	40	41	43	44	37	46
34	24	43.4	3.29	40	41	43	46	48	38	50
35–36	26	46.6	2.36	44	45	46	48	50	43	53
37–38	18	48	3.77	**43**	45	48	50	52	42	55

The values in bold characters correspond to aberrant results. Please refer to the comment at the beginning of „Detailed Results of Biometry for Each Parameter Studied", p. 86.

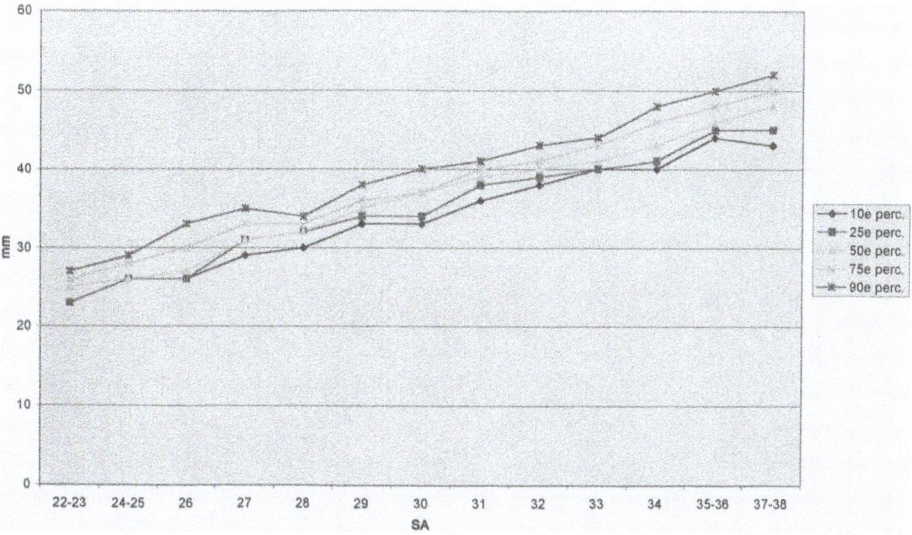

Surface of the Vermis

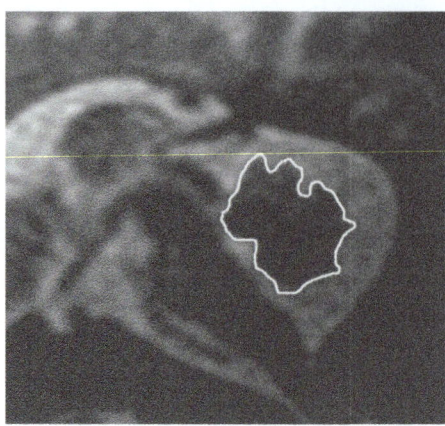

WG	Cohort	Average	SD	10th perc.	25th perc.	50th perc.	75th perc.	90th perc.	Min.	Max.
28	5	180	34.9	148	150	177	200	217	146	229
29	9	181.5	28.59	158	160	**168**	**190**	223	151	231
30	16	212.1	34.67	164	190	216	228	257	159	274
31	16	**209.6**	29.13	178	190	**204**	220	**242**	168	282
32	21	240.7	34.39	196	210	250	269	276	165	287
33	14	259.5	41.64	221	235	259	288	300	174	336
34	15	259.1	23.68	228	248	261	**269**	**287**	215	303
35–36	24	310.9	52.67	266	273	295	346	372	240	456
37–38	10	337.7	57.46	276	295	336	359	375	274	470

The values in bold characters correspond to aberrant results. Please refer to the comment at the beginning of „Detailed Results of Biometry for Each Parameter Studied", p. 86.

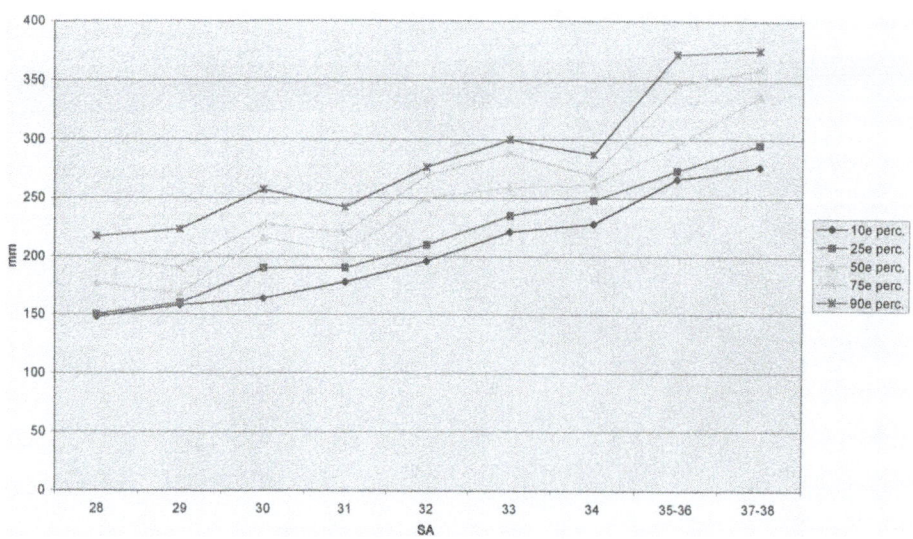

Anteroposterior Interopercular Distance

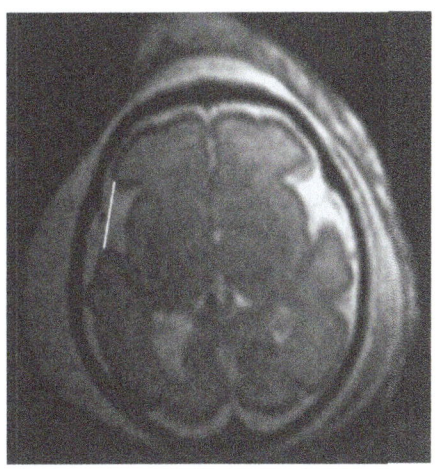

WG	Cohort	Average	SD	10th perc.	25th perc.	50th perc.	75th perc.	90th perc.	Min.	Max.
22–23	6	11.8	1.45	11	12	12	13	13	10	13
24–25	7	11.7	2.1	10	10	13	14	15	10	16
26	4	13.2	3.83	10	10	12	14	15	10	15
27	12	12	1.73	10	**11**	12	13	14	9	15
28	10	10.6	1.9	9	9	10	12	13	8	14
29	16	10.4	1.25	9	**10**	10	11	12	8	12
30	24	9.6	1.44	8	9	10	10	11	6	12
31	17	8.2	1.25	7	8	8	9	10	6	11
32	19	8.1	1.51	6	7	8	9	10	5	11
33	18	7.4	1.81	5	6	7	8	9	5	11
34	20	7.4	1.78	5	6	**8**	**9**	9	5	10
35–36	22	5.8	1.92	4	4	6	8	8	3	10
37–38	12	5.2	2.04	3	4	5	6	7	3	9

The values in bold characters correspond to aberrant results. Please refer to the comment at the beginning of „Detailed Results of Biometry for Each Parameter Studied", p. 86.

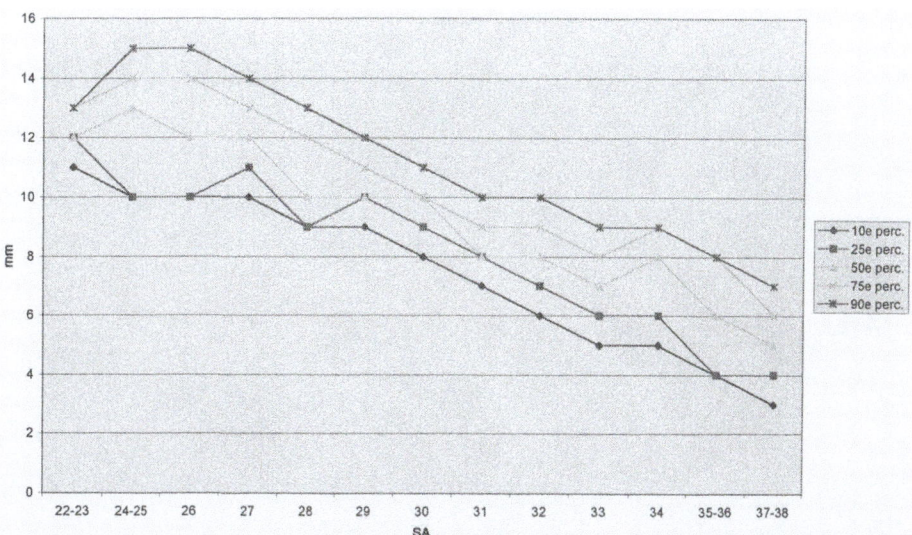

Craniocaudal Interopercular Distance

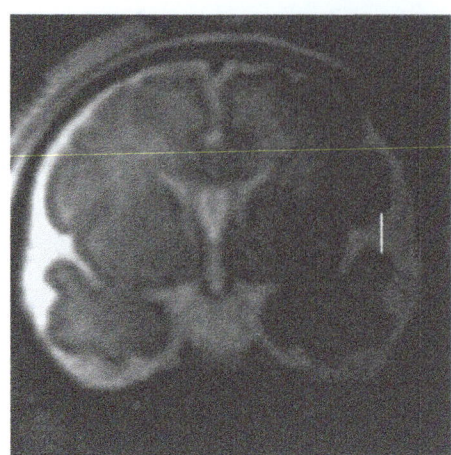

WG	Cohort	Average	SD	10th perc.	25th perc.	50th perc.	75th perc.	90th perc.	Min.	Max.
22–23	5	7.6	1.82	7	7	8	8	9	5	10
24–25	7	6.9	1.27	5	6	7	7	8	5	9
26	4	5.5	1.29	5	5	5	6	6	4	7
27	11	4.5	1.27	3	3	4	5	6	2	6
28	7	3.6	1.27	2	3	4	4	5	2	5
29	14	3.5	0.53	3	3	4	4	**4**	3	4
30	24	3.6	1.06	2	3	4	5	5	2	5
31	18	3.2	1.29	2	2	3	4	5	2	6
32	17	2.4	1.2	1	2	3	3	**4**	1	4
33	18	2.7	0.77	2	2	3	3	**4**	1	4
34	20	2.2	0.83	1	2	2	3	3	1	4
35–36	19	1.7	0.88	1	1	2	2	3	1	3
37–38	11	1.6	0.86	1	1	1	2	3	1	3

The values in bold characters correspond to aberrant results. Please refer to the comment at the beginning of „Detailed Results of Biometry for Each Parameter Studied", p. 86.

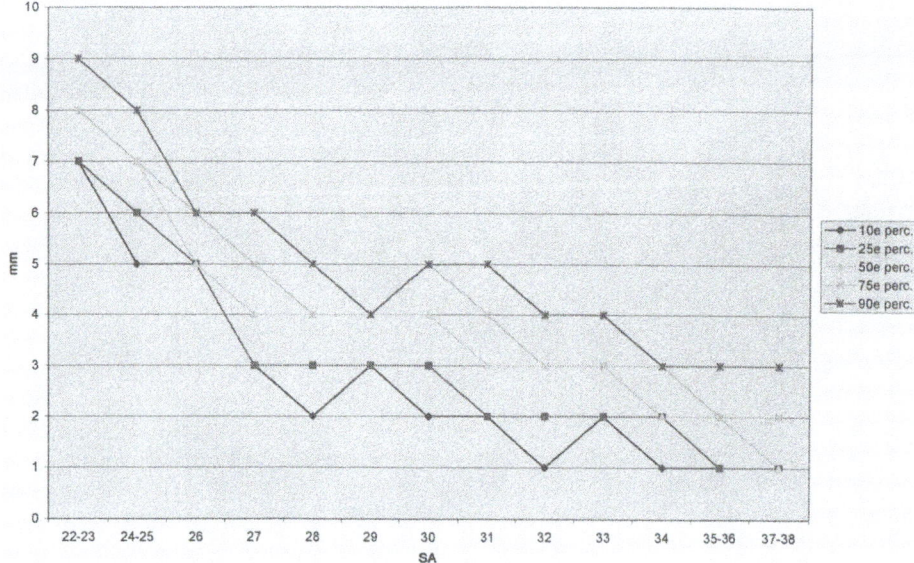

Atrial Diameter

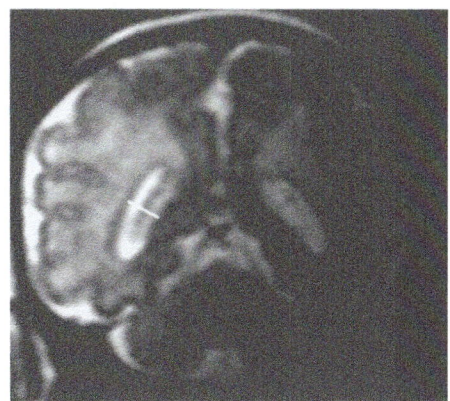

WG	Cohort	Average	SD	10th perc.	25th perc.	50th perc.	75th perc.	90th perc.	Min.	Max.
22–23	7	6.7	1.24	5	5	6	8	9	4	10
24–25	7	7.5	1.7	5	7	7	9	9	4	10
26	5	8	1.49	6	7	8	9	10	6	10
27	16	5.2	2.14	4	5	5	7	9	4	10
28	9	6.3	2.56	3	5	5	8	10	2	10
29	16	6	2.04	3	4	6	7	8	2	10
30	23	6.5	1.98	3	6	6	8	9	2	10
31	21	6.7	1.93	4	5	7	8	10	3	10
32	21	7	1.84	5	6	7	8	9	3	10
33	20	6.7	1.8	4	6	6	8	9	3	10
34	20	6.4	2.14	4	5	6	8	9	3	10
35–36	27	6.3	1.94	4	5	6	8	9	2	10
37–38	18	6.7	1.83	4	5	7	8	9	2	10

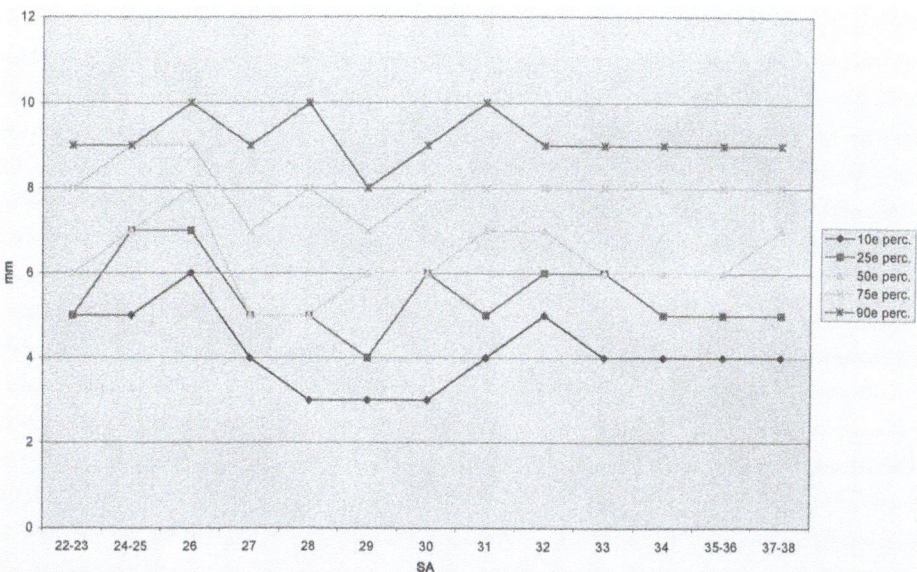

Atriocerebral Index (AD/Cerebral BPD)

WG	Average BPD	Average AD	Ratio (%)
22–23	49	6.7	13.6
24–25	51.8	7.5	14.4
26	57.8	8	13.8
27	59.4	5.2	8.7
28	61.3	6.3	10.2
29	65.7	6	9.1
30	69	6.5	9.4
31	70.5	6.7	9.5
32	72.4	7	9.6
33	77.7	6.7	8.6
34	76.7	6.4	8.3
35–36	81.2	6.3	7.7
37–38	83.6	6.7	8

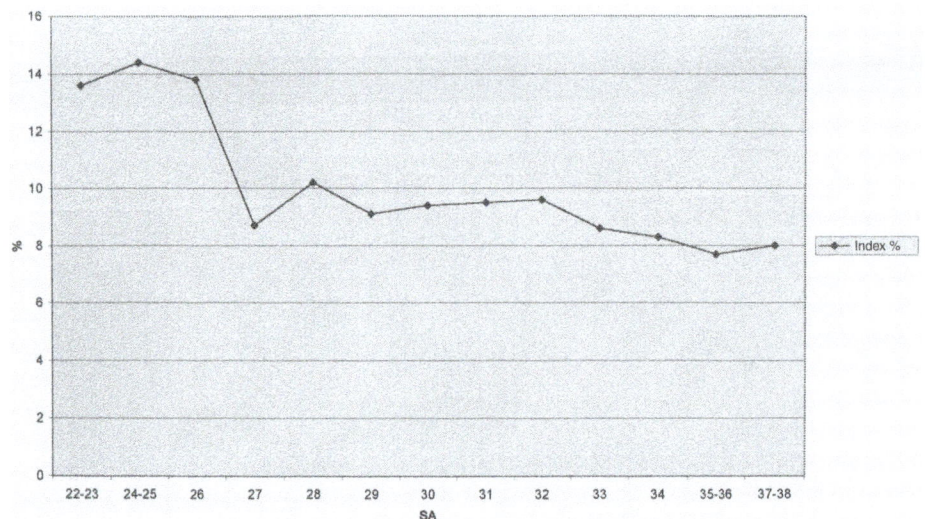

Lateral Diameter of the 3rd Ventricle

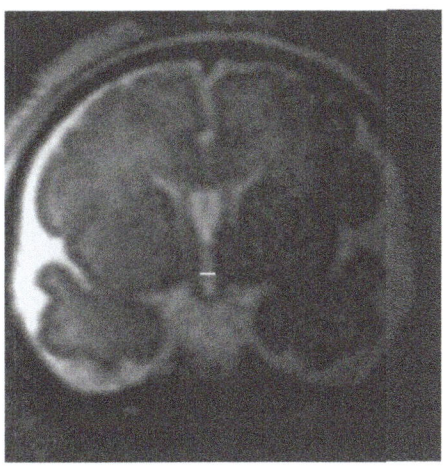

WG	Cohort	Average	SD	10th perc.	25th perc.	50th perc.	75th perc.	90th perc.	Min.	Max.
22–23	6	2.6	1.21	1.5	2	2.5	3	3.5	1	4
24–25	6	2.7	0.8	2	2	2.5	3	3	2	3.5
26	4	3.6	0.94	3	3	3	4	4.5	2	4.5
27	12	2.4	0.78	1.5	2	2.5	3	3	1	5
28	8	2.5	0.6	2	2	2	3	3	2	3.5
29	11	2.6	0.49	2	2	3	3	3	2	3
30	24	2.5	0.82	2	2	2.5	3	4	1	4
31	18	2.7	0.57	2	2.5	3	3	3.5	2	4
32	16	2.5	0.45	2	2	2.5	3	3	2	3
33	15	2.8	0.63	2	2.5	3	3	3.5	2	4
34	17	2.9	0.78	2	2	3	3	3.5	2	5
35–36	20	2.5	0.57	2	2	2	3	3	1.5	3.5
37–38	13	3	0.64	2	3	3	3	4	2	4

This measurement is not very precise, as it concerns a very small structure. However, despite some fluctuations the values are relatively constant throughout the pregnancy. The third ventricle (DV3)/cerebral BPD index indicates that this structure becomes smaller and smaller in proportion to the fetal brain.

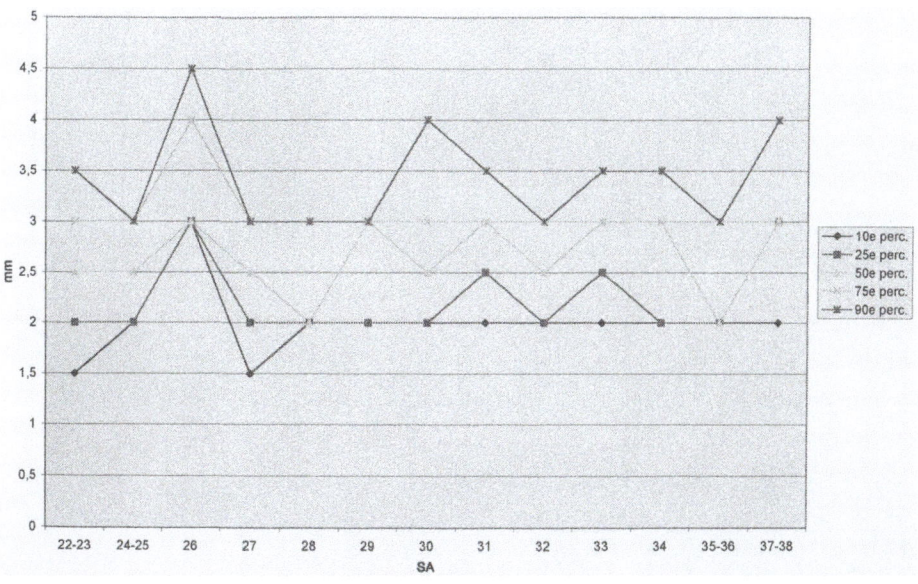

DV3/Cerebral BPD Index

WG	Average cerebral BPD	Average DV3	Ratio (%)
22–23	49	2.6	5.3
24–25	51.8	2.7	5.2
26	57.8	3.6	6.2
27	59.4	2.4	4
28	61.3	2.5	4
29	65.7	2.6	3.9
30	69	2.5	3.6
31	70.5	2.7	3.8
32	72.4	2.5	3.4
33	77.7	2.8	3.6
34	76.7	2.9	3.7
35–36	81.2	2.5	3
37–38	83.6	3	3.5

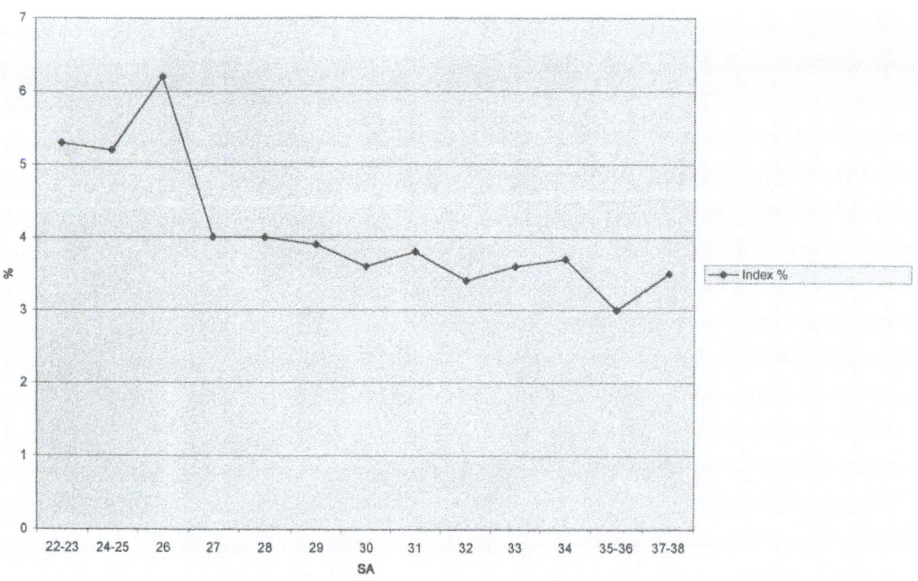

Anteroposterior Diameter of the 4th Ventricle

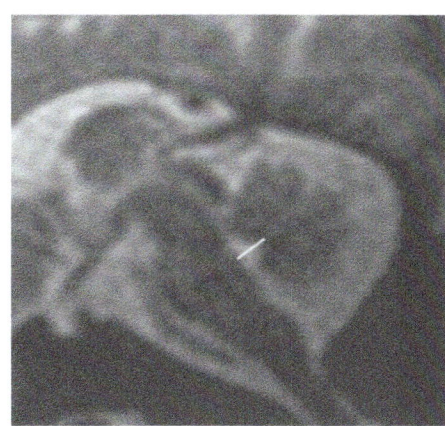

WG	Cohort	Average	SD	10th perc.	25th perc.	50th perc.	75th perc.	90th perc.	Min.	Max.
22–23	6	3.6	0.57	2	3	3.5	4	4	2	4
24–25	6	4.5	0.63	3	3.5	4	5	5	3	6
26	4	5.2	1.25	4	5	5	5.5	6.5	4	7
27	10	3	0.78	2	2.5	3.5	4	4.5	2	5
28	9	4.5	0.88	4	4	5	5	5	3	5
29	12	4.4	0.93	3	4	5	5	5.5	3	6
30	24	4.4	1.01	3	4	4	5	6	3	6
31	17	4.6	0.89	4	4	5	5	5	3	6
32	16	4.9	0.62	4	4.5	5	5	6	4	6
33	16	5.1	0.98	4	5	5	6	6	3	7
34	17	5	0.89	4	4	5	6	6	4	7
35–36	22	5.3	0.78	4	4	5	6	7	4	7
37–38	14	5.4	0.95	5	5	5	6	7	3	7

This measurement is not very precise, as it concerns a very small structure. A discreet growth of the fourth ventricle is noticed during the pregnancy. This growth remains proportional to that of the brain, as is shown by the DV4/FOD Index after 28 WG.

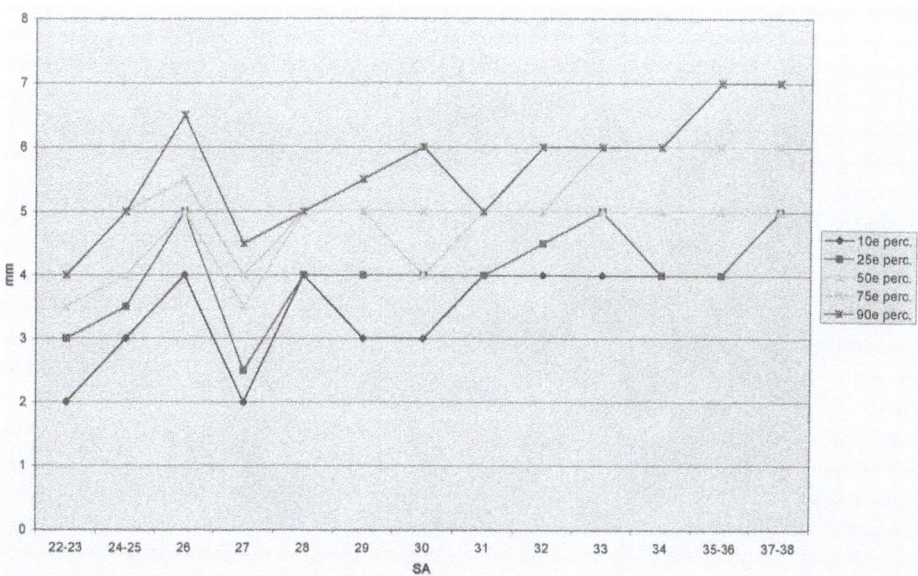

DV4/FOD Index

WG	Average cerebral FOD	Average DV4	Ratio (%)
22–23	67.5	3.6	5.3
24–25	69.7	4.5	6.4
26	76.8	5.2	6.7
27	81.3	3	3.7
28	81.5	4.5	5.5
29	85.3	4.4	5.1
30	89.2	4.4	4.9
31	91	4.6	5
32	93.4	4.9	5.2
33	97	5.1	5.2
34	99	5	5
35–36	102.2	5.3	5.1
37–38	103	5.4	5.2

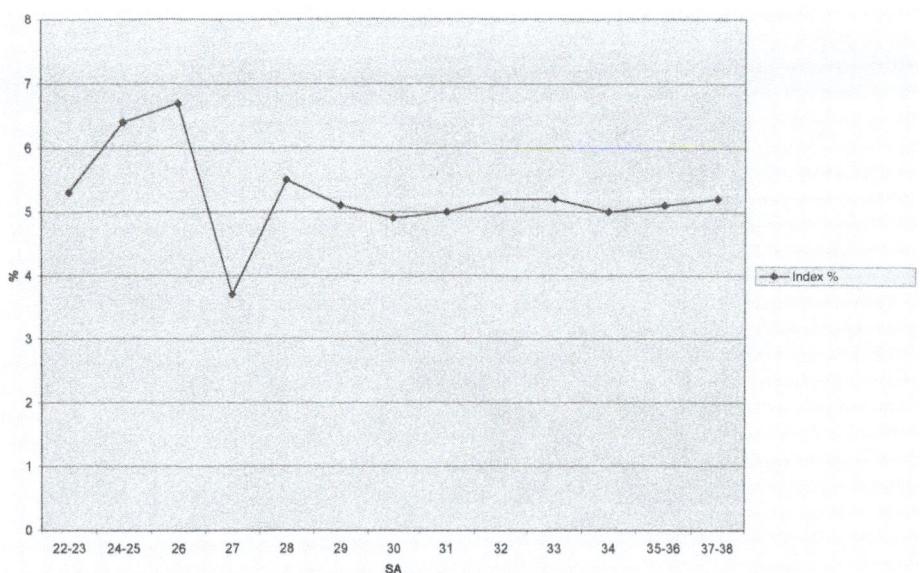

Detailed Results of Gyration for Each Sulcus Observed

The tables presented below show the population studied for each sulcus and each week's gestation, i.e. the number of fetuses where the slices concerning a given sulcus were interpretable. The number of fetuses where the sulcus was actually visualized appears next to the corresponding percentage shown in brackets. The notion of detectability does not appear in these tables, since all the other details are provided. Two two-entry summary tables are presented after these results. They provide an overview of the presence, in 75%–100% of cases and in 100% of cases, of the various sulci between 22 and 38 weeks of gestation.

Table 1. Interhemispheric fissure

WG	Number of fetuses	Sulci present
22–23	5	5 (100%)
24–25	5	5 (100%)
26	5	5 (100%)
27	12	12 (100%)
28	11	11 (100%)
29	18	18 (100%)
30	24	24 (100%)
31	21	21 (100%)
32	25	25 (100%)
33	20	20 (100%)
34	24	24 (100%)
35	17	17 (100%)
36	10	10 (100%)
37–38	18	18 (100%)

Table 2. Lateral sulcus

WG	Number of fetuses	Sulci present
22–23	8	8 (100%)
24–25	7	7 (100%)
26	5	5 (100%)
27	16	16 (100%)
28	11	11 (100%)
29	18	18 (100%)
30	24	24 (100%)
31	21	21 (100%)
32	25	25 (100%)
33	20	20 (100%)
34	24	24 (100%)
35	17	17 (100%)
36	11	11 (100%)
37–38	18	18 (100%)

Table 3. Internal parieto-occipital fissure

WG	Number of fetuses	Sulci present
22–23	7	6 (85.71%)
24–25	6	6 (100%)
26	5	5 (100%)
27	15	15 (100%)
28	10	10 (100%)
29	18	18 (100%)
30	24	24 (100%)
31	21	21 (100%)
32	25	25 (100%)
33	19	19 (100%)
34	23	23 (100%)
35	16	16 (100%)
36	10	10 (100%)
37–38	15	15 (100%)

Table 4. Hippocampal fissure

WG	Number of fetuses	Sulci present
22–23	6	6 (100%)
24–25	7	7 (100%)
26	4	4 (100%)
27	12	12 (100%)
28	9	9 (100%)
29	17	17 (100%)
30	24	24 (100%)
31	21	21 (100%)
32	23	23 (100%)
33	19	19 (100%)
34	23	23 (100%)
35	16	16 (100%)
36	9	9 (100%)
37–38	16	16 (100%)

Table 5. Callosal sulcus

WG	Number of fetuses	Sulci present
22–23	6	5 (82.82%)
24–25	6	6 (100%)
26	5	5 (100%)
27	11	11 (100%)
28	9	9 (100%)
29	17	17 (100%)
30	23	23 (100%)
31	20	20 (100%)
32	24	24 (100%)
33	19	19 (100%)
34	21	21 (100%)
35	16	16 (100%)
36	9	9 (100%)
37–38	15	15 (100%)

Table 6. Calcarine fissure

WG	Number of fetuses	Sulci present
22–23	6	4 (66.66%)
24–25	4	3 (75%)
26	5	5 (100%)
27	14	14 (100%)
28	11	11 (100%)
29	16	16 (100%)
30	24	24 (100%)
31	21	21 (100%)
32	24	24 (100%)
33	20	20 (100%)
34	23	23 (100%)
35	17	17 (100%)
36	10	10 (100%)
37–38	15	15 (100%)

Table 7. Cingular sulcus

WG	Number of fetuses	Sulci present
22–23	6	4 (66.6%)
24–25	6	6 (100%)
26	5	5 (100%)
27	14	14 (100%)
28	10	10 (100%)
29	18	18 (100%)
30	24	24 (100%)
31	21	21 (100%)
32	25	25 (100%)
33	20	20 (100%)
34	21	21 (100%)
35	16	16 (100%)
36	9	9 (100%)
37–38	15	15 (100%)

Table 8. Marginal sulcus

WG	Number of fetuses	Sulci present
22–23	5	2 (40%)
24–25	6	2 (33.33%)
26	5	3 (60%)
27	11	9 (81.81%)
28	9	8 (88.88%)
29	17	17 (100%)
30	23	23 (100%)
31	20	20 (100%)
32	24	24 (100%)
33	19	19 (100%)
34	21	21 (100%)
35	15	15 (100%)
36	9	9 (100%)
37–38	15	15 (100%)

Table 9. Central sulcus

WG	Number of fetuses	Sulci present
22–23	5	1 (20%)
24–25	3	1 (33.33%)
26	4	3 (75%)
27	10	10 (100%)
28	9	9 (100%)
29	15	15 (100%)
30	23	23 (100%)
31	20	20 (100%)
32	21	21 (100%)
33	16	16 (100%)
34	20	20 (100%)
35	13	13 (100%)
36	9	9 (100%)
37–38	14	14 (100%)

Table 10. Precentral sulcus

WG	Number of fetuses	Sulci present
22–23	6	0 (0%)
24–25	5	0 (0%)
26	3	2 (66.66%)
27	12	9 (75%)
28	10	9 (90%)
29	14	14 (100%)
30	20	20 (100%)
31	19	19 (100%)
32	21	21 (100%)
33	14	14 (100%)
34	19	19 (100%)
35	13	13 (100%)
36	9	9 (100%)
37–38	14	14 (100%)

Table 11. Postcentral sulcus

WG	Number of fetuses	Sulci present
22–23	6	0 (0%)
24–25	4	0 (0%)
26	3	1 (33.33%)
27	12	6 (50%)
28	11	9 (81.81%)
29	15	15 (100%)
30	21	21 (100%)
31	20	20 (100%)
32	21	21 (100%)
33	15	15 (100%)
34	19	19 (100%)
35	13	13 (100%)
36	9	9 (100%)
37–38	14	14 (100%)

Table 12. Intraparietal sulcus

WG	Number of fetuses	Sulci present
22–23	7	0 (0%)
24–25	6	1 (16.66%)
26	5	2 (40%)
27	11	8 (72.72%)
28	9	9 (100%)
29	17	17 (100%)
30	23	23 (100%)
31	20	20 (100%)
32	23	23 (100%)
33	20	20 (100%)
34	22	22 (100%)
35	14	14 (100%)
36	8	8 (100%)
37–38	13	13 (100%)

Table 13. Collateral sulcus

WG	Number of fetuses	Sulci present
22–23	6	1 (16.66%)
24–25	7	3 (42.85%)
26	4	3 (75%)
27	12	10 (83.33%)
28	9	9 (100%)
29	17	17 (100%)
30	24	24 (100%)
31	21	21 (100%)
32	23	23 (100%)
33	19	19 (100%)
34	23	23 (100%)
35	16	16 (100%)
36	9	9 (100%)
37–38	16	16 (100%)

Table 14. Superior (posterior) temporal sulcus

WG	Number of fetuses	Sulci present
22–23	5	0 (0%)
24–25	6	0 (0%)
26	4	2 (50%)
27	13	11 (84.61%)
28	10	10 (100%)
29	17	17 (100%)
30	24	24 (100%)
31	21	21 (100%)
32	24	24 (100%)
33	20	20 (100%)
34	23	23 (100%)
35	16	16 (100%)
36	9	9 (100%)
37–38	16	16 (100%)

Table 15. Superior (anterior) temporal sulcus

WG	Number of fetuses	Sulci present
22–23	6	0 (0%)
24–25	6	0 (0%)
26	4	0 (0%)
27	12	0 (0%)
28	10	0 (0%)
29	17	2 (11.76%)
30	24	1 (4.16%)
31	21	12 (57.14%)
32	24	22 (91.66%)
33	20	19 (95%)
34	23	23 (100%)
35	16	16 (100%)
36	9	9 (100%)
37–38	16	16 (100%)

Table 16. Inferior temporal sulcus

WG	Number of fetuses	Sulci present
22–23	6	0 (0%)
24–25	6	0 (0%)
26	4	0 (0%)
27	12	1 (8.33%)
28	9	1 (11.11%)
29	17	4 (23.53%)
30	23	13 (56.52%)
31	21	14 (66.66%)
32	22	18 (81.81%)
33	19	17 (84.21%)
34	23	23 (100%)
35	16	16 (100%)
36	9	9 (100%)
37–38	16	16 (100%)

Table 17. External occipitotemporal sulcus

WG	Number of fetuses	Sulci present
22–23	6	0 (0%)
24–25	6	0 (0%)
26	5	0 (0%)
27	12	0 (0%)
28	9	1 (11.11%)
29	17	4 (22.22%)
30	21	10 (47.61%)
31	20	13 (65%)
32	22	16 (72.72%)
33	19	16 (84.21%)
34	23	23 (100%)
35	15	15 (100%)
36	9	9 (100%)
37–38	16	16 (100%)

Table 18. Superior frontal sulcus

WG	Number of fetuses	Sulci present
22–23	7	0 (0%)
24–25	5	2 (40%)
26	4	1 (25%)
27	12	8 (66.66%)
28	9	6 (66.66%)
29	17	17 (100%)
30	23	23 (100%)
31	20	20 (100%)
32	22	22 (100%)
33	18	18 (100%)
34	20	20 (100%)
35	16	16 (100%)
36	9	9 (100%)
37–38	14	14 (100%)

Table 19. Inferior frontal sulcus

WG	Number of fetuses	Sulci present
22–23	7	0 (0%)
24–25	6	1 (16.66%)
26	5	1 (20%)
27	13	8 (61.54%)
28	8	5 (62.5%)
29	15	14 (93.33%)
30	23	23 (100%)
31	20	20 (100%)
32	22	22 (100%)
33	18	18 (100%)
34	20	20 (100%)
35	15	15 (100%)
36	9	9 (100%)
37–38	14	14 (100%)

Table 20. Secondary cingular sulci

WG	Number of fetuses	Sulci present
22–23	7	0 (0%)
24–25	7	0 (0%)
26	5	0 (0%)
27	12	0 (0%)
28	11	0 (0%)
29	18	0 (0%)
30	24	4 (16.66%)
31	21	11 (52.38%)
32	23	13 (56.56%)
33	20	15 (75%)
34	19	16 (84.21%)
35	16	16 (100%)
36	10	10 (100%)
37–38	15	15 (100%)

Table 21. Insular sulci

WG	Number of fetuses	Sulci present
22–23	7	0 (0%)
24–25	7	0 (0%)
26	5	0 (0%)
27	16	0 (0%)
28	11	0 (0%)
29	17	0 (0%)
30	23	0 (0%)
31	20	2 (10%)
32	23	10 (43.48%)
33	18	8 (44.44%)
34	19	15 (78.94%)
35	13	12 (92.30%)
36	10	10 (100%)
37–38	14	14 (100%)

Table 22. Secondary occipital sulci

WG	Number of fetuses	Sulci present
22–23	8	0 (0%)
24–25	7	0 (0%)
26	5	0 (0%)
27	15	0 (0%)
28	11	0 (0%)
29	18	0 (0%)
30	24	0 (0%)
31	20	2 (10%)
32	25	10 (40%)
33	17	7 (41.17%)
34	20	15 (75%)
35	14	13 (92.85%)
36	10	10 (100%)
37–38	14	14 (100%)

Table 23. Presence of the different sulci (in 75%–100% of cases) by stage

	22–23 WG	24–25 WG	26 WG	27 WG	28 WG	29 WG	30 WG	31 WG	32 WG	33 WG	34 WG	35 WG	36 WG	37–38 WG
Interhemispheric fissure	+	+	+	+	+	+	+	+	+	+	+	+	+	+
Lateral sulcus	+	+	+	+	+	+	+	+	+	+	+	+	+	+
Internal parieto-occipital fissure	+	+	+	+	+	+	+	+	+	+	+	+	+	+
Hippocampal fissure	+	+	+	+	+	+	+	+	+	+	+	+	+	+
Pericallosal sulcus	+	+	+	+	+	+	+	+	+	+	+	+	+	+
Calcarine fissure	−	+	+	+	+	+	+	+	+	+	+	+	+	+
Cingular sulcus	−	+	+	+	+	+	+	+	+	+	+	+	+	+
Marginal sulcus	−	−	−	+	+	+	+	+	+	+	+	+	+	+
Central sulcus	−	−	+	+	+	+	+	+	+	+	+	+	+	+
Precentral sulcus	−	−	−	+	+	+	+	+	+	+	+	+	+	+
Postcentral sulcus	−	−	−	−	+	+	+	+	+	+	+	+	+	+
Intraparietal sulcus	−	−	−	−	+	+	+	+	+	+	+	+	+	+
Collateral sulcus	−	−	+	+	+	+	+	+	+	+	+	+	+	+
Superior (posterior) temporal sulcus	−	−	−	+	+	+	+	+	+	+	+	+	+	+
Superior (anterior) temporal sulcus	−	−	−	−	−	−	−	−	+	+	+	+	+	+
Inferior temporal sulcus	−	−	−	−	−	−	−	−	+	+	+	+	+	+
External occipitotemporal sulcus	−	−	−	−	−	−	−	−	−	+	+	+	+	+
Superior frontal sulcus	−	−	−	−	−	+	+	+	+	+	+	+	+	+
Inferior frontal sulcus	−	−	−	−	−	+	+	+	+	+	+	+	+	+
Secondary cingular sulci	−	−	−	−	−	−	−	−	−	+	+	+	+	+
Insular sulci	−	−	−	−	−	−	−	−	−	−	+	+	+	+
Secondary occipital sulci	−	−	−	−	−	−	−	−	−	−	+	+	+	+

Table 24. Presence of the different sulci (in 100% of cases) by stage

Table 24. Presence of the different sulci (in 100% of cases) by stage

	22–23 WG	24–25 WG	26 WG	27 WG	28 WG	29 WG	30 WG	31 WG	32 WG	33 WG	34 WG	35 WG	36 WG	37–38 WG
Interhemispheric fissure	+	+	+	+	+	+	+	+	+	+	+	+	+	+
Lateral sulcus	+	+	+	+	+	+	+	+	+	+	+	+	+	+
Internal parieto-occipital fissure	–	+	+	+	+	+	+	+	+	+	+	+	+	+
Hippocampal fissure	+	+	+	+	+	+	+	+	+	+	+	+	+	+
Pericallosal sulcus	–	+	+	+	+	+	+	+	+	+	+	+	+	+
Calcarine fissure	–	+	+	+	+	+	+	+	+	+	+	+	+	+
Cingular sulcus	–	+	+	–	+	+	+	+	+	+	+	+	+	+
Marginal sulcus	–	–	–	–	–	+	+	+	+	+	+	+	+	+
Central sulcus	–	–	–	+	+	+	+	+	+	+	+	+	+	+
Precentral sulcus	–	–	–	–	–	+	+	+	+	+	+	+	+	+
Postcentral sulcus	–	–	–	–	+	+	+	+	+	+	+	+	+	+
Intraparietal sulcus	–	–	–	–	+	+	+	+	+	+	+	+	+	+
Collateral sulcus	–	–	–	–	+	+	+	+	+	+	+	+	+	+
Superior (posterior) temporal sulcus fissure	–	–	–	–	+	+	+	+	+	+	+	+	+	+
Superior (anterior) temporal sulcus	–	–	–	–	–	–	–	–	–	–	+	+	+	+
Inferior temporal sulcus	–	–	–	–	–	–	–	–	–	–	+	+	+	+
External occipitotemporal sulcus	–	–	–	–	–	–	–	–	–	–	+	+	+	+
Superior frontal sulcus	–	–	–	–	+	+	+	+	+	+	+	+	+	+
Inferior frontal sulcus	–	–	–	–	–	–	+	+	+	+	+	+	+	+
Secondary cingular sulci	–	–	–	–	–	–	–	–	–	–	–	+	+	+
Insular sulci	–	–	–	–	–	–	–	–	–	–	–	–	+	+
Secondary occipital sulci	–	–	–	–	–	–	–	–	–	–	–	+	+	+

Detailed Results for Myelination in Each Area

We used the same method here as for sulci. One column shows the population studied and the other gives the percentage of presence of a T1 hypersignal. In our series, this hypersignal was constantly absent from 22 to 38 weeks of gestation in the semi-oval centres, the nucleus caudatus and the anterior limb of the internal capsule. We therefore did not deem it useful to show these results in tables.

Table 27. Myelination of the pons (tegmentum excluded)

WG	Number of fetuses	T1 hypersignal
22–23	5	0 (0%)
24–25	4	0 (0%)
26	4	0 (0%)
27	11	11 (100%)
28	8	0 (0%)
29	14	0 (0%)
30	18	0 (0%)
31	17	1 (5.88%)
32	19	1 (5.26%)
33	14	0 (0%)
34	16	0 (0%)
35	11	1 (9.09%)
36	9	1 (11.11%)
37–38	12	2 (16.66%)

Table 25. Myelination of the vermis

WG	Number of fetuses	T1 hypersignal
22–23	4	1 (25%)
24–25	4	1 (25%)
26	4	2 (50%)
27	10	7 (75%)
28	6	5 (83.33%)
29	14	11 (78.57%)
30	21	19 (90.47%)
31	20	16 (80%)
32	18	18 (100%)
33	13	12 (92.31%)
34	14	14 (100%)
35	10	10 (100%)
36	8	8 (100%)
37–38	14	14 (100%)

Table 28. Myelination of the tegmentum

WG	Number of fetuses	T1 hypersignal
22–23	5	3 (60%)
24–25	4	3 (75%)
26	4	4 (100%)
27	11	11 (100%)
28	8	8 (100%)
29	14	14 (100%)
30	18	18 (100%)
31	17	17 (100%)
32	19	19 (100%)
33	14	14 (100%)
34	16	16 (100%)
35	11	11 (100%)
36	9	9 (100%)
37–38	12	12 (100%)

Table 26. Myelination of the middle cerebellar peduncles

WG	Number of fetuses	T1 hypersignal
22–23	4	1 (25%)
24–25	4	1 (25%)
26	4	2 (50%)
27	10	6 (80%)
28	6	5 (83.33%)
29	14	11 (78.57%)
30	21	19 (90.47%)
31	20	18 (90%)
32	18	18 (100%)
33	13	13 (100%)
34	14	14 (100%)
35	10	10 (100%)
36	8	8 (100%)
37–38	14	14 (100%)

Table 29. Myelination of the posterior limb of the internal capsule (in its medial portion)

WG	Number of fetuses	T1 hypersignal
22–23	5	0 (0%)
24–25	5	0 (0%)
26	4	0 (0%)
27	10	0 (0%)
28	9	0 (0%)
29	14	0 (0%)
30	23	3 (13.04%)
31	17	2 (11.76%)
32	23	7 (30.43%)
33	16	7 (43.75%)
34	20	10 (50%)
35	11	7 (63.64%)
36	10	9 (90%)
37–38	13	12 (92.30%)

Table 30. Myelination of the posterior limb of the internal capsule (in its lateral portion)

WG	Number of fetuses	T1 hypersignal
22–23	5	0 (0%)
24–25	5	0 (0%)
26	4	0 (0%)
27	9	0 (0%)
28	9	0 (0%)
29	14	1 (7.14%)
30	21	8 (38.09%)
31	19	12 (63.16%)
32	23	16 (69.56%)
33	16	14 (87.5%)
34	20	19 (95%)
35	11	11 (100%)
36	10	10 (100%)
37–38	13	13 (100%)

Table 32. Myelination of the globus pallidus

WG	Number of fetuses	T1 hypersignal
22–23	5	0 (0%)
24–25	7	0 (0%)
26	4	0 (0%)
27	13	0 (0%)
28	9	0 (0%)
29	14	0 (0%)
30	23	4 (17.39%)
31	17	4 (23.53%)
32	23	8 (34.78%)
33	16	11 (68.75%)
34	20	17 (85%)
35	11	8 (76.72%)
36	10	9 (90%)
37–38	13	12 (92.30%)

Table 31. Myelination of the thalamus

WG	Number of fetuses	T1 hypersignal
22–23	5	0 (0%)
24–25	7	0 (0%)
26	4	0 (0%)
27	13	0 (0%)
28	9	0 (0%)
29	14	0 (0%)
30	23	0 (0%)
31	17	0 (0%)
32	23	0 (0%)
33	16	0 (0%)
34	20	0 (0%)
35	11	0 (0%)
36	10	1 (10%)
37–38	13	2 (15.38%)

Table 33. Myelination of the putamen

WG	Number of fetuses	T1 hypersignal
22–23	5	0 (0%)
24–25	7	0 (0%)
26	4	0 (0%)
27	13	0 (0%)
28	9	0 (0%)
29	14	0 (0%)
30	23	0 (0%)
31	17	1 (5.88%)
32	23	0 (0%)
33	16	0 (0%)
34	20	0 (0%)
35	11	0 (0%)
36	10	2 (20%)
37–38	13	1 (7.69%)

Comments on the Results

Biometry

From a biometrical viewpoint, fetal brain development is gradual and steady. The brain is proportionally very voluminous in the embryo and accounts for 1/10–1/7 of the body weight during the last trimester of pregnancy, whereas it only represents 1/50 of an adult's weight. The cerebellum, on the contrary, represents 1/25 of the brain's weight in newborns vs 1/15–1/10 for adults [51].

Until now, the cerebral biometric data available for fetuses have been provided by fetopathological or sonographic studies.

Fetopathological studies are based on the analysis of fixed brains, in which certain parameters are estimated: total weight, weight of the brain stem and cerebellum, fronto-occipital diameter, frontotemporal height, and biparietal diameter.

The fronto-occipital diameter, according to Larroche [51, 52], measures 80 mm at 28 weeks of gestation, 90 mm at 32 weeks of gestation, 100 mm at 34 weeks of gestation, 110 mm at 36 weeks of gestation and 120 mm at 40 weeks of gestation. These values are a little higher on the left than on the right in 50% of cases, the opposite being observed in 30% of cases. In the remaining 20% of cases, the values are identical on both sides. Similar values are obtained with MRI, except at 36 weeks of gestation where the values are approximately 10 mm lower than in fetopathology. It can be said that the number of fetuses studied is not given in the articles cited above [51, 52] and that there are only three fetuses in the group representing 36–37 weeks of gestation in the Fees-Higgins and Larroche atlas, where the figures tally with our results.

According to Larroche, the FOD is a good index of fetal brain maturation from 28 weeks of gestation. The measurements of the maximum biparietal diameter in the Fees-Higgins and Larroche atlas [53] for the few fetuses in the age group of 36–37 weeks of gestation tally on average with our data for biparietal diameter.

Fetopathological examinations do not provide measurements of either the pericerebral space or the ventricular system. We have found no fetopathological biometric data for the cerebellum, except in one study [54], which gives values for the vermis's height on fixed brains in proportion to the size of the fetus. These values tally with ours.

Sonographic studies on fetal brain biometry give no indication of the cerebral biparietal diameter. Sonographic measurement of the bone BPD (from the external table of the most superficial parietal bone to the internal table of the deepest parietal bone) is close to the MRI measurement of the bone BPD between the two internal tables of the parietal bones. Our values are lower than those obtained in sonography by a few millimetres, which can partly be explained by our voluntarily not taking into account the thickness of the skull in order to be able to estimate the pericerebral space by measuring the difference between bone and cerebral BPD. It must be remembered that the true BPD is the cerebral BPD, which cannot be measured by sonography. The ratio of bone BPD minus cerebral BPD/bone BPD (craniocerebral index) decreases progressively throughout pregnancy, which shows the decrease in pericerebral space.

The fronto-occipital diameter is generally not measured in sonographic examinations. Standards have been published [55], with the FOD measured on an axial slice at the level of the thalami where the skull is longest, from the frontal bone to the occipital bone. The sonographic values are always somewhat higher than ours, which is not surprising since, as for the bone BPD, the sonographic FOD takes into account the skull and the pericerebral space. In a study conducted on 22 fetuses with no suspected CNS abnormalities, BPD and head circumference measurements were obtained with MRI in a manner similar to the ultrasonographic technique and a significant correlation was found between both measurements [56].

The size of the lateral ventricles has been exhaustively studied in sonography [57–60]. The measurement is generally made on an axial or a coronal slice perpendicular to the axis of the ventricle at the level of the atrium. In sonography, it often proves very difficult to measure the ventricle closest to the probe because of artefacts hindering the visibility of the most superficial cerebral structures. All the studies cited were carried out during the last two trimesters of pregnancy; they all found the ventricular diameter to be relatively stable throughout pregnancy. According to Patel et al. [57], a difference may exist on the size of the atrium between the sexes, this value being slightly higher for males. Fetus sex was not taken into account in our study. We have excluded the fetuses whose AD was greater than 10 mm from the study, as this value is generally considered the upper limit of the atrial diameter [61]. According to a study conducted with MRI in 23 normal fetuses (with atrial measurement obtained in the axial plane image through the thalamic nuclei just below the plane of the BPD measurement), the MRI mean atrial measurements are slightly smaller than ultrasonographic measurements, but the cut-off value for ventriculomegaly on MRI is also greater than 10 mm [62]. The study of the AD/cerebral BPD index shows a distinct decrease in this value between 22 and 29 weeks of gestation, meaning that the AD remains stable as the brain grows.

Measurement of the AD by MRI has the advantage over sonography that it is possible whatever the position of the fetus's head and the ventricle measured. The ventricle closest to the surface is as clearly visible as the deepest one.

A study on a large number of fetuses during the second and third trimesters of pregnancy by Hertzberg et al. [63] has provided measurements of the 3rd ventricle. The average diameter is relatively constant between 12 and 28 weeks of gestation at approximately 1 mm; it then increases but is never higher than 1.9 mm. A diameter exceeding 3.5 mm can be considered abnormal. Our average values are a little higher, but do not exceed 3 mm on average and 4 mm for the maximum values. This small difference can probably be explained by the much sharper visualization of the 3rd ventricle in MRI, and also the great uncertainty of the measurement of such a small structure whatever the technique used. The DV3 becomes smaller and smaller in proportion to the cerebral BPD (DV3/cerebral BPD index) owing to brain growth.

The same remarks apply to the measurement of the 4th ventricle, carried out by the same team [64] in sonography on a large series of axial slices. The anteroposterior diameter of the 4th ventricle was 3.5 mm ± 1.3 and its width was 3.9 mm ± 1.7. We measured the anteroposterior diameter of the 4th ventricle on a midline sagittal slice and its value was 4.5 mm ± 2.5 mm. The DV4 and FOD grow proportionally after 28 weeks of gestation, as shown by the DV4/FOD index.

Our study of the transverse cerebellar diameter gave values compatible with the sonographic biometrical data, except at 35–36 and 37–38 weeks of gestation, where our figures are lower than the sonographic data by a few millimetres [65]. The later the stage, the greater the artefacts caused by the petrous part of the temporal bone and the less precise the sonographic measurement is as a result. This probably explains the discordance noted in the end of pregnancy between the sonographic and the MRI measurements.

The anteroposterior diameter of the vermis was estimated in sonography on premature babies of less than 32 weeks of gestation [66], on anterior or posterior transfontanellar slices. The sonographic values are all higher than ours by a few millimetres. It is highly probable that, concerning the vermis, the spatial resolution is better in MRI than in sonography.

The surface of the vermis was measured by Birnholz [67] on transfontanellar slices on premature babies aged from 26 weeks of gestation and on babies born at term. The vermis was assimilated to an ellipsis. Hence, the technique and conditions of measurement were very different from ours, and it seems difficult to compare the results. Even more than for linear measurements, measurements of the surface of the vermis should be used with caution, as evidenced by the large number of aberrant values appearing in bold characters. Only an order of magnitude is given here, and it seems clear that as the studies multiply there is great variability, both between and within the groups of observers, in the way such measurements are taken. As we have already pointed out in Chap. 3, the spatial resolution currently does not allow each one of the nine lobules composing the vermis to be considered separately.

The length of the corpus callosum was measured in sonography on transfontanellar slices [68]. Our values are concordant except at 32–33 weeks of gestation, where we found higher values. The small sizes of the representative cohorts for each week in our study should be stressed; this is even more pronounced in Malinger's study. Growth of the corpus callosum is linear during the second trimester and slows down in the third trimester [68]. Our data also indicate that the corpus callosum's growth is proportionally slower than the brain's (LCC/FOD index). It should furthermore be noted that the corpus callosum is more clearly delimited on a transfontanellar sonography than in MRI, although the former method is not always applicable due to the closing of the fontanelle window. At the moment, the spatial resolution of MRI seems insufficient to correctly analyse this structure, because of partial volume effects on the callosal sulcus. As we have already pointed out in Chap. 3, measuring its thickness with any precision is illusory.

Gyration

Gyration is the creasing of the telencephalic surface. This phenomenon appears late in fetal development. It is first observed at the 2nd month of intrauterine life; the primary sulci develop parallel to the growth of the future cerebral hemispheres, and this phenomenon is closely linked to the earliest phases of cerebral ontogenesis: neurogenesis and neuronal migration. The secondary sulci develop at the same time as the synaptogenesis begins in the cortical plate. The appearance of tertiary sulci is contemporary to the activity-dependent synaptic remodelling phenomena [69]. The cortical creasing as it exists in adults is not generally observed before the end of the 1st year of life [70].

Neurofetopathologists hold gyration to be a good indicator of fetal brain maturation. Moreover, good knowledge of the normal fetal gyration greatly facilitates the diagnosis of certain pathologies using imaging techniques.

The primary sulci are the first indentations appearing on the brain surface. Initially, the sulci are shallow and their banks are round. They later grow deeper and the banks become angular. In parallel, the distance between any two adjacent sulci decreases progressively [71]. The maturation of the brain – by the appearance, following an established chronology, of the various sulci – and the maturation of the sulci themselves are therefore concomitant. The secondary sulci correspond to ramifications of the primary sulci. They are initially rectilinear and develop a V-shaped ending. Their later ramifications are the tertiary sulci [72]. The dates secondary and tertiary sulci appear are also relatively established; their topography, on the contrary, is highly variable from one individual to another. Fetal gyration has been essentially studied in neurofetopathology, in sonography and very little in MRI.

Neurofetopathological Studies

We will essentially consider three studies [50, 51, 73]. On methodology, it must be remembered that the gestational age is established from the date of the last menstrual period for Chi [50] and Larroche [51]. Dorovini-Zis takes into account the cranial perimeter, the size of the embryo (vertex-heel length), and the body and brain weight.

Chi studied 597 photographs of brains and 207 slice series of brains from fetuses aged from 10 to 44 weeks of gestation. He made slice series between 15 and 30 μm in thickness: the photographs studied were of slices ranging in thickness from 2 to 5 mm. He held a sulcus to be present when he could observe a distinct indentation on the cerebral surface in 25 %–50 % of brains (depending on the number of fetuses studied). Generally, the sulci are present in 75 %–100 % of cases 2 weeks after that date. No difference was noted between the two sexes. On the other hand, he noted a delay of 2–3 weeks between 19 and 32 weeks of gestation in twins when compared to monofetal pregnancies. After 33 weeks of gestation, this difference disappears. Chi's study also clearly shows an asymmetry in the maturation of the hemispheres: the superior frontal and temporal sulci and the secondary sulci appear 1–2 weeks earlier on the left side than on the right. The opposite is very rarely observed. Moreover, the internal part of the superior temporal gyrus develops more towards the back on the left side; it is also more vertical on this side than on the right, so that the planum temporale is larger on the left side.

The chronology of the appearance of the various sulci in neuroanatomy according to Chi and in MRI according to our study is presented in the table below.

Chronology of appearance of the various sulci in neuroanatomy and in MRI (the gestational age is in weeks of gestation)

Sulci	Neuroanatomy[a]	MRI[b]
Calcarine fissure	16	22-23
Cingular	18	22–23
Central	20	24–25
Superior temporal	23	26
Collateral	23	24–25
Precentral	24	26
Postcentral	25	26
Superior frontal	25	24–25
Intraparietal	26	26
Inferior frontal	28	28
Inferior temporal	30	30
External occipitotemporal	30	30
Secondary insular	34	32

[a] According to Chi [50].
[b] According to our study.

Dorovini-Zis [73] studied 80 brains from 22 weeks of gestation to 1 month of life. Thickness of the slices is not indicated. Only five brains of 33 (studied with the specific aim of finding asymmetries) presented an asymmetry in the maturation of the hemispheres. In three cases, the development was earlier on the right of the superior temporal sulcus.

In her atlas [53], Larroche offers no precision on the number of fetuses on which the results were established. She mentions three control fetuses in each gestational age group. Thirty-micrometre-thick slice series were made.

We have noted differences between the three studies [50, 51, 53, 73], particularly regarding the appearance date of the various sulci. For instance, the calcarine fissure appears at 16 weeks of gestation for Chi, at 18 weeks of gestation for Larroche; the central sulcus appears at 20 weeks of gestation for Chi and Larroche, and at 24 weeks of gestation for Dorovini-Zis. According to Larroche, the superior temporal sulcus appears at 28 weeks of gestation and is a very reliable morphological criterion of gestational age, whereas to Chi it is detectable from 23 weeks of gestation.

The secondary sulci appear at 32 weeks of gestation according to Chi, between 28 and 30 weeks of gestation for Dorovini-Zis; the tertiary sulci appear at 36 weeks of gestation for Chi and at 40 weeks of gestation for Dorovini-Zis.

These discrepancies may be attributable to the different techniques used by these authors (in Chi's opinion); in any event, they stress the difficulty of establishing gyration atlases that can be reliable by a 1- or 2-week margin. It can furthermore be noted that these neurofetopathological studies are made on a relatively limited number of specimens, which also probably explains the differences observed between the different series.

Sonographic Studies

Several articles have studied gyration in sonography [74–76]. The earlier few were analysed by Naidich [72]. Most of these articles dealt with examinations carried out on premature babies [74, 75]. It is obvious that the quality of the sonographies greatly influences the visibility of cerebral sulci and that the choice of a pelvic or endovaginal approach is quite important in antenatal studies. We therefore prefer to draw on one of the more recent articles [76]. Many things hinder the sonographic study of gyration such as the impossibility of obtaining a transfontanellar

window, the fineness of pericerebral spaces and the reverberations on the calvaria. Monteguado [76] retrospectively analysed sulci by endovaginal sonography on 262 fetal brains. Pregnancies were all monofetal; their term was determined by the date of the last menstrual period and an early sonography. Some coronal and sagittal slices were made by transfontanellar sonography and therefore do not correspond to the neuroanatomical data, since these are oriented obliquely in a fan shape from the fontanelle. These figures correspond to the gestational age at which each sulcus is observed for the first time; the article does not state the percentage concerned. The opercularization of the sylvian fissure is visible on coronal and parasagittal slices between 23 and 35 weeks of gestation.

As we can see, numerous sulci are not easily analysed in fetal sonography; this article deals chiefly with the study of the internal surface of the hemispheres. The inferior surface of the brain was not explored, thus excluding the collateral and external occipitotemporal sulci. Visualization of the brain's convexity is difficult in sonography, and only tangential slices can be obtained, by inclining the probe greatly. Analysis of the central, precentral and postcentral sulci is quite difficult. The frontal sulci, although not studied in this work, can be visualized clearly if the pericerebral space is large enough. The secondary sulci are described at the level of the cingular sulcus at around 30–40 weeks of gestation.

The poor spatial resolution of sonography, the retrospective nature of this study and the poor reflectivity of a mere indentation on the cortical surface account for the late appearance of sulci in sonography when compared to neuroanatomical studies.

MRI Studies

The MRI study of gyration was done in vitro [70], in vivo after birth [71], and in vivo in the antenatal period [77–80].

The study conducted by Hansen et al. [70] involved 136 set fetal brains and three fresh brains aged from 6 to 28 weeks of gestation, with a 1.5 T MRI unit (T1- and T2-weighted slices). The gestational age was estimated from the craniocaudal length and the biparietal diameter. This was a global study of the fetal brain, and thus not exclusively dedicated to gyration, but also to the analysis of various anatomical elements of the brain. The description of gyration is rather cursory. It only differentiates three steps: a step where the brain is smooth before the 5th month of pregnancy, a period between the 5th and the 8th months where the principal sulci appear, and the last month, characterized by the growing complexity of the sulci and convolutions. No indication was given as to the date each sulcus appears.

Van der Knapp [71] analysed the gyration in 39 living premature babies aged 30–37 weeks of gestation at the time of the MRI, and five children aged between 38 and 42 weeks of gestation at the time of their death. These are all relatively old fetuses, and the article essentially deals with the progression of sulci maturation in various cerebral territories, which has been described in the beginning of the comments on gyration. This progressive burying of the sulci into the cortical mantle and the modifications of their edges are primarily observed in the frontoparietal region around the central sulcus, then in the internal occipital region, in the parietal region (except for the central sulcus), in the occipital region (except on the internal face) and in the posterior temporal region, and finally in the anterior frontal and temporal regions.

Very few studies have dealt with the in vivo antenatal gyration [77–80] so far because of the difficulty of obtaining cohorts of normal fetuses in fetal MRI. Levine's article [77] includes twin and single pregnancies, MRIs done on pregnant women (slices not orthogonal to the fetus), and MRIs dedicated to the fetus. The cohorts of fetuses do not exceed two to seven fetuses in each age group, and the sulci are considered present if at least half of the sulci in each group are effectively observed in the age group where they are supposed to be present. These differences in methodology with our atlas render any comparison between the two studies rather difficult.

Our results show that, in MRI, the best correlation between a sulcus and the gestational age is obtained for the sulci detectable after 28 weeks of gestation. The later a sulcus appears anatomically, the shorter the delay in appearance of this sulcus on MRI slices (see the table on p. 117). The following sulci are the most precise references: frontal (superior and inferior), inferior temporal, postcentral, intraparietal, external occipitotemporal and insular. At 34 weeks of gestation, the primary sulci and most secondary sulci are already present. After this stage, the narrowness of pericerebral space hinders visibility of the sulci. *Therefore, the interval during which fetal MRI best studies gyration is between 28 and 34 weeks of gestation.* Another technical limitation is the thickness of the slices used, which is at best 3 mm, far from the

15–30 µm of the neuroanatomical slices. It seems certain that the spatial resolution can only be altered by this inconsistency, contributing to the discrepancies observed between the anatomy series and the date of appearance of the sulci in MRI.

The study of gyration therefore appears to be an indispensable step in the analysis of the fetal brain, as is biometry. It is an indisputable contribution of fetal MRI, since with MRI the analysis of sulci benefits from a much better consistency and precision than in sonography.

Myelination

This atlas starts at 22 weeks of gestation, after the phase of neuronal proliferation, and at a date when the neuronal migration is almost complete (see Appendix for the germinal zone). Myelination is the last phase of cerebral maturation. It begins during the second trimester of fetal life and continues long after birth. Preceding myelination is a phase of vascularization and a proliferation of the glial cells, which contain the lipidic precursors of myelin. This is called the premyelination phase. Myelin is characterized by its richness in lipids and to a lesser extent in proteins. Myelination is therefore accompanied by an increase in the brain's lipid and protein content, while its water content decreases.

Myelination of the fetal brain has long been studied in fetopathology [81] and is regarded, like gyration, as an indicator of fetal cerebral maturation. The chronology and topography of fetal myelination were particularly studied by Larroche [52, 82], whose work is based to a large extent on Luxol coloration, which identifies the phospholipid constituent of myelin. Myelination progresses according to a precisely defined sequence, along a caudocranial axis, in a centrifugal manner in the brain; it appears in the central nervous system first in the sensory system and then in the motor system. Where Luxol coloration is accomplished, myelination is observed: in the internal part of the globus pallidus at 26 weeks of gestation, in the external part of the globus pallidus at 32 weeks of gestation, and in the ventrolateral nucleus of the thalamus at 38 weeks of gestation [82].

More recently, the myelination phenomenon was studied using an immunohistochemical method that provokes a reaction of the myelin basic protein (a component of myelin) [83, 84]. Using this method, myelin is detected earlier than with Luxol coloration. It appears at 25 weeks of gestation in the globus pallidus, the internal capsule, posterior limb, and the ventral lateral nucleus of the thalamus, at 35 weeks of gestation in the striatum and the pre- and postcentral gyri, and at 37 weeks of gestation in the anterior limb of the internal capsule, and the optic radiations.

Myelination has been widely studied in MRI on newborns and during the 1st year of life [85–91]. Relatively few articles deal with the in vivo [78, 92, 93] or in vitro [94] myelination of fetuses. MRI as an imaging method is particularly well adapted to the study of myelination, since the biochemical modifications contemporary to this phenomenon are reflected by variations of the cerebral parenchyma's signal. Actually, the physiopathology of these variations is still debatable. The T1 hypersignal is widely considered to correspond to an increase in the cholesterol and glycolipid content accompanying the formation of myelin and to an interaction of these constituents with free water's hydrogen, which results in an increase in the quantity of bound water [95]. It was, however, also suggested that this hypersignal could correspond to an increase in cellular density [92].

Our results tally with Girard's [92], who finds a T1 hypersignal at as early as 23 weeks of gestation in the tegmentum (myelination of the sensory fibres) and from 31 weeks of gestation in the posterior limb of the internal capsule. However, the study does not distinguish between the lateral posterior limb and the middle posterior limb. We have not, however, found any T1 hypersignal in the semi-oval nucleus until 37–38 weeks of gestation, whereas Girard observed it at 35 weeks of gestation (in three fetuses).

Brisse [94] noted that the basal ganglia that share the same embryological origins (i. e. the neostriatum for the caudate nucleus and the putamen, and the paleostriatum for the ventral lateral nucleus of the thalamus and the globus pallidus) have the same signal in MRI. He found signal modifications contemporary to those observed by labelling the myelin basic protein [83, 84], with T1 hypersignals from 27 weeks of gestation in the thalamus and the globus pallidus, and from 34 weeks of gestation in the putamen and the caudate nucleus. These hypersignals appear much later in our study, but the qualities of examinations carried out in vitro and in vivo are not comparable, and furthermore this study is based on a small cohort (n = 5) of fetuses examined in vitro.

Appendix

In the present chapter, we wish to provide the reader with a detailed description of the aspect of certain cerebral structures, which were not systematically studied on each one of the fetuses in this atlas, but which nonetheless are all particularly interesting in the study of the fetal brain.

Pituitary Gland

The pituitary gland of the fetus, as is also observed on newborns until they reach 6–8 weeks, appears convex towards the top and globally hyperintense. No distinction can be made between the anterior and the posterior parts of the pituitary gland (arrow) (Fig. 1).

The mother's pituitary hormones do not pass through the placenta; the fetus is therefore entirely dependent on its own hormonal secretions. The fetal pituitary gland grows very quickly, and high levels of the various hormones secreted by the anterior pituitary gland are observed in fetuses during the last two trimesters of pregnancy. Histochemical studies have reported an intense development activity and differentiation of the pituitary cells throughout pregnancy. This may result in an increase in protein synthesis activity, which would account for the T1 hyperintensity of the anterior pituitary gland [95–97]. On the T2-weighted midline sagittal slice (slice no. 1, pp 66, 67), the pituitary stalk is discernible in most cases.

Optic Chiasm

The optic chiasm is clearly visible on the T2-weigthed midline sagittal slice (slice no. 1, pp 66, 67), and sometimes also on a coronal slice (arrow) (Figs. 2, 3).

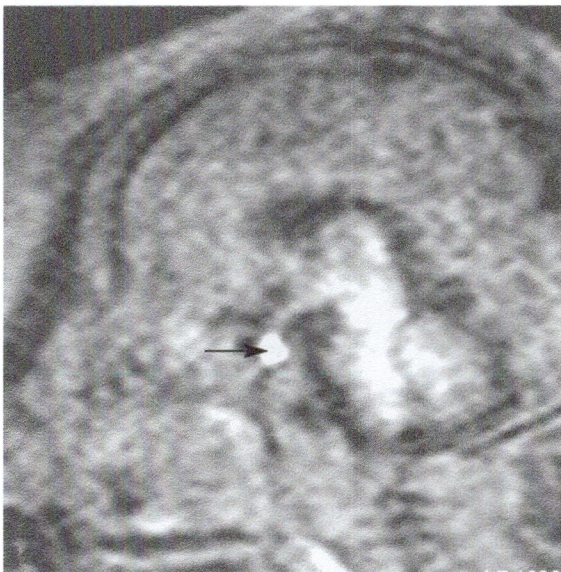

Fig. 1. Pituitary gland. T1-weighted midline sagittal slice at 35 weeks of gestation

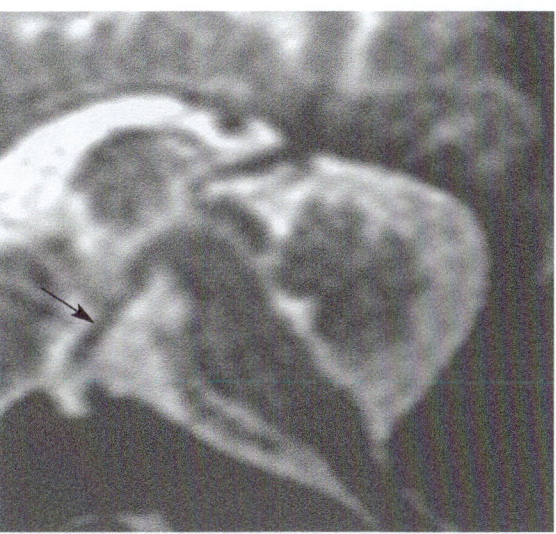

Fig. 2. Optic chiasm. T1-weighted midline sagittal slice at 35 weeks of gestation

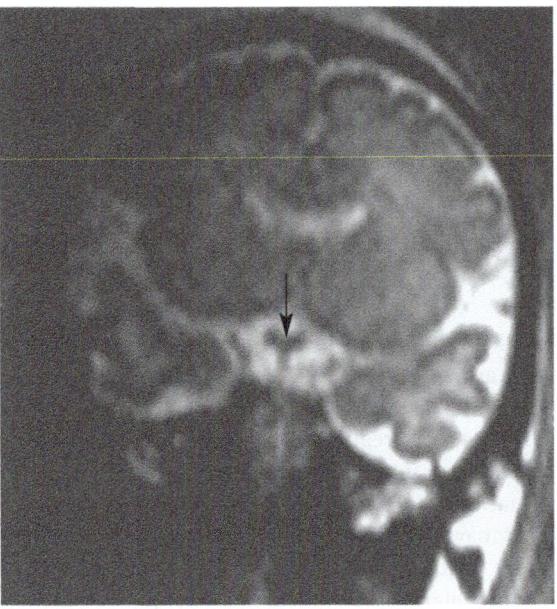

Fig. 3. Optic chiasm. T2-weighted anterior coronal slice at 32 weeks of gestation

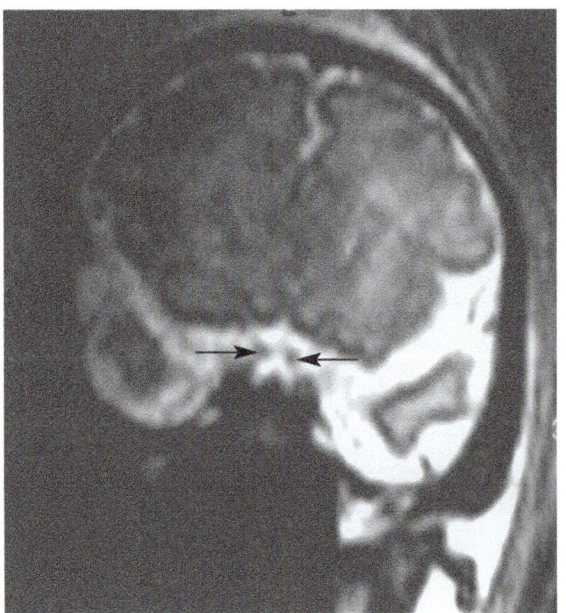

Fig. 4. Optic nerves. T2-weighted anterior coronal slice at 32 weeks of gestation

It is a small structure in fetuses and the MRI spatial resolution precludes establishing size standards for the chiasm; the optic nerves are not always visible. These may be visualized on a T2-weighted coronal slice (arrows) (Fig. 4).

Abnormalities of the optic tract (and notably septo-optic dysplasia) cannot be diagnosed at present because of the limitations in spatial resolution.

Brain Stem

The brain stem is clearly visible on the midline sagittal slice (slice no. 1, pp 66, 67) and on the axial slice at the level of the fourth ventricle (slice no. 8, pp 80, 81). Myelination of the pons was studied on the latter.

It is important to quantify the relative growth of the posterior fossa structures in fetal MRI. The contrast between the hypointense brain stem–vermis group and the hyperintense posterior fossa provides a good segmentation of these structures (slice no. 1, pp 66, 67). The line between the origin of the vein of Galen and the mamillary bodies marks the upper limit of the brain stem. The lower limit passes through the anterior and posterior points of the foramen magnum. The surfaces of the brain stem and vermis can then be assessed by planimetry and semi-automatic segmentation (Fig. 5).

The surface of the brain stem/surface of the vermis ratio can be evaluated: 1.56 at 28 weeks of gestation and 1.22 at 39 weeks of gestation. The growth of the vermis is slightly greater than that of the brain

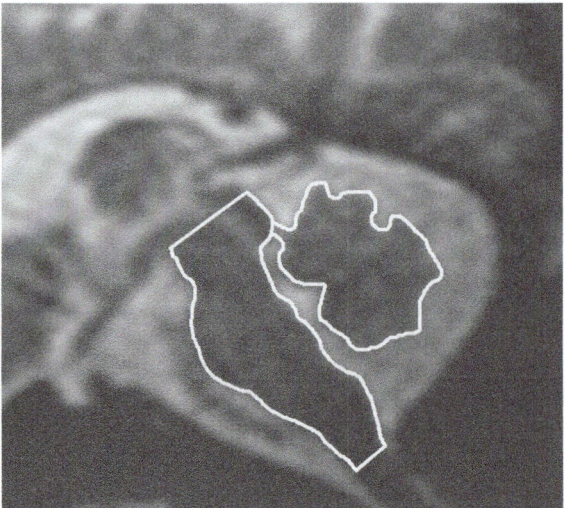

Fig. 5. Assessment of the surfaces of the brain stem and vermis. T2-weighted midline sagittal slice at 35 weeks of gestation

stem [98]. The biometric aspect aside, the brain stem's morphology ought to be considered as well, since this is rather difficult to appreciate in sonography (with the notable exception of the cerebral peduncles). In particular, it seems important to check whether the bump of the pons is indeed present.

Orbital Face of the Frontal Lobes

The sulci on the orbital face of the frontal lobes are considered as good late-stage markers of fetal maturation. In neurofetopathology [50], the olfactory sulci start developing at 16 weeks of gestation, but are only actually recognizable until 25 weeks of gestation; they delimit the gyrus rectus. As early as 28 weeks of gestation, Chi observed the progressive development of the orbital sulci, which divide the orbital faces of the frontal lobes into the medial and lateral orbital gyri. After 36 weeks of gestation, a subdivision in anterior and posterior orbital gyri becomes visible.

These various sulci can be visualized in postnatal examinations, on premature babies, using transfontanellar sonography or MRI [72]. Their visibility is, however, quite uncertain in MRI, since it is, as for other sulci, hindered by the development of the secondary sulci and the fineness of pericerebral spaces. The olfactory bulbs may be seen on very anterior T2-weighted coronal slices (Fig. 6).

The olfactory sulci hold great interest as late-stage markers of fetal maturation, but they should also be analysed where a pathology of the midline is suspected, in order to rule out arhinencephalia (Fig. 7).

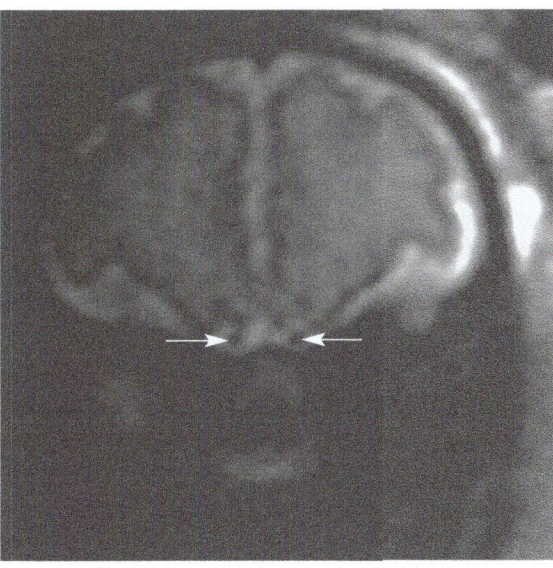

Fig. 6. T2-weighted anterior coronal slice at 35 weeks of gestation. Olfactory bulbs (*arrows*)

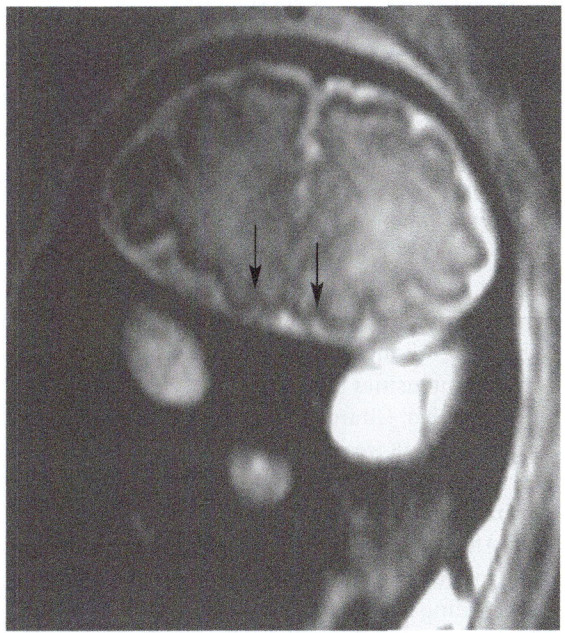

Fig. 7. T2-weighted anterior coronal slice at 35 weeks of gestation. Olfactory sulci (*arrows*)

Cerebral Mantle

This atlas starts at 22 weeks of gestation, at a stage where the neuroblasts from the germinal layer are about to complete their migration by successive waves towards the brain surface. At around 26–28 weeks of gestation, a few immature cells remain in the periventricular regions. The aspect of the fetal cerebral mantle has been studied in vitro [94, 99] and in vivo [92].

The variable aspect of the intermediate zone, which is divided in MRI into two or three layers, depending on the observer, probably results from the great variation in neuronal migration waves with time and from one individual to another; they are also unequally close to the germinal zone [94].

Consequently Brisse [94] has individualized four layers, in vitro at 22 weeks of gestation, in T1 and from depth to surface:

- The germinal zone (hyperintense)
- A layer of migrating cells of intermediate signal
- An intermediate zone with a low cell content (hypointense)
- The cortex (hyperintense)

At 27 weeks of gestation, three layers are differentiated; the intermediate zone, hypointense, corresponds to the white matter. At 34 weeks of gestation, the germinal zone has disappeared and only two layers (white matter and cortex) remain.

In vitro, Chong [99] found five distinct layers of different intensities between 16 and 18 weeks of gestation. In vivo, Girard [92] identified five layers between 23 and 28 weeks of gestation: the three central layers correspond to migrating cells surrounded by two intermediate zones: a deep zone and a surface zone. After 28 weeks of gestation, only the cortex and white matter remain visible.

According to Girard, the T1 hypersignal of the germinal zone, migrating cells and cortex correspond to zones of high cell content.

The no. 8 slices at 22–23, 27 and 31 weeks of gestation (Figs. 8–10) are a good illustration of the progressive disappearance of the germinal zone which, although initially visible as a T1 hypersignal around the atria (black arrows), is hardly discernible at 27 weeks of gestation and ceases to be individualized at 31 weeks of gestation. The cortical ribbon, however, remains clearly visible in T1 hypersignal (white arrows).

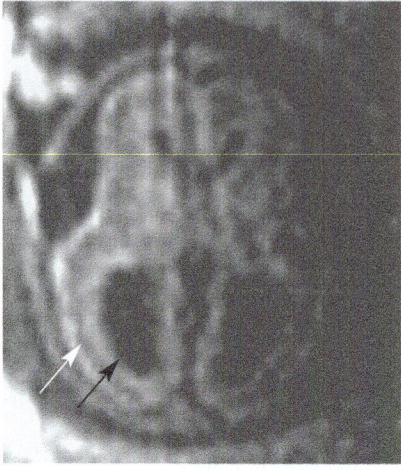

Fig. 8. Slice no. 8 at 22–23 weeks of gestation

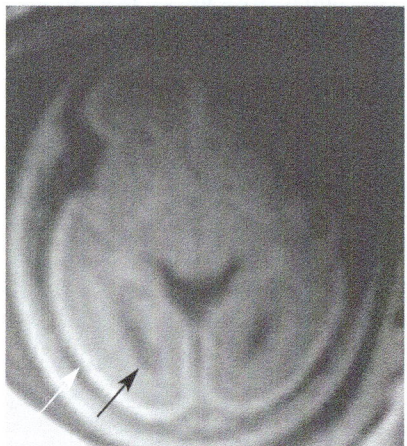

Fig. 9. Slice no. 8 at 27 weeks of gestation

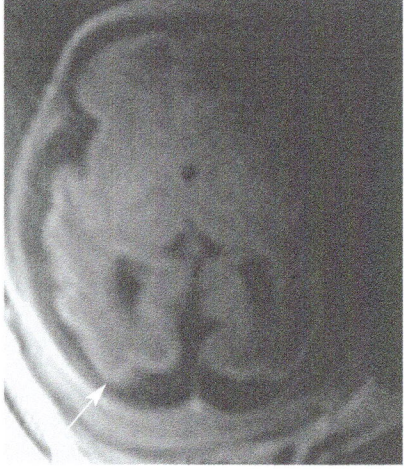

Fig. 10. Slice no. 8 at 31 weeks of gestation

References

1. Smith FW, Adam AH, Phillips WDP (1983) NMR imaging in pregnancy (letter). Lancet 1:61–62
2. Myers C, Duncan KR, Gowland PA, Johnson IR, Baker PN (1998) Failure to detect intrauterine growth restriction following in utero exposure to MRI. Br J Radiol 71:549–551
3. Elster AD (1994) Questions and answers. AJR 162: 1493–1497
4. The National Radiological Protection Board ad hoc advisory group on nuclear magnetic resonance clinical imaging (1983) Revised guidelines on acceptable limits of exposure during nuclear magnetic resonance clinical imaging. Br J Radiol 56:974–977
5. Huisman TAGM, Martin E, Kubik-Huch R, Marincek B (2002) Fetal magnetic resonance imaging of the brain: technical considerations and normal brain development. Eur Radiol 12:1941–1951
6. Ertl-Wagner B, Lienemann A, Strauss A, Reiser MF (2002) Fetal magnetic resonance imaging: indications, technique, anatomical considerations and a review of fetal abnormalities. Eur Radiol 12:1931–1940
7. Levine D (2001) Magnetic resonance imaging in prenatal diagnosis. Curr Opin Pediatr 13:572–578
8. Yamashita Y, Namimoto T, Abe Y, Takahashi M, Iwamasa J, Miyazaki K, Okamura H (1997) MR Imaging of the fetus by a HASTE sequence. AJR 168:513–519
9. Levine D, Hatabu H, Gaa J, Atkinson MW, Edelman RR (1996) Fetal anatomy revealed with fast MR sequences. AJR 167:905–908
10. Nitz WR (2002) Fast and ultrafast non-echo-planar MR imaging techniques. Eur Radiol 12:2866–2882
11. Chung HW, Chen CY, Zimmerman RA, Lee KW, Lee CC, Chin SC (2000) T2-weighted fast MR imaging with true FISP versus HASTE: comparative efficacy in the evaluation of normal fetal brain maturation. AJR 175:1375–1380
12. Penzkofer AK, Pfluger T, Pochmann Y, Meissner O, Leinsinger G (2002) MR Imaging of the brain in pediatric patients: diagnostic value of HASTE sequences. AJR 179:509–514
13. Sugahara T, Korogi Y, Hirai T, Hamatake S, Ikushima I, Shigematu Y, Takahashi M (1997) Comparison of HASTE and segmented-HASTE sequences with a T2-weighted fast spin-echo sequence in the screening evaluation of the brain. AJR 169:1401–1410
14. Patel MR, Klufas RA, Alberico RA, Edelman RR (1997) Half-Fourier acquisition single-shot turbo spin-echo (HASTE) MR: comparison with fast spin-echo MR in diseases of the brain. Am J Neuroradiol 18:1635–1640
15. Guo WY, Chang CY, Wong TT, Sheu MH, Cheng HC, Chen SJ, Hung JH (2001) A comparative MR and pathological study on fetal CNS disorders. Childs Nerv Syst 17:512–518
16. Duchêne M, Caldas JGMP, Benoudiba F, Cerri GG, Doyon D (2002) Comparative study of MR sequences to detect cavernous angiomas. J Radiol 83:1843–1846
17. Neil JJ, Shiran SI, McKinstry RC, Schefft GL, Snyder AZ, Almli CR, Akbudak E, Aronovitz JA, Miller JP, Lee BCP, Conturo TE (1998) Normal brain in human newborns: apparent diffusion coefficient and diffusion anisotropy measured by using diffusion tensor MR imaging. Radiology 209:57–66
18. Hüppi PS, Maier SE, Peled S, Zientara GP, Barnes PD, Jolesz FA, Volpe JJ (1998) Microstructural development of human newborn cerebral white matter assessed in vivo by diffusion tensor magnetic resonance imaging. Pediatr Res 44:584–590
19. Righini A, Bianchini E, Parazzini C (2003) Apparent diffusion coefficient determination in normal fetal brain: a prenatal MR imaging study. AJNR Am J Neuroradiol 24:799–804
20. Bui T, Daire Jl, Alberti C, Elmaleh M, Garel C, Luton D, Hassan M, Sebag G (2003) Microstructural development of fetal brain assessed in utero by diffusion tensor imaging. Pediatr Radiol 33:526
21. Marcos HB, Semelka RC, Worawattanakul S (1997) Normal placenta: gadolinium-enhanced, dynamic MR imaging. Radiology 205:493–496
22. Palacios Jaraquemada JM, Bruno C (2000) Gadolinium-enhanced MR imaging in the differential diagnosis of placenta accreta and placenta percreta. Radiology 216:610–611
23. Garel C, Brisse H, Sebag G, Elmaleh M, Oury JF, Hassan M (1998) Magnetic resonance imaging of the fetus. Pediatr Radiol 28:201–211
24. Garel C, Sebag G, Hornoy P, Elmaleh M, Hassan M (2000) Imagerie par résonance magnétique fœtale. Encycl Med Chir, Radiodiagnostic-Urologie-Gynécologie, 34–760-A-10
25. Garel C, Sebag G, Brisse H, Elmaleh M, Oury JF, Hassan M (1996) Imagerie par résonance magnétique chez le fœtus. Presse Med 25:452–456
26. Yamashita Y, Namimoto T, Abe Y, Takahashi M, Iwamasa J, Miyazaki K, Okamura H (1997) MR imaging of the fetus by a haste sequence. AJR 168:513–519
27. Yuh WTC, Nguyen HD, Fisher DJ, Tali ET, Gao F, Simonson TM, Kao SC, Weiner CP (1994) MR of fetal central nervous system abnormalities. AJNR 15:459–464
28. Girard N, Raybaud C, Dercole C, Boubli L, Chau C, Cahen S, Potier A, Gamerre M (1993) In vivo MRI of the fetal brain. Neuroradiology 35:431–436
29. Revel MP, Pons JC, Lelaidier C, Fournet P, Vial M, Musset D, Labrune M, Frydman R (1993) Magnetic resonance imaging of the fetus: a study of 20 cases performed without curarization. Prenat Diagn 13:775–799
30. Resta M, Spagnolo P, Dicuonzo F, Palma M, Florio C, Greco P, D'addario V, Vimercati A, Selvaggi L, Caruso G, Clemente R (1994) La risonanza magnetica del feto. Parte I: Tecnica d'esame ed anatomia normale dell' encefalo. Riv Neuroradiol 7:53–65

31. Lair-Milan F, Gelot A, Baron JM, Lewin F, Andre C, Adamsbaum C (1997) IRM encéphalique anténatale. Etude rétrospective à propos de 34 examens. J Radiol 78:499–505

32. Elmaleh M, Stempfle N, Hassan M, Vuillard E, Oury JF (1993) Evaluation des espaces péricérébraux du cerveau foetal en IRM anténatale : utilisation d'une séquence ultra-rapide à 0.5 T (abstract). Rev Im Med 5:S58

33. Levine D, Hatabu H, Gaa J, Atkinson MW, Edelman RR (1996) Fetal anatomy revealed with fast MR sequences. AJR 167:905–908

34. Sonigo P, Rypens F, Carteret M, Delezoide AL, Brunelle F (1998) MR imaging of fetal cerebral anomalies. Pediatr Radiol 28:212–222

35. Sonigo P, Rypens F, Carteret M, Brunelle F (1995) IRM cérébrale foetale dans le diagnostic anténatal des agénésies du corps calleux. Med Foet Echogr Gynécol 24:19–22

36. Brisse H, Sebag G, Fallet C, Elmaleh M, Garel C, Rossler L, Vuillard E, Oury JF, Hassan M (1998) IRM anténatale des agénésies calleuses : étude de 20 cas avec corrélations neuropathologiques. J Radiol 79:659–666

37. Revel MP, De Laveaucoupet J, Saada P, Delezoide AL, Musset D, Labrune M (1993) Echographie et IRM des malformations sous-tentorielles foetales (abstract). Rev Im Med 5: S333

38. Rypens F, Sonigo P, Elmaleh A, Lallemand D, Delezoide AL, Narcy F, Brunelle F (1995) Rôle de l'IRM cérébrale fœtale dans le diagnostic anténatal des anomalies de gyration et de migration neuronale (abstract). J Radiol 76:743

39. Rypens F, Sonigo P, Aubry MC, Delezoide AL, Cessot F, Brunelle F (1996) Prenatal MR diagnosis of a thick corpus callosum. AJNR 17:1918–1920

40. De Coudenhove S, Sonigo P, Carteret M, Sayegh N, Sambourg C, Brunelle F (1996) Apport de l'IRM dans le diagnostic prénatal des kystes arachno sus-tentoriels (abstract). J Radiol 77:986

41. Revel MP, Morel MP, Musset D, Frydman R, Labrune M (1993) Echographie et IRM des dilatations ventriculaires anténatales (abstract). Rev Im Med 5:S333

42. Koga Y, Tahara Y, Kida T, Matumoto Y, Negishi H, Fujimoto S (1997) Prenatal diagnosis of congenital unilateral hydrocephalus. Pediatr Radiol 27:319–320

43. Sonigo P, Sayegh N, Carteret M, De Coudenhove S, Sambourg C, Brunelle F (1996) Rôle de L'IRM cérébrale foetale dans le diagnostic antenatal des microcéphalies (abstract). J Radiol 77:846

44. Brisse H, Fallet C, Sebag G, Garel C, Elmaleh M, Vuillard E, Blot P, Evrard P, Hassan M (1997) In utero MRI: diagnosis of antenatal brain ischemia (abstract). Pediatr Radiol 27:465

45. Reiss I, Gortner L, Möller J, Gehl HB, Baschat AA, Gembruch U (1996) Fetal intracerebral hemorrhage in the second trimester: diagnosis by sonography and magnetic resonance imaging. Ultrasound Obstet Gynecol 7:49–51

46. Brisse H, Garel C, Sebag G, Elmaleh M, Fallet C, Vuillard E, Hassan M (1996) Diagnostic d'une hyperintensité focale en pondération T1 en IRM cérébrale foetale (abstract) J Radiol 77:846

47. Sonigo P, Elmaleh A, Fermont L, Delezoide AL, Mirlesse V, Brunelle F (1996) Prenatal MRI diagnosis of fetal cerebral tuberous sclerosis. Pediatr Radiol 26:1–4

48. Campi A, Scotti G, Filippi M, Gereveni S, Strigimi F, Lasjaunias P (1996) Antenatal diagnosis of vein of Galen aneurysmal malformation: MR study of fetal brain and post-natal follow-up. Neuroradiology 38:87–90

49. Huisman TA, Wisser J, Martin E, Kubik-Huch R, Marincek B (2002) Fetal magnetic resonance imaging of the central nervous system: a pictorial essay. Eur Radiol 12:1952–1961

50. Chi JG, Dooling EC, Gilles FH. Gyral development of the human brain. Ann. Neurol. 1977 ; 1:86–93

51. Larroche JC (1981) Critères morphologiques du développement du système nerveux central du fœtus humain. J Neuroradiol 8:93–108

52. Larroche JC (1977) Developmental pathology of the neonate. Excerpta Medica, Amsterdam, pp 320–327

53. Fees-Higgins A, Larroche JC (1987) Le développement du cerveau foetal humain. Atlas anatomique INSERM. CNRS, Masson, Paris

54. Dunn HL (1921) The growth of the central nervous system in the human fetus as expressed by graphic analysis and empirical formulae. J Comp. Neurol 33:405–491

55. Guihard-Costa AM, Larroche JC (1995) Fetal biometry: growth charts for practical use in fetopathology and antenatal ultrasonography. Fetal Diagn Ther 10:215–278

56. Reichel TF, Ramus RM, Caire JT, Hynan LS, Magee KP, Twickler DM (2003) Fetal central nervous system biometry on MR imaging. AJR 180:1155–1158

57. Patel MD, Goldstein RB, Tung S, Filly RA (1995) Fetal cerebral ventricular atrium: difference in size according to sex. Radiology 194:713–715

58. Hilpert PL, Hall BE, Kurtz AB (1995) The atria of the fetal lateral ventricles: a sonographic study of normal atrial size and choroid plexus volume. AJR 164:731–734

59. Browning PD, Laorr A, McGahan JP, Krasny RM, Cronan MS (1994) Proximal fetal cerebral ventricle: description of US technique and initial results. Radiology 192:337–341

60. Farrell TA, Hertzberg BS, Kliewer MA, Harris L, Paine SS (1994) Fetal lateral ventricles: reassessment of normal values for atrial diameter at US. Radiology 193:409–411

61. Filly RA, Goldstein RB (1994) The fetal ventricular atrium: fourth down and 10 mm to go. Radiology 193:315–317

62. Twickler DM, Reichel T, McIntire DD, Magee KP, Ramus RM (2002) Fetal central nervous system ventricle and cisterna magna measurements by magnetic resonance imaging. Am J Obstet Gynecol 187:927–931

63. Hertzberg BS, Kliewer MA, Freed KS, Mc Nally PJ, DeLong DM, Bowie JD, Kay HH (1997) Third ventricle: size and appearance in normal fetuses through gestation. Radiology 203:641–644

64. Baumeister LA, Hertzberg BS, Mc Nally PJ, Kliewer MA, Bowie JD (1994) Fetal fourth ventricle: US appearance and frequency of depiction. Radiology 192:333–336

65. Callen PW (1994) Ultrasonography in obstetrics and gynecology, 3rd edn. W.B. Saunders, Philadelphia

66. Cuddihy SL, Anderson NG, Wells JE, Darlow BA (1999) Cerebellar vermis diameter at cranial sonography for assessing gestational age in low-birth-weight infants. Pediatr Radiol 29:589–594

67. Birnholz JC (1982) Newborn cerebellar size. Pediatrics 70: 284–287

68. Malinger G, Zakut H (1993) The corpus callosum: normal fetal development as shown by transvaginal sonography. AJR 161:1041–1043

69. Gelot A (1999) La giration : développement in utero. Lettres à la rédaction/Gynécologie. JEMU 20:67–68

70. Hansen PE, Ballesteros MC, Soila K, Garcia L, Howard JM (1993) MR imaging of the developing human brain. Part 1. Prenatal development. Radiographics 13:21–36

71. Van der Knaap MS, Van Wezel-Meijler G, Barth PG, Barkhof F, Ader HJ, Valk J (1996) Normal gyration and sulcation in preterm and term neonates: appearance on MR images. Radiology 200:389–396

72. Naidich TP, Grant JL, Altman N, Zimmerman RA, Birchansky SB, Braffman B, Daniel JL (1994) The developing cerebral surface. Neuroimaging Clin N Am 4:201–240

73. Dorovini-Zis K, Dolman CL (1977) Gestational development of brain. Arch Pathol Lab Med 101:192–195

74. Huang CC (1991) Sonographic cerebral sulcal development in premature newborns. Brain Dev 13:27–31

75. Murphy NP, Rennie J, Cooke RW (1989) Cranial ultrasound assessment of gestational age in low birthweight infants. Arch Dis Child 64:569–572

76. Monteagudo A, Timor-Tritsch IE (1997) Development of fetal gyri, sulci and fissures: a transvaginal sonography study. Ultrasound Obstet Gynecol 9:222–228

77. Levine D, Barnes PD (1999) Cortical maturation in normal and abnormal fetuses as assessed with prenatal MR imaging. Radiology 210:751–758

78. Lan LM, Yamashita Y, Tang Y, Sugahara T, Takahashi M, Ohba T, Okamura H (2000) Normal fetal brain development: MR imaging with a half-Fourier rapid acquisition with relaxation enhancement sequence. Radiology 215:205–210

79. Garel C, Chantrel E, Brisse H, Elmaleh M, Luton D, Oury JF, Sebag G, Hassan M (2001) Fetal cerebral cortex: normal gestational landmarks using prenatal MR imaging. AJNR Am J Neuroradiol 22:184–189

80. Adamsbaum C, Gelot A, André C, Baron JM (2001) Atlas d'IRM du cerveau fœtal. Masson, Paris

81. Flechsig P (1920) Anatomie des menschlichen Gehirns und Rückenmarks auf myelogenetisher Grundlage. Georg Thieme, Leipzig, pp 9–37

82. Larroche JC (1966) The development of the central nervous system during intra-uterine life. In: Falkner F (ed) Human development. Saunders, Philadelphia, pp 57–276

83. Hasegawa M, Houdou S, Mito T, Takashima S, Asanuma K, Ohno T (1992) Development of myelination in the human fetal and infant cerebrum: a myelin basic protein immunohistochemical study. Brain Dev 14:1–6

84. Tanaka S, Mito T, Takashima S (1995) Progress of myelination in the human fetal spinal nerve roots, spinal cord and brainstem with myelin basic protein immunohistochemistry. Early Hum Dev 41:49–59

85. Lee BC, Lipper E, Nass R, Ehrlich ME, De Ciccio-Bloom E, Auld PA (1986) MRI of the central nervous system in neonates and young children. Am J Neuroradiol 7:605–616

86. Holland BA, Haas DK, Norman D, Brant Zawadzki M, Newton TH (1986) MRI of normal brain maturation. Am J Neuroradiol 7:201–208

87. McArdle CB, Richardson CJ, Nicholas DA, Mirfakhraee M, Hayden CK, Amparo EG (1987) Developmental features of the neonatal brains: MR imaging. I. Gray-white matter differentiation and myelination. Radiology 162:223–229

88. Barkovich AJ, Kjos BO, Jackson DE, Norman D (1988) Normal maturation of the neonatal and infant brain: MR imaging at 1.5 T. Radiology 166:173–180

89. Dietrich RB, Bradley WG, Zarogoza EJ, Oto RJ, Tatra RK, Wilson GH, Kangarloo H (1988) MR evaluation of early myelination patterns in normal and developmentally delayed infants. AJNR 150:889–896

90. Van der Knapp MS, Valk J (1990) MR imaging of the various stages of normal myelination during the first year of life. Neuroradiology 31:459–470

91. Girard N, Raybaud C, Du Lac P (1991) MRI study of brain myelination. J Neuroradiol 18:291–307

92. Girard N, Raybaud C, Poncet M (1995) In vivo MR study of brain maturation in normal fetuses. AJNR 16:407–413

93. Wang Z, Chen J, Qin Z, Zhang J (1998) The research of myelinization of normal fetal brain with magnetic resonance imaging. Chin Med J 111:71–74

94. Brisse H, Fallet C, Sebag G, Nessmann C, Blot P, Hassan M (1997) Supratentorial parenchyma in the developing fetal brain: in vitro MR study with histologic comparison. AJNR 18:1491–1497

95. Barkovich AJ (2000) Normal development of the neonatal and infant brain, skull and spine. In: Pediatric neuroimaging, 3rd edn. Lippincot Williams and Wilkins, Philadelphia

96. Wolpert SM, Osborne M, Anderson M, Runge VM (1988) The bright pituitary gland. A normal MR appearance in infancy. AJNR 9:1–3

97. Tien RD, Kucharczyk J, Bessette J, Middleton M (1992) MR imaging of the pituitary gland in infants and children: changes in size, shape and MR signal with growth and development. AJR 158:1151–1154

98. Mestdagh P, Daire JL, Elmaleh M, Garel C, Claude I, Robert Y, Hassan M, Sebag G (2002) Quantitative growth of the brainstem: a semiautomated MR study in fetuses. J Neuroradiol 29:1S225–1S233

99. Chong BW, Babcook CJ, Salamat MS, Nemzek W, Kroeker D, Ellis WG (1996) A magnetic resonance template for normal neuronal migration in the fetus. Neurosurgery 39:110–116

PART II

Imaging the Pathological Fetal Brain

Pathology of the Midline

Corpus Callosum Dysgenesis

Corpus Callosum Agenesis

Corpus callosum agenesis (CCA) is a relatively frequent malformation. Its exact prevalence in the population is still unknown, as CCA can be completely asymptomatic. This prevalence essentially depends on the population studied and the diagnostic method used and varies between 0.3 % and 0.7 % in the general population (diagnosis by encephalography [1], and hence on selected cases). It reaches 2 %–3 % for patients showing mental retardation (diagnosis by computed tomography [2]). CCA accounts for 3 %–5 % of all nervous system malformations detected by antenatal ultrasonography (US) and for approximately 50 % of all malformations of the midline [3].

Embryology Overview

The corpus callosum is one of the three commissures forming a junction between the cerebral hemispheres. Between the 6th and 8th weeks of development, the dorsal part of the primitive lamina terminalis (in the region of the anterior neuropore) thickens and transforms into the lamina reuniens. Between the 8th and the 11th weeks, the future anterior commissure at the front and fornical commissure at the back form. Formation of the corpus callosum starts later, in the 11th week, by the formation of the genu at the front. Growth of the corpus callosum follows that of the hemispheres and reproduces the winding motion of the cerebral vesicles. The body, isthmus and splenium are successively formed; the most anterior part, or rostrum, is formed last, between 18 and 20 weeks [4, 5].

The crossing of axons from one hemisphere to the other is preceded by the setting up of glial slings, which depends on chemical factors.

In most cases, CCA is not strictly speaking an agenesis, but rather a dysgenesis, since the neurons whose axons should form the corpus callosum are present but unable to cross the midline because of the alteration of a recognition protein; they form bundles of Probst on the internal aspect of the homolateral hemisphere [6, 7]. In some rare forms of the pathology, the commissural fibres are absent. Other hypotheses have been put forward concerning the physiopathology of CCAs. They could result from the absence of progression of callosal neurons associated either with extrinsic causes (lipoma, interhemispheric cyst) or disorders in neuronal migration and intracortical disposition linked with a global anomaly of gyration and corticogenesis [7]. The partial absence of corpus callosum can also be linked to a clastic lesion, in which case the bundles of Probst are absent.

Moreover, hypoplasia of the corpus callosum can be associated with inherited metabolic diseases such as nonketotic hyperglycinaemia, propionic acidaemia, methyl malonic acidaemia, maternal phenylketonuria or anomalies of the Krebs cycle such as fumarase deficiency and pyruvate dehydrogenase or decarboxylase deficiency. In these diseases, hypoplasia of the corpus callosum might proceed from a late destruction of the corpus callosum [8].

Postnatally, as early as in the first weeks of life, an important loss of callosal axons is observed prior to myelination.

Signs of CCA in Ultrasonography

Standards for the length and thickness of the corpus callosum at the levels of the genu, body and splenium were established in US, by the endovaginal approach, in an already rather old study [9] made on fetuses aged between 18 and 42 weeks of gestation.

The US study, done at best in the three planes of space, indicates [10–12]:

- A direct sign:
  - The corpus callosum not visible, which should normally be observed at 18–20 weeks of gestation

But above all:
- Indirect signs:
  - Absence of septum pellucidum
  - Broadening of the occipital horns (colpocephaly) and of the ventricular atria
  - Parallelism of the lateral ventricles
  - Internal concavity and excessive distance between the frontal horns
  - Ascension of the third ventricle
  - Radial disposition of the sulci on the internal aspects of the hemispheres
  - Absence of visibility in colour Doppler imaging of the loop formed by the pericallosal artery

These signs are not always present, and the position of the fetus's head sometimes makes it impossible to obtain slices in the three planes. This probably partially explains the frequent false-negative diagnoses of CCA with US. Indeed, in a recent study [13], ultrasonography made it possible to visualize CCA directly in only four cases out of 14.

In another recent series [14], six cases of CCA out of 14 were detected by ultrasonography, seven others were suspected (including one false-positive case). In our own experience, 16 cases of CCA out of 20 were correctly diagnosed with ultrasonography [15].

This variation in sensitivity from one series to another concerning the positive diagnosis of CCA is very probably due to the US examinations not always being conducted by referring sonographers. Moreover, the examination conditions (maternal wall, position of the fetal head, use of the endovaginal approach) are not always stated.

Contribution of MRI to the Antenatal Diagnosis of CCA

As in ultrasonography, we use MRI to answer three questions:

- Is there CCA?
- Is this CCA complete?
- Are there any other associated abnormalities?

Several general articles on fetal MRI [16–19] report cases of CCA, but the MRI symptomatology is not de-

scribed, and the contribution of MRI when compared to US is not specified. Three recent articles evaluated the contribution of MRI to the diagnosis of CCA:

The first one [13] investigating 14 cases correlates antenatal MR images with postnatal neuroradiological examinations in four cases, and with fetopathological examinations in four other cases. The second article [14] reports 14 CCA cases and compares fetal MRI data with postnatal MRI in five cases and with neuropathological examinations in eight cases. The third article [15] contrasts antenatal MRI with postnatal MRI in two cases and with neuropathological examinations in 18 cases. We will essentially refer to these last two articles. Since the article based on our own experience [15] was published, our series has grown larger and currently includes 58 cases of CCA.

MRI Seems Efficient in the Positive Diagnosis of CCA

The direct sign, i.e. the corpus callosum is not visible, is found in most cases (Figs. 1, 2).

The indirect signs are identical to the US signs and, as in US, they are not always present, particularly the radial pattern of sulci at early stages. The importance of T2-weighted axial and coronal slices should be stressed, as they contribute greatly to diagnosis.

A significant ventricular dilatation could hide the parallelism of lateral ventricles or the internal concavity of the frontal horns. It must be noted that the diagnosis of CCA in MRI is possible even at early stages (from 21, 5 [15] or 22 weeks of gestation [14]).

Whether the CCA is complete or not is difficult to see in US [10], and in this field the contribution of MRI is indisputable [14, 15] (Figs. 2, 3). Taking axial slices at the level of the corpus callosum genu is indispensable. Errors are possible, however, notably on the hypertrophy of the anterior columns of the fornix, which can be erroneously interpreted as a genu of the corpus callosum. On the contrary, MRI may fail to detect the persistence of a very small anterior part of the corpus callosum.

Fig. 1 a–f. Isolated complete corpus callosum agenesis: fetus at ▶ 27 weeks of gestation. a, b Antenatal US. Coronal slices at the level of the frontal horns (a), of the temporal lobes (b). c, d Antenatal MRI. T2-weighted coronal slices at the same levels as a and b. e, f Corresponding macroscopic views. Note the typical steer horn configuration of the lateral ventricles, whose horns present an internal concavity. The ascent of the third ventricle is visible, as well as voluminous Probst bundles (*arrows*) inside the lateral ventricles. No other cerebral abnormality is detected

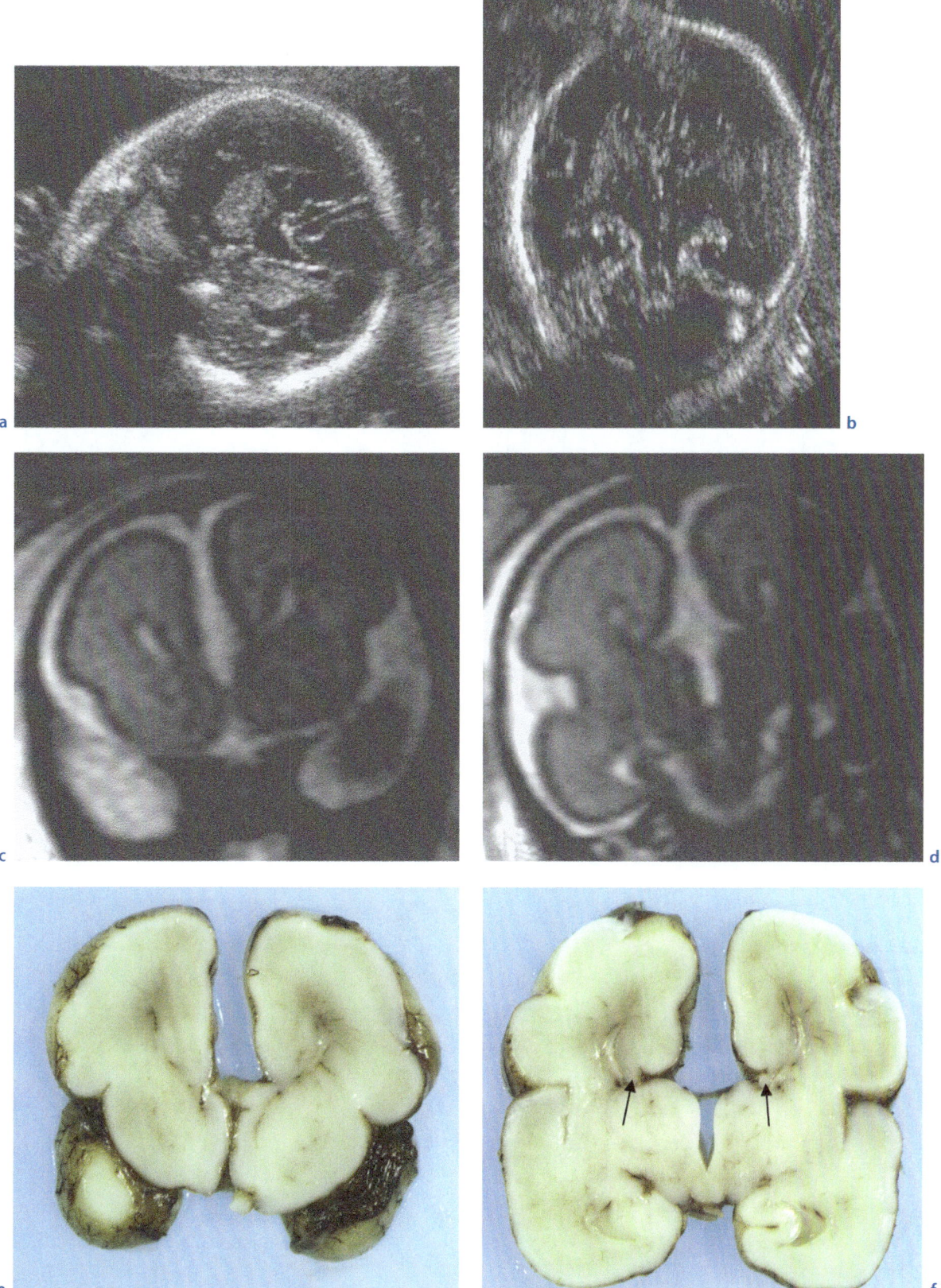

Fig. 2 a–c

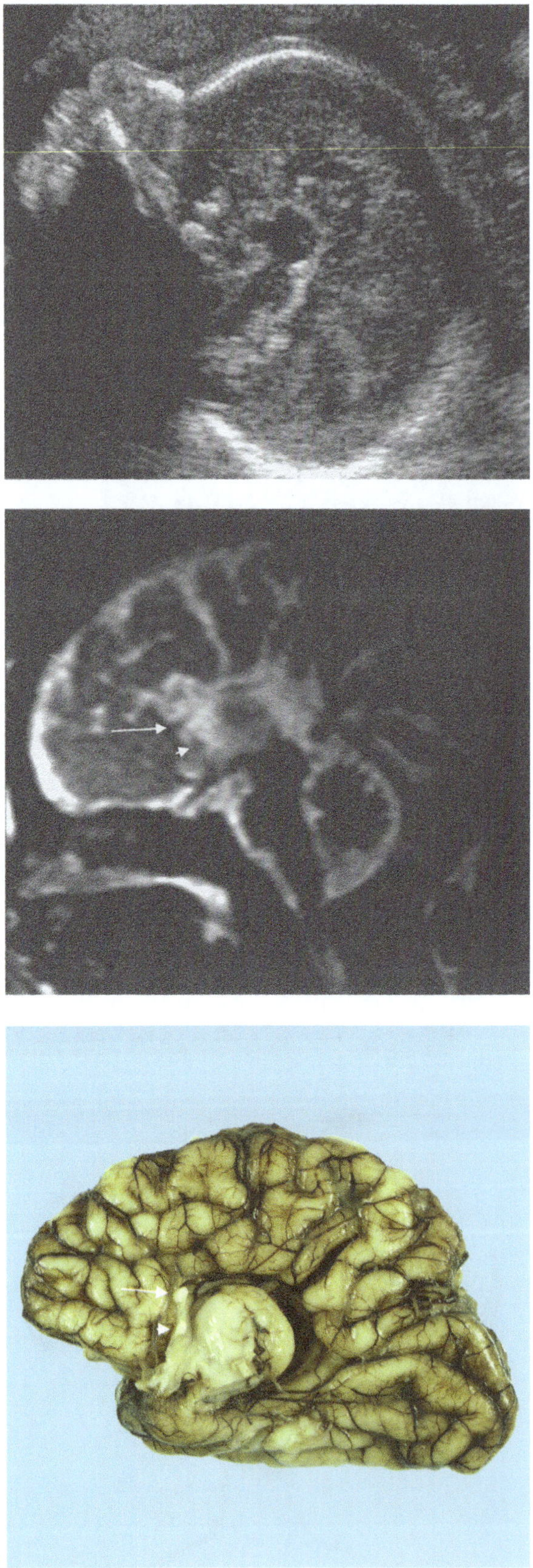

a

b

c

Fig. 3 a–c

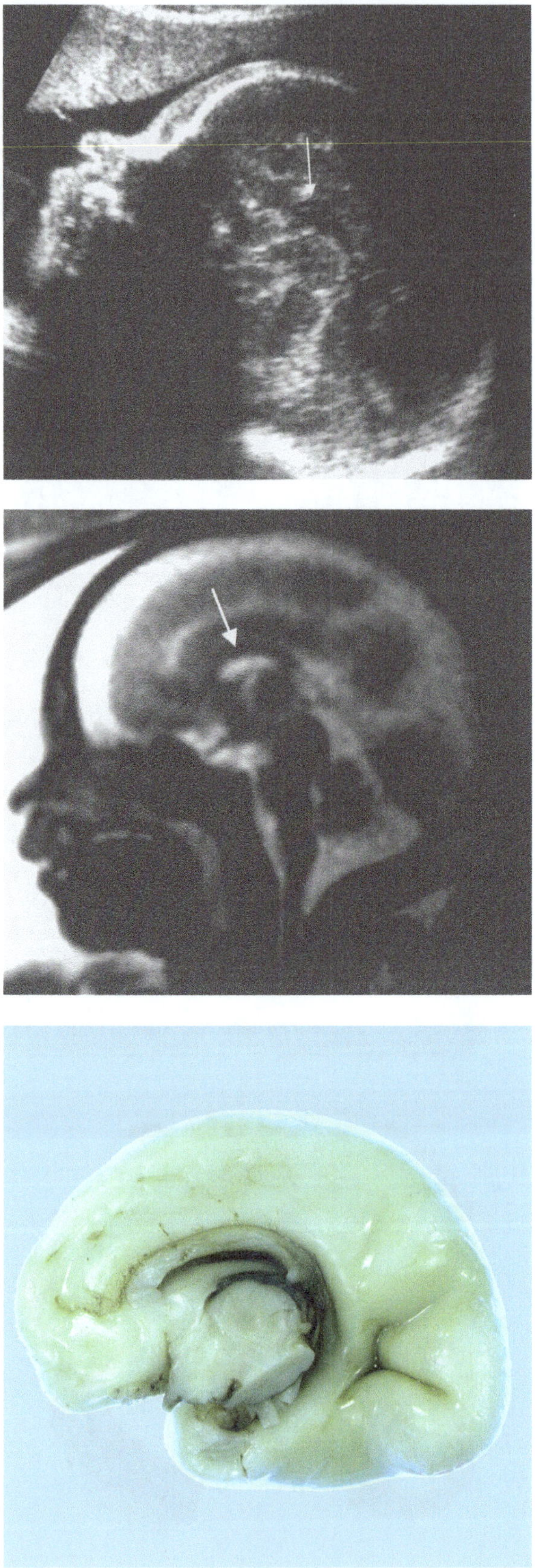

a

b

c

◀ **Fig. 2 a–c.** Isolated quasi-complete CCA. Midline sagittal slice. **a** Antenatal US. Fetus at 25 weeks of gestation. **b** Antenatal MRI. Fetus at 34 weeks of gestation. **c** Macroscopic view, same fetus as on (**b**), at 35 weeks of gestation. The corpus callosum, which is normally visible as a whole on this slice as early as 20 weeks of gestation, is absent. In US, one should be careful not to mistake the anterior columns of the fornix for a corpus callosum. The radial pattern of the sulci on the internal aspect of the hemispheres is seen clearly on the MRI slice presented and on the macroscopic view. It is not visible on **a**, as the fetus is too young. On MRI and fetopathological slices, a very small part of the corpus callosum genu (*arrow*) is visible at the front, directly above the anterior white commissure (*arrowhead*)

Fig. 3 a–c. Isolated partial CCA. Fetus at 28 weeks of gestation. Midline sagittal slice. **a** Antenatal US. **b** Antenatal MRI. The genu and body of the corpus callosum are present (*arrow*). The splenium is absent. It is nearly impossible to individualize the rostrum in imaging at this stage, but the absence of rostrum is established on macroscopic examination (**c**). **c** Fetus at 25 weeks of gestation. Macroscopic view. The rostrum and splenium are absent

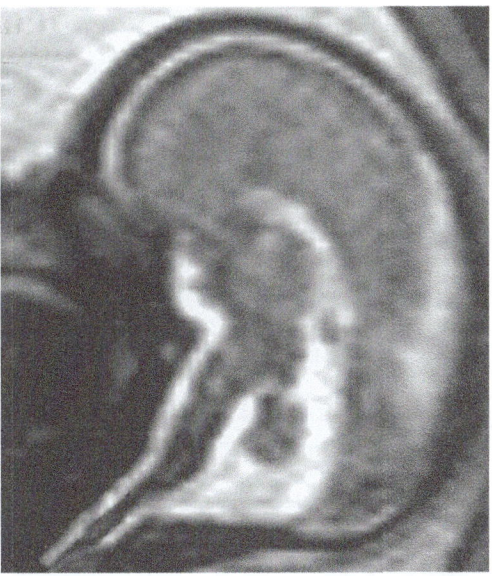

a

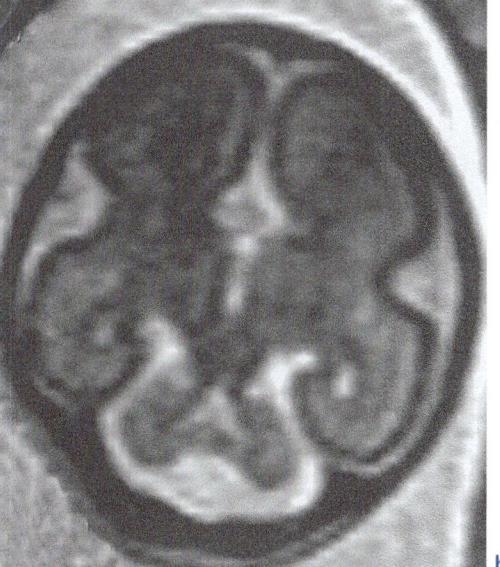

b

The Search for Associated Abnormalities Is Essential

From one series to another, the occurrence rate of such abnormalities varies between 50% and 85% [20–22]. We will here only consider CCA-associated cerebral abnormalities. In our initial study [15], MRI examinations led to the diagnosis of CCA with associated abnormalities in 11 cases out of 15, and identified accurately 15 of the 33 associated intracranial abnormalities. Abnormalities of the posterior fossa included a Dandy-Walker malformation, cerebellum and/or brain stem hypoplasia (Fig. 4), Arnold Chiari malformation and several cases of cerebellum heterotopia [9, 13–15]. Because of their small size, the latter are not more easily identified in MRI than in US and are only found in neuropathological examinations. Moreover, their prognostic signification is debatable. The search for abnormalities of the posterior cerebral fossa is based on morphological and biometrical criteria [23, 24], described in Chap. 12.

The CCA-associated abnormalities at the supratentorial level are for the most part gyration abnormalities (Figs. 4–6), which are not easily characterized on the internal aspects of the hemispheres (possibly a primitive CCA-associated abnormality or an abnormality secondary to CCA). In this field too, the contribution of MRI is indisputable [14, 15, 25]. MRI can also reveal abnormalities in supratentorial neuronal migration (see Chap. 9).

Hypoxaemic–ischaemic lesions can also be observed. They are best seen on T1-, T2- and T2*-

Fig. 4 a, b. Complete CCA associated with abnormalities of gyration and of the posterior fossa. Trisomy 18. Fetus at 25 weeks of gestation. Fetal MRI. **a** Midline sagittal slice. The brain stem is abnormally thin. The bulge of the pons is absent. The dimensions (height and anteroposterior diameter) of the vermis are lower than standard. **b** Coronal slice at the level of the temporal horns. The cerebellum is abnormally small (the transverse diameter is below standard). The posterior part of the superior temporal sulcus is not yet visible. Opercularization of the sylvian fissures is normally more advanced at this stage

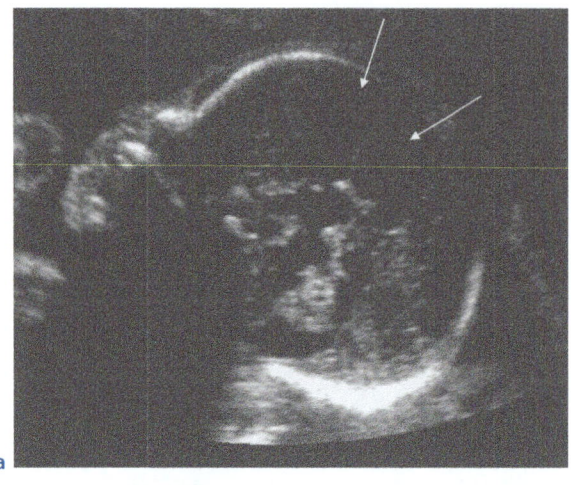

a

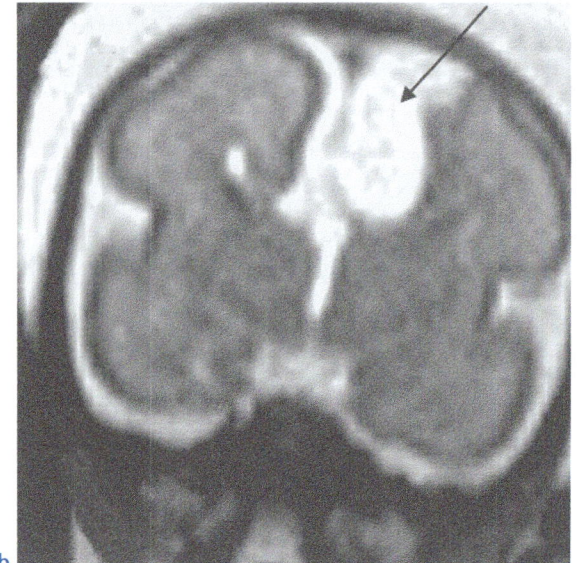

b

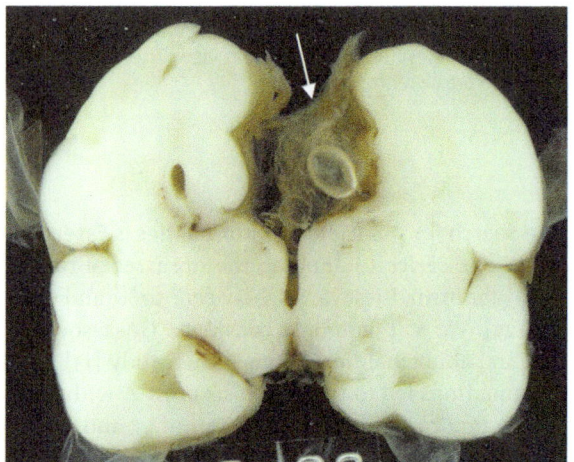

c

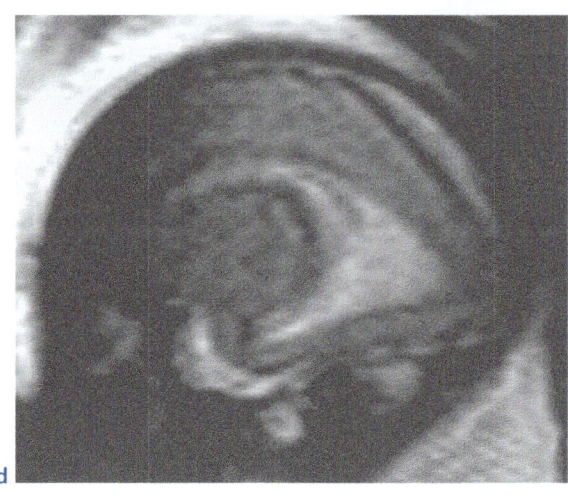

d

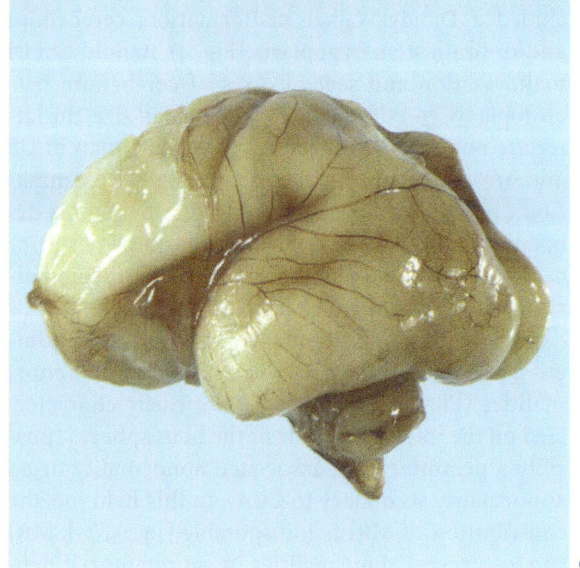

e

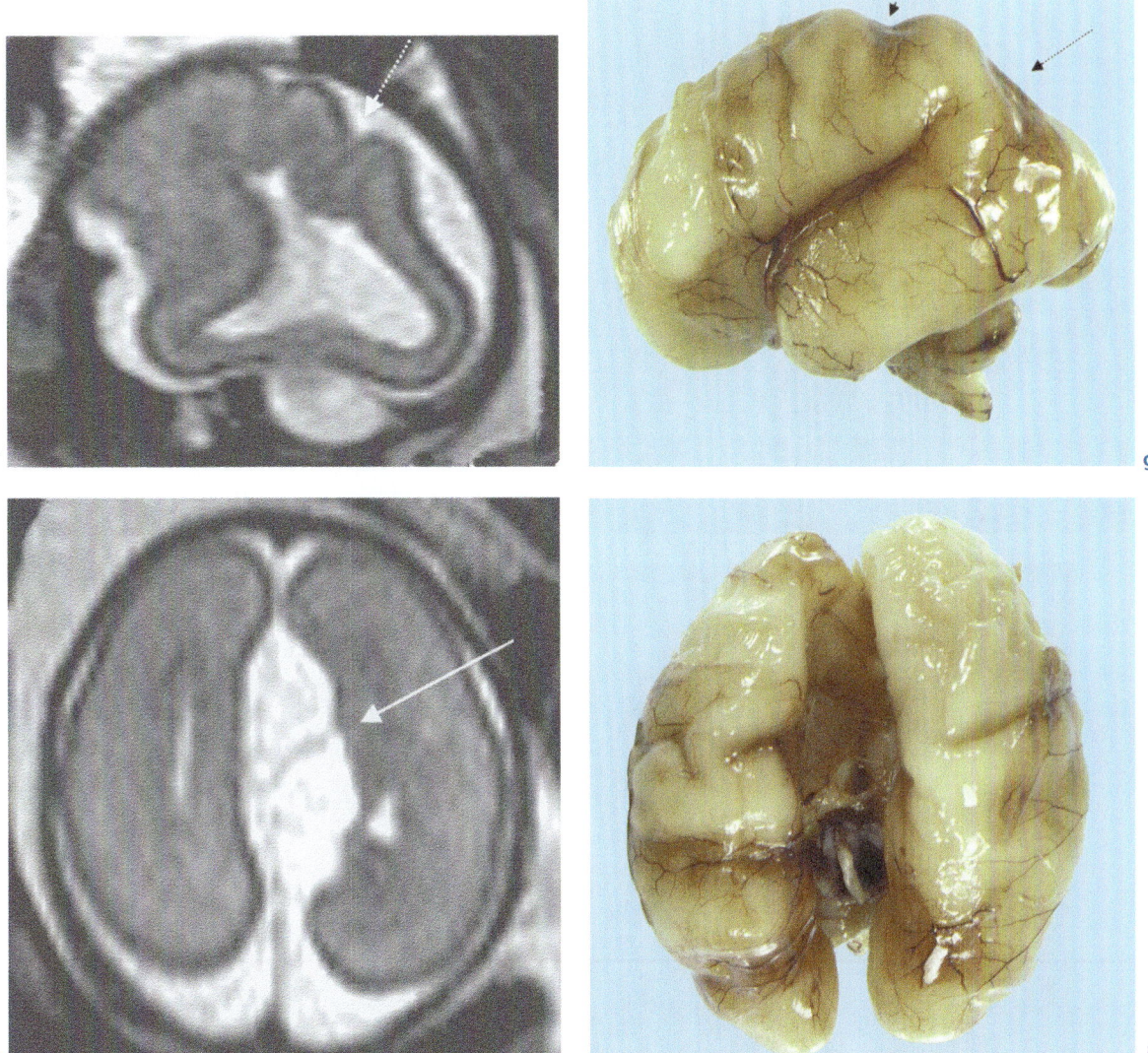

Fig. 5a–i. Partial CCA associated with paramedian cysts and gyration abnormalities. Fetus at 26 weeks of gestation. **a** Midline sagittal US slice. The paramedian cysts are clearly visible (*arrows*). They are separated by a septum. Coronal MRI slice (**b**), macroscopic view (**c**). Left paramedian cyst (*arrow*). **d–g** Parasagittal MRI slices at the level of the atria (**d, f**) and homolateral external views (**e, g**). On the right side (**d, e**), gyration is normal for the stage. On the left side (**f, g**), presence of abnormal parietal sulci (*dotted arrows*). Note the abnormal outline of the lateral ventricle under the abnormal sulcus (**f**). Axial MRI slice at the level of the vertex (**h**) and top view (**i**). Both paramedian cysts are clearly visible (*arrow*) and separated by a septum in MRI. They are collapsed on macroscopic examination, on which the abnormalities of frontal gyration are apparent

weighted sequences [15] (see Chap. 14). In this context, the absence of corpus callosum corresponds to destruction rather than agenesis (Fig. 6).

Progressive ventricular dilatation or arrhinencephaly can also be associated with CCA [10, 15, 20].

CCA is frequently associated (in 35 out of 105 CCA cases [26]) with an interhemispheric cyst (Fig. 6), although it is not, strictly speaking, an associated abnormality since the cyst might be the primitive abnormality, in which case CCA is only the consequence of a mechanical interruption of the corpus callosum's formation [27, 28].

These cysts belong to various histological types (neuroepithelial, arachnoid, etc.) and can be classi-

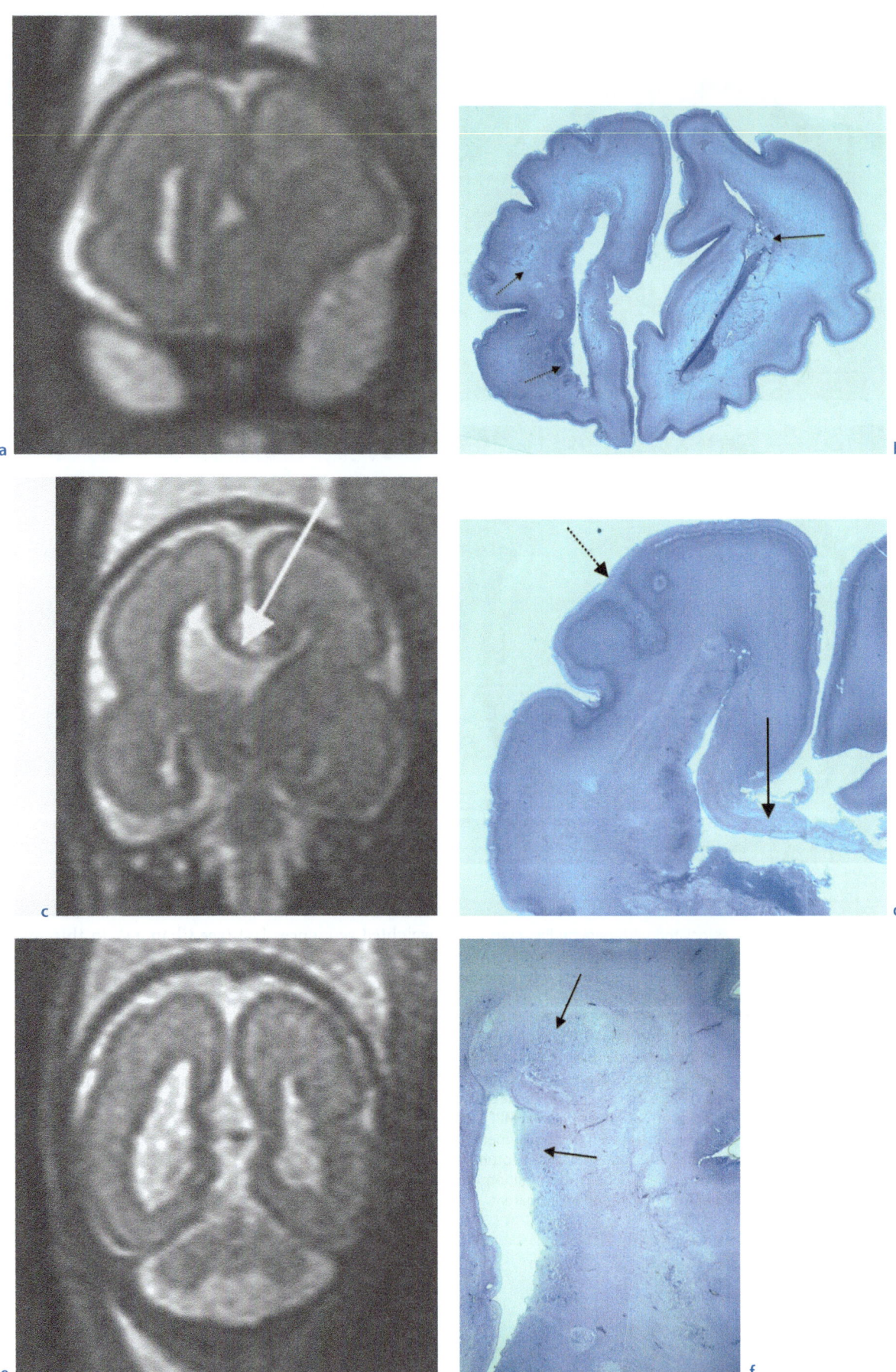

◄ **Fig. 6 a–f.** Partial destruction of the corpus callosum with periventricular heterotopias and gyration abnormalities in a hypoxic–ischaemic context. **a, b** Anterior coronal MRI slice at 28 weeks of gestation (**a**) and histological slice at 29 weeks of gestation (same fetus). The right frontal horn is dilated. A voluminous heterotopia (*arrow*) is observed on the left side, while on the right side ischaemic lesions of the white matter and germinal zone are visible (*dotted arrows*). **c, d** More posterior coronal MRI slices at 28 weeks of gestation (**c**) and corresponding histological slice at 29 weeks of gestation (**d**). The corpus callosum is visible at this level (*arrow*), but the leaves of the septum are probably destroyed. Opercularization of the sylvian fissures is very abnormal for this stage. Frontal gyration is abnormal (extra sulcus on the right side) (*dotted arrow*) and temporal gyration is delayed (absence of superior temporal sulcus). Also note the clastic ventricular dilatation, particularly on the right side, with destruction of the germinal zone. **e, f** Posterior coronal MRI slice at the level of the atria at 28 weeks of gestation (**e**) and slightly anterior histological slice at 29 weeks of gestation (**f**). The atria are parallel to each other in relation with the absence of corpus callosum, and the right atrium is dilated. The outlines of the ventricles are indented by neuronal heterotopias (*arrows*), the presence of which is confirmed by the histological examination (**f**)

fied by whether they communicate with the ventricular system, are associated with other cerebral malformations, or are uni- or multilocular. They correspond to different clinical presentations [29].

MRI offers good visibility of these cysts and has the advantage over ultrasonography of better distinguishing between cases of third-ventricle expansion and other formations independent of the ventricular system [15]. The intracystic septa are as clearly visible as in US.

Prognosis

The prognosis of callosal ageneses is still a rather controversial subject, because of the small size of cohorts in series studying the follow-up of children who present this malformation and the significant number of possible variables associated with CCA.

Furthermore, the neurological state of children with CCA is of course very different in the series for which the patients were recruited on cerebral imaging data (examination justified by neurological signs) [30, 31] and in the much rarer series that study the postnatal follow-up of children who were diagnosed with CCA in the antenatal or perinatal periods [32–35]. The most severe complications are mental retardation (CAA was found in 2%–3% of mentally handicapped patients [12]) and epilepsy.

It stands to reason that for children whose CCA is part of a more complex context (chromosomal abnormality, Mendelian syndrome, metabolic disease), the prognosis of CCA is closely linked to that of these various disorders.

Most authors make no difference, as far as the subsequent prognosis is concerned, between complete CCA and partial CCA. However, a recent study [32] reports a worse prognosis for the complete forms of CCA, which could be explained by greater involvement of the neuronal functions.

The fetus's sex bears prognostic significance for some [36], in the sense that female sex may be the only antenatal sign of an Aicardi's syndrome, of worse prognosis. Other authors [32] believe that there is no significant relation between the fetus's sex and the prognosis.

A number of sonographic criteria that are transposable to MRI are held to be of bad prognosis [22]: progressive ventricular dilatation or dilatation exceeding 13 mm, cranial perimeter under –2 standard deviations, and cerebellar hypoplasia. For other authors [12], on the contrary, ventricular dilatation less than 14 mm is a factor of poor prognosis, as are the asymmetry of the ventricles and the upward displacement of the third ventricle. It should be noted, however, that these conclusions are based on the follow-up of very small cohorts (fewer than 15 children).

There is nonetheless one point of consensus in the literature: the prognosis of CCA associated with other abnormalities of the central nervous system is poor [11, 20, 32, 35, 36], which tends to show how fundamental it is to perform a fetal MRI upon discovering apparently isolated CCA in ultrasonography. Delayed development is observed in approximately 15% of children with isolated CCA [12, 15, 20, 22] and in 56% of children showing an associated abnormality (intra- or extracranial) [20]. In the antenatal period, the greatest difficulty lies in diagnosing such associated abnormalities. Notably, when a CCA is detected early, gyration abnormalities may only appear at a much later stage, making it difficult to wait until 32–34 weeks of gestation to perform an MRI examination and reach a decision concerning the pursuit of pregnancy [33].

To conclude, let us cite the special case of CCA associated with giant or paramedian interhemispheric arachnoid cysts. Studies on small series (three children [27] and 11 children [37]) suggest that the clinical neurological disorder might be rather mild, or even absent in some cases.

Thick Corpus Callosum: Corpus Callosum Lipoma

Thick Corpus Callosum

The antenatal detection of a thick corpus callosum is exceptional. Standards for thickness of the fetal corpus callosum have been established in US by the endovaginal approach [9] but not in MRI, on account of an insufficient spatial resolution and the small size of the structure. Thickness of the genu and splenium must not exceed 5 mm, and the corpus should not be more than 3 mm thick.

To the best of our knowledge, only one observation of a thick corpus callosum, made with US at 24 weeks of gestation, was confirmed in fetal MRI [38]. MRI examination confirmed the diagnosis at 33 weeks of gestation and also found opercular dysplasia, polymicrogyria and subependymal neuronal heterotopias.

The prognosis of cases of thick corpus callosum has yet to be determined, although it certainly depends on the associated abnormalities.

Corpus Callosum Lipoma

Corpus callosum lipoma is a rare entity. Its occurrence rate is not known: 1/1,700 individuals [39] or 1/2,500–25,000 autopsies [40].

The lipoma, it is suggested, results from an abnormal differentiation of the primitive meninges [5]. The interhemispheric fissure is the most frequent location of intracranial lipomas. The term 'corpus callosum lipoma' is inadequate, for the lipoma is actually distinct from the corpus callosum. It is actually almost always associated with a generally partial [40] lack of development of the corpus callosum (hypogenesis or agenesis) [5].

Several cases have been reported in antenatal US, where the lipoma appears as a hyperechoic mass of variable thickness, nodular or curvilinear shape in the interhemispheric fissure. A recent series [40] reports the observation of five cases of corpus callosum lipoma in fetal MRI; the lipoma is hyperintense on T1-weighted slices and hypointense on T2-weighted slices. MRI is useful as it assesses the lipoma's expansion better, the precise type of corpus callosum abnormality encountered, and also allows the search for associated abnormalities (notably in gyration).

The prognosis is variable, depending on the callosal abnormalities and other associated malforma-tions; in 50 % of cases, the corpus callosum lipoma is asymptomatic [41]. Headaches, epilepsy (in 50 % of cases in the second decade), mental retardation and psychological disorders may be observed [40, 41]. A corpus callosum lipoma may also be observed as part of Goldenhar's syndrome.

Holoprosencephaly and Absence of Septum Pellucidum

Holoprosencephaly

The term 'holoprosencephaly' refers to a vast group of cerebral malformations of a common embryological origin. The occurrence rate of holoprosencephaly in the north of England, assessed in a recent study, is of 1.2/10,000 births, including fetal losses and terminations of pregnancy after 20 weeks of gestation [42]. This rate is much higher (41/10,000) if embryos are taken into account [43], which tends to suggest that holoprosencephaly often coincides with miscarriage during the first trimester of pregnancy.

Embryology Overview and Classification

The prosencephalon separates into two parts, the telencephalon (caudate nuclei, putamen and cerebral hemispheres) and the diencephalon (thalami, hypothalamus and pallidi), around the 32nd day. The separation of the telencephalon into two cerebral hemispheres begins between the 32nd and the 34th day. Holoprosencephaly results from a lack of cleavage of the prosencephalon in the longitudinal (between the di- and telencephalon) and transversal (in two distinct hemispheres) directions [5].

The result of this is a large range of facial and/or cerebral malformations of very different phenotypes, which are usually sorted into several categories. This distinction is actually artificial, since all the intermediary forms not strictly belonging to any of these subgroups are observed, as the separation of the hemispheres and the formation of the falx cerebri progresses from the occipital to the frontal pole. Thus, we can distinguish between three types.

Alobar Holoprosencephaly. In such cases, the falx cerebri, interhemispheric fissure and corpus callosum are absent. There is a single large ventricle forming a voluminous dorsal cyst; the cerebral parenchyma is present at the front, in the periphery of this single ventricle. The thalami appear fused, as the separation of the two structures has not occurred. The third ventricle, as a result, is absent.

Semilobar Holoprosencephaly. The interhemispheric fissure and falx cerebri are partly present at the back. At the front, a fusion and a lack of development of the brain are observed. There are some callosal fibres in the region of the splenium, although there is no anatomical corpus callosum. The thalami are partially fused.

Lobar Holoprosencephaly. The third ventricle is completely formed, the frontal horns only partially; the temporal horns are neatly individualized. The callosal fibres of the corpus callosum body and of the splenium are present. The falx cerebri is present at the front, although it is sometimes poorly developed. The frontal lobes are hypoplastic. The existence of a common border between lobar holoprosencephaly and septo-optic dysplasia is established.

All forms of holoprosencephaly share an anatomical characteristic: the absence of the fornix and septum pellucidum [44, 45]. Moreover, holoprosencephaly is often associated with hypoplasia, or aplasia (arrhinencephalia), of the olfactory tract and bulbs [46].

The most severe forms of facial dysmorphy are generally associated with alobar holoprosencephaly, although this is not always the case and craniofacial abnormalities may be significantly dissociated from cerebral abnormalities [46, 47].

Furthermore, there is a particular form of holoprosencephaly (syntelencephaly) in which the hemispheres are only fused in their median part, where an absence of corpus callosum is noted [48, 49].

In a series of 258 cases of holoprosencephaly reported by Odent et al. [50], 39% of holoprosencephaly cases were linked with a cytogenetic abnormality, 20% were syndromic with a normal karyotype and 41% were isolated.

Holoprosencephaly is genetically heterogeneous. Several chromosomal abnormalities have been reported. Additionally, mutations of the Sonic hedgehog (SHH) gene have been observed in association with a wide spectrum of abnormalities of the midline. The analysis of the segregation of familial forms of the disease is compatible with an autosomal dominant transmission with variable penetrance (82% for major forms). The proportion of sporadic cases is estimated at 68% [51, 52]. Maternal diabetes is a teratogenic factor responsible for holoprosencephaly,

with a risk of 1%–2% for children of diabetic mothers [46].

Signs in Ultrasonography

The diagnosis of holoprosencephaly is based on an association of various intracranial and facial abnormalities. All types of intermediary phenotypes between major facial malformations (cyclopia, proboscis) and simple hypotelorism with or without labio-palatine cleft may be observed. According to various studies, such facial malformations are present in 54% [46] to 65% or even 80% of cases [53]. They should immediately attract attention and call for a search for the associated intracranial abnormalities, which essentially consist in a single ventricle, the fusion of the thalami and the absence of the interhemispheric fissure. Moreover, these fetuses often display microcephaly, or more exceptionally macrocephaly, depending on the size of the dorsal cyst [45, 53].

Actually, essentially the semilobar and alobar forms are diagnosed in US. Their prognosis is such that these abnormalities ought to be detected as early as possible, thus ideally at a stage where fetal MRI examination cannot be done. The earliest diagnoses reported have been made at 13–14 weeks of gestation [45, 53]. In a recent epidemiological study of 48 cases [42], the average age of detection was 20 weeks of gestation; in another study of 12 cases, the average age was 23 weeks of gestation [45]. It seems that three-dimensional US does not change the diagnosis of holoprosencephaly, although it gives a more precise idea of its seriousness and extent than two-dimensional US [47].

In the different series we have reported, the antenatal diagnosis of holoprosencephaly was made at a later stage for some of the fetuses studied, and even in the last trimester for six of them [42]. Some holoprosencephalies had been mistakenly interpreted as ventricular dilatations, encephalocoeles or intracerebral cysts.

Distinguishing between the semilobar and alobar forms in US is, however, quite difficult, and the detection of the lobar form is all but uncertain [45, 53].

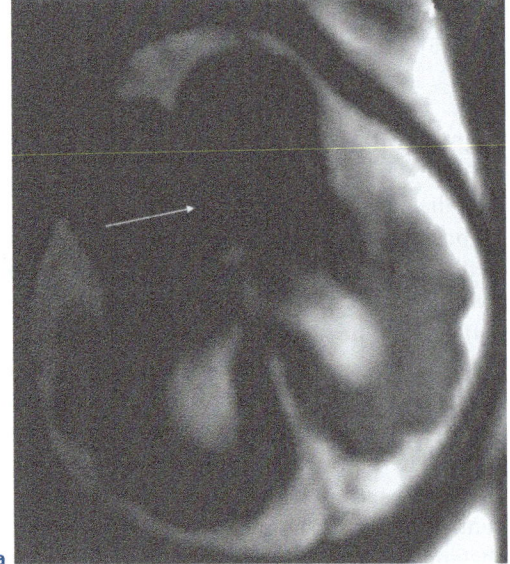

a

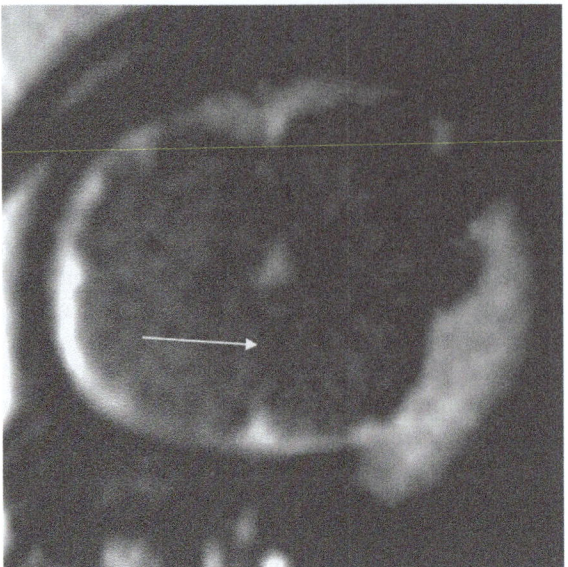

b

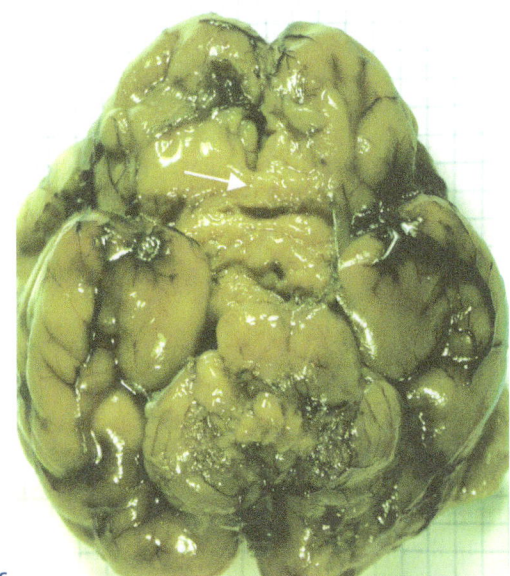

c

Fig. 7 a–c. Lobar holoprosencephaly. On US at 29 weeks of gestation, the fetus showed a bilateral cleft lip and palate, hypotelorism and left microphthalmia. **a, b** Fetal MR image. T2-weighted axial (**a**) and anterior coronal (**b**) slices. The posterior part of the ventricles is mildly dilated. The frontal horns are scarcely visible (not at all on these shots). The interhemispheric fissure is not complete at the front. The frontal lobes are fused (*arrow*). **c** Macroscopic inferior view corresponding to **a**, showing the partial fusion of the frontal lobes (*arrow*)

Contribution of Fetal MRI to the Antenatal Diagnosis of Holoprosencephaly

A few cases of holoprosencephaly have been reported in fetal MRI series [16–18], but the contribution of MRI to these diagnoses, and often the type of holoprosencephaly observed, were not stated.

One article [54] reports two cases of holoprosencephaly, one semilobar and one lobar form, the diagnoses of which had been suggested by US and confirmed with MRI, although only the anatomical resolution was improved.

In our experience (seven cases), MRI is very rarely used. Indeed, as mentioned above, the diagnosis of holoprosencephaly with US is in most cases made at a much earlier stage.

The main advantage of MRI lies in the recognition of lobar forms, as the fusion of the frontal lobes is sometimes very limited and therefore difficult to evaluate in sonography (Fig. 7). In such cases, MRI examinations are recommended on the basis of extracerebral symptoms (hypotelorism, microcephaly, labiopalatine cleft). It is therefore essential to take very anterior coronal slices in order to observe the fusion of the frontal lobes.

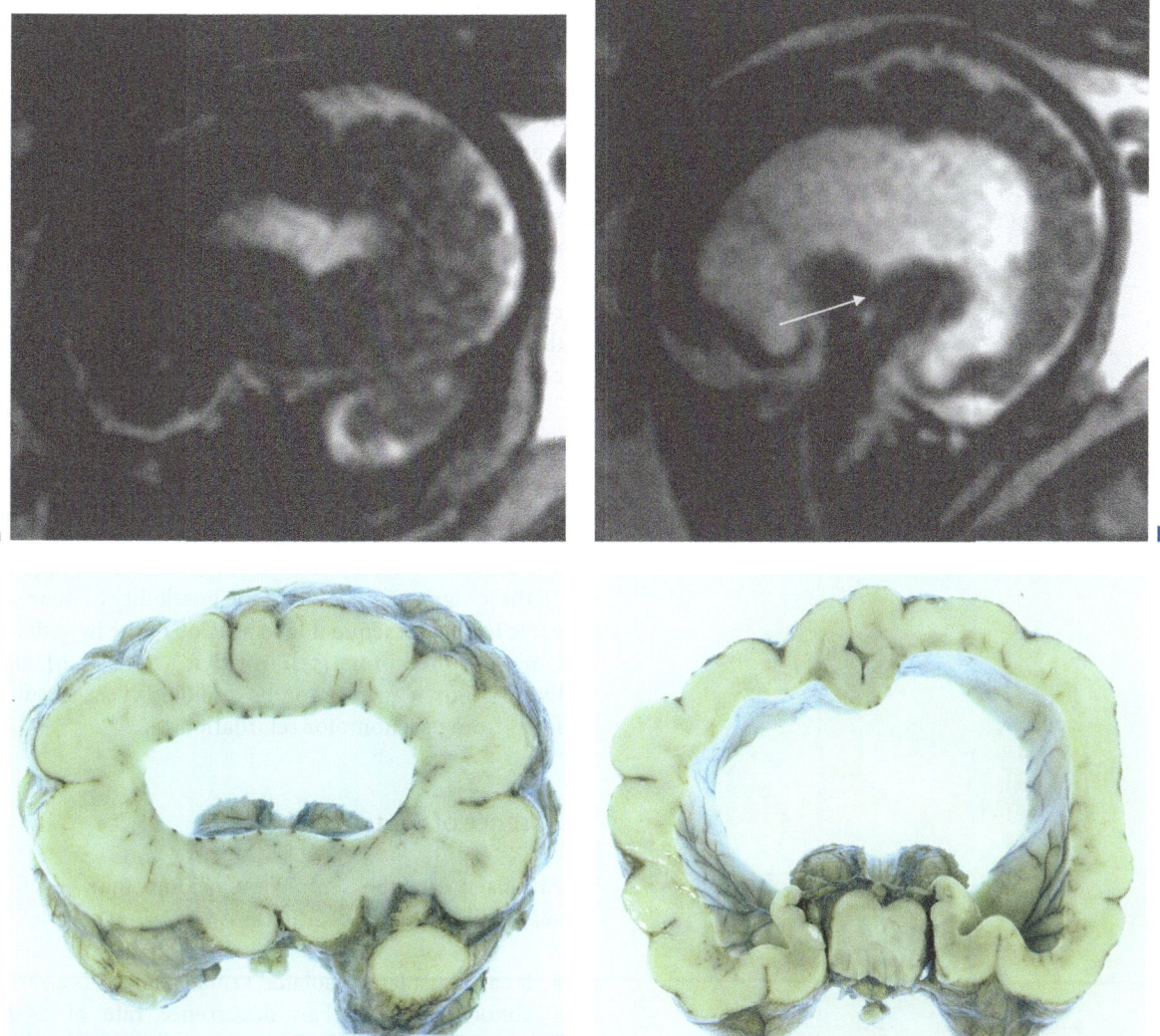

Fig. 8a–d. Alobar holoprosencephaly. **a, b** Fetus aged 40 weeks of gestation sent to MRI for a major hydrocephaly detected on US, with no facial malformations except for left microphthalmia. Fetal MR image; T2-weighted coronal slices. **a** Anterior slice showing the absence of interhemispheric fissure and the single ventricle at the front. **b** Posterior slice. Typical appearance of the single ventricle, with no interhemispheric fissure. The cortex is visible on the periphery. The thalami are fused (*arrow*). The third ventricle has not developed. **c, d** Macroscopic views at 35 weeks of gestation corresponding to **a** and **b**. **d** A primitive interhemispheric fissure can be seen

Moreover, the single ventricle of near-term fetuses may be difficult to recognize, and can be mistaken for substantial ventricular dilatation. Reverberation artefacts on the calvaria in US sometimes make it difficult to observe the absence of falx cerebri or to see the cerebral parenchyma being pressed back in the periphery, whereas these phenomena are easily seen in MRI (Fig. 8).

Another interesting contribution of MRI is that made to the diagnosis of arrhinencephaly (Fig. 9). Indeed, in common practice, the olfactory sulci and bulbs are observed on very anterior coronal slices, at the inferior aspect of the frontal lobes [24], but the number of series studied is still insufficient to fully appreciate the predictive value of the absence of these structures in MRI.

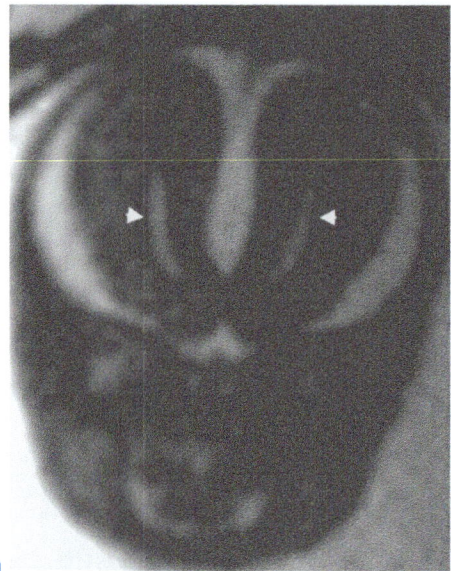

a

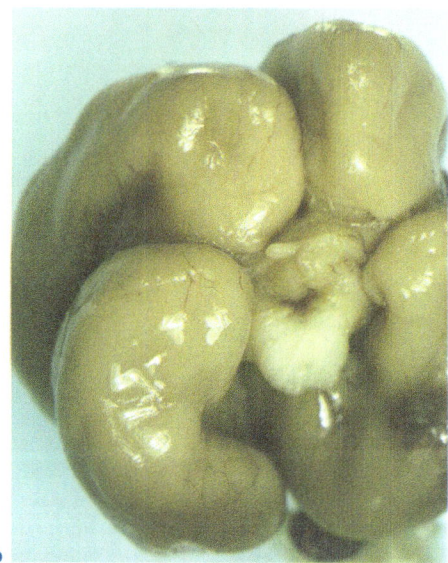

b

Fig. 9 a, b. Arrhinencephaly. Fetus at 24 weeks of gestation suffering from Fryns syndrome, with total CCA and cerebellar hypoplasia at the cerebral level. **a** Fetal MR image. Anterior coronal slice. The frontal horns (*arrowheads*) are distant from one another and have an internal concavity (corpus callosum agenesis). The olfactory bulbs are not visible. **b** Macroscopic view showing the absence of olfactory bulbs

Prognosis

Even where holoprosencephaly is not included in a particular symptomatic framework or accompanied by a chromosomal abnormality, its prognosis is generally very poor. Not only do facial abnormalities usually predict cerebral malformations, but there also seems to be a correlation between the cerebral abnormalities and the neurological prognosis [45].

The severity of holoprosencephaly seems to be directly linked to the degree of frontal development of the brain and the degree of anterior extension of the callosal fibres [5].

The alobar forms have a catastrophic prognosis, most of the children dying in utero or during the 1st year of life [45]. However, even the lobar forms, the prognosis of which is more uncertain, are accompanied by mental retardation with neurological sequelae, and olfactory and visual abnormalities [45]. To these signs may be added the possibility of neurogenic hypernatraemia due to a lesion of the hypothalamic osmoreceptors [55]. In Odent's series [50], all living children aged 3 months or older (33 cases) suffered from psychomotor retardation.

Absence of Septum Pellucidum

An absence of the septum pellucidum may be observed in a number of situations:

- It can be isolated. Isolated septal agenesis is a rare abnormality, with an occurrence rate of 2–3/10,000 individuals [56].
- It may be associated with other malformations, notably with corpus callosum agenesis.
- It may be associated with an abnormality of the visual tract. Septo-optic dysplasia was first described by Morsier in 1956. It consists in a combination of clinical (anosmia, hypothalamic deficiency, optic nerve hypoplasia) and imaging (septal agenesis) data [5, 57]. Septo-optic dysplasia is sometimes considered to be a minor form of holoprosencephaly. It is mostly sporadic, although certain forms might result from a mutation of the *HESX1* gene [58, 59].
- The septum pellucidum may also have been ruptured because of severe hydrocephaly (aqueductal stenosis, Chiari II malformation) [56].
- Finally, the absence of the septum pellucidum may be associated with hypoxic–ischaemic lesions such as schizencephaly [57].

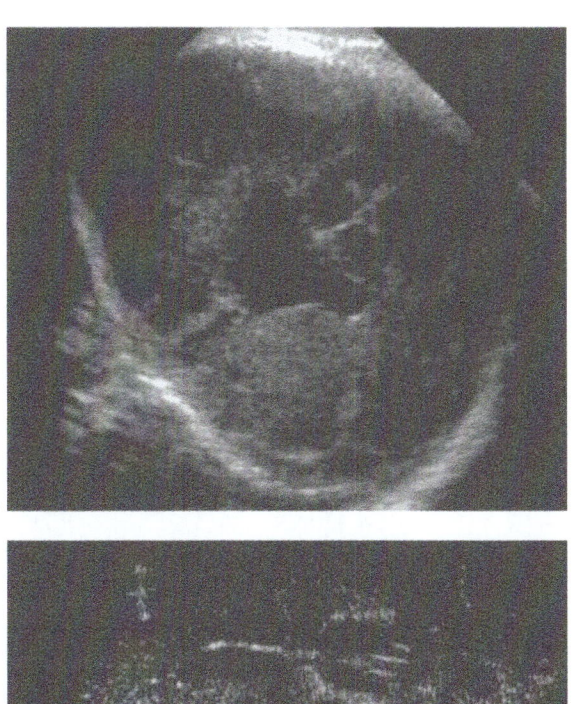

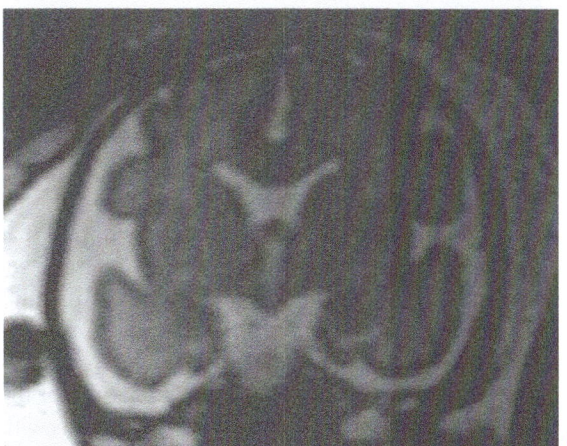

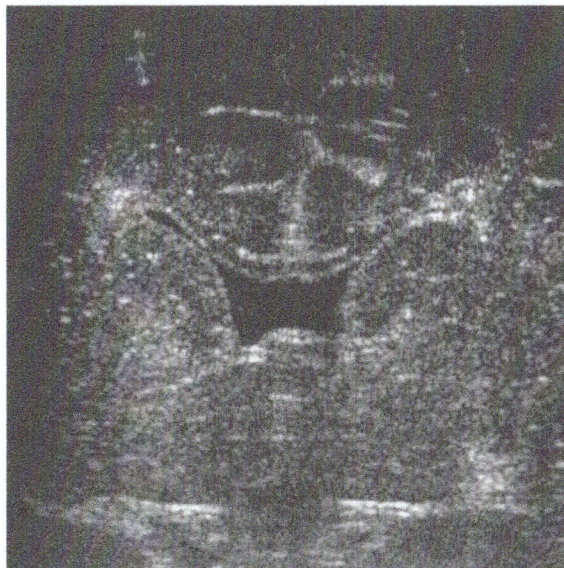

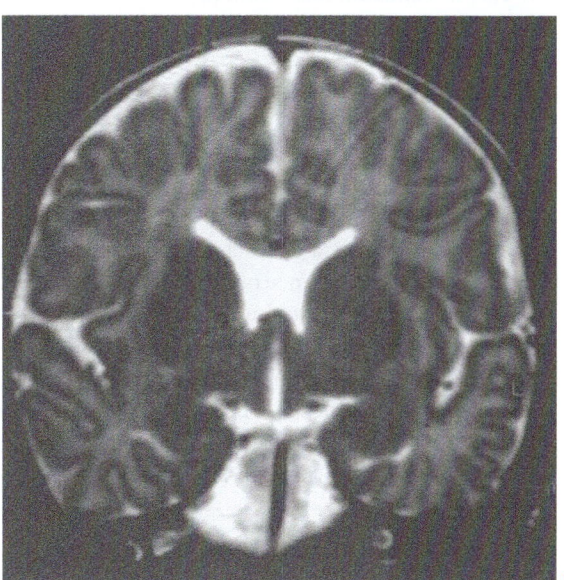

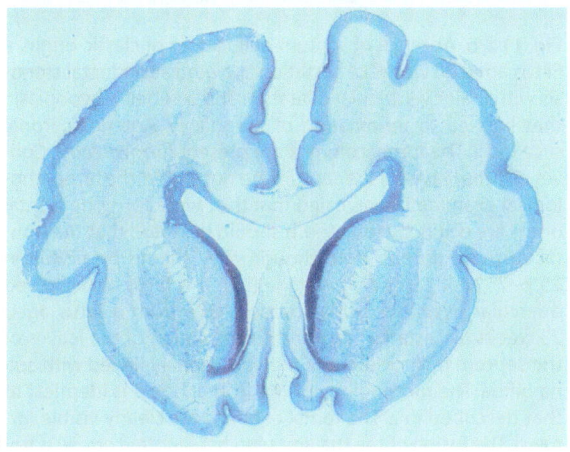

Fig. 10 a–e. Septal agenesis. **a, b** Fetus at 27 weeks of gestation. Typical pattern of septal agenesis on anterior coronal slices in US (**a**) and in MRI (**b**). The characteristic square frontal horns are observed. Fetal MRI has detected no associated abnormality. **c, d** Same child in postnatal period, in transfontanellar sonography at 2 days (**c**) and in MRI at 2 months (**d**). Postnatal MRI found no other abnormality. **e** Histological slice of septal agenesis in a fetus at 26 weeks of gestation. The leaves of the septum are absent. The frontal horns are not separated

Embryology Overview

The primitive lamina terminalis (located in the region of the anterior neuropore) thickens to become the lamina reuniens on the midline. The portion of the lamina terminalis situated between the future commissure of the fornix and the corpus callosum primordium is to become the septum pellucidum, the seat of two distinct phenomena. A cavitation that corresponds to the cavum septi between the two leaves of the septum pellucidum appears on the midline. Additionally, the septum pellucidum appears stretched and thinned because of the different rates at which the corpus callosum and commissure of the fornix grow. These phenomena are synchronous with the corpus callosum formation [4].

Signs in Ultrasonography

The diagnosis of septal agenesis is a sonographic diagnosis that involves coronal slices. The symptomatology is the same in ante- and postnatal US. The frontal horns display a characteristic square pattern that is a direct consequence of the absence of septum, and hence not specific to any given cause. The position of the fornix is abnormally low [56] (Fig. 10).

The ventricles are thin in the isolated primitive forms of septal agenesis, whereas they are dilated where the absence of septum results from the rupture of its leaves, which occurs in some cases of hydrocephaly (Fig. 11).

Contribution of Fetal MRI to the Diagnoses of Septal Agenesis and Septo-optic Dysplasia

In our experience (seven cases of isolated septal agenesis and six cases of septum destruction), MRI contributes little new information compared with US to the diagnosis of septal agenesis. The symptomatology is the same in MRI and US. On coronal slices, the fornix is lowered and the roofs of the lateral ventricles are abnormally horizontal (Fig. 10). On axial slices, a loss of the anterior concavity of the frontal horns is visible. The advantage of MRI in the diagnosis of septal agenesis lies in the improved visibility, on sagittal slices, and in comparison with US, of the motion of the fornix to the horizontal. The fornix is attached to the posteroinferior surface of the corpus callosum (Fig. 12). Here, MRI is mainly used in the search for

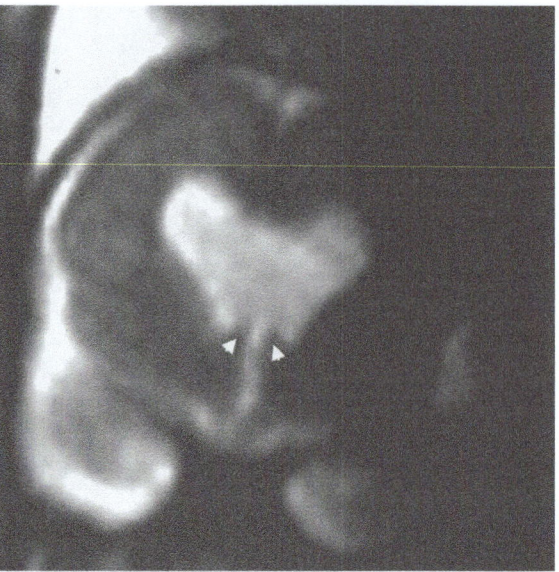

a

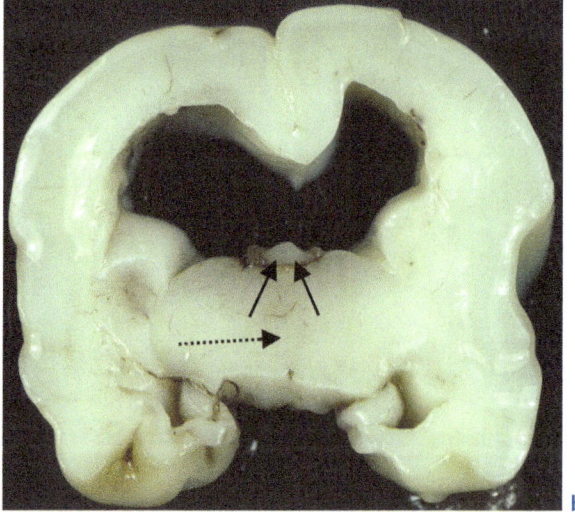

b

Fig. 11 a, b. Absence of septum pellucidum of clastic origin. **a** Fetus aged 28 weeks of gestation showing aqueductal stenosis with major ventricular dilatation and cerebellar hypoplasia that has led to termination of pregnancy. Anterior coronal slice in T2. The fornix columns are present (*arrowheads*). Conversely, the leaves of the septum are not visible; the fetopathological examination revealed that they were torn. The frontal horns are distinctly rounded. It should be noted that the frontal sulci are absent, even though they should be visible in 25%–75% of cases at this stage [24]. This fetus also showed opercular dysplasia. **b** Macroscopic slice from a fetus aged 23 weeks of gestation showing a destruction of the leaves of the septum pellucidum due to hydrocephaly linked with spina bifida. The morphology of the frontal horns is identical to that described in **a**. The fornix columns are clearly visible (*arrows*). The fusion of the thalami seen here (*dotted arrow*) is frequently observed in cases of spina bifida

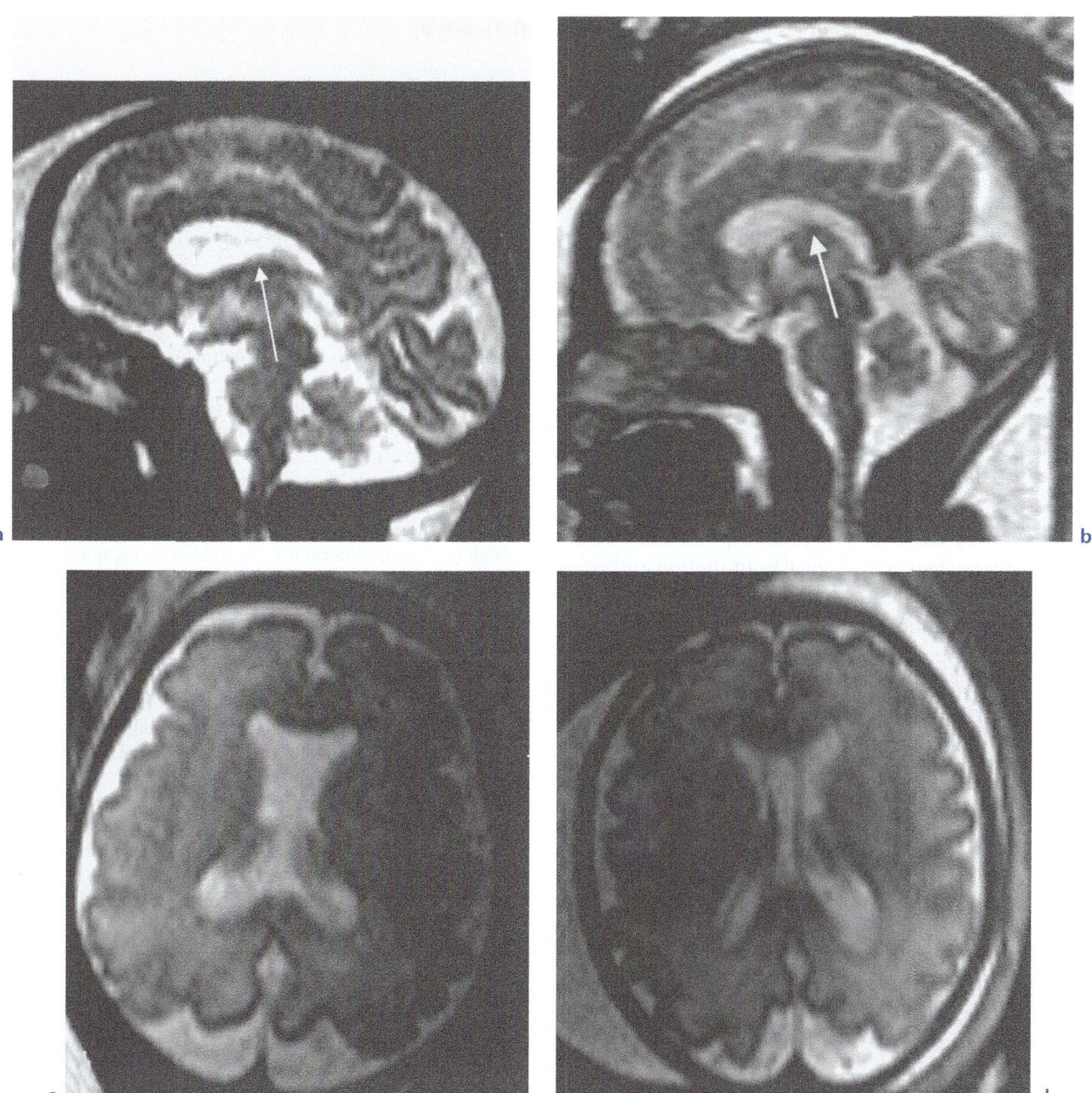

Fig. 12 a–d. Isolated agenesis of the septum. Position of the fornix. Fetus at 32 weeks of gestation. **a** T2-weighted midline sagittal slice. The fornix (*arrow*) lies abnormally low when compared with a control fetus at the same stage (**b**). **c** T2-weighted axial slice at the level of the lateral ventricles showing the loss of their anterior concavity. **d** Control fetus at the same stage

potential abnormalities associated with septal agenesis, which are more easily diagnosed with MRI than US.

Very anterior coronal slices ought to be acquired, notably to look for olfactory sulci and bulbs. In addition to arrhinencephaly, which is potentially associated with septal agenesis, pathologies such as schizencephaly and grey matter heterotopia should be looked for, but also signs of bleeding in case of clastic destructive activity. Ectopic neurohypophysis has never been reported in fetal MRI.

Although the optic nerve and chiasma are visible in MRI [24], this technology cannot provide arguments in favour of a diagnosis of septo-optic dysplasia in cases of apparently isolated septal agenesis. Indeed, the spatial resolution presently cannot establish reliable standards for the sizes of these structures; it is therefore impossible to gather conclusive evidence of hypoplasia with MRI. But above all, and even in postnatal cases, hypoplasia of the optic tract is only detected in imaging in about half of the patients suffering from septo-optic dysplasia. MRI is not sensitive to mild degrees of hypoplasia of the optic nerve [56, 60]. These facts account for the great difficulty encountered in establishing an antenatal prognosis for this kind of abnormality.

Prognosis

In general, patients with isolated septal agenesis have a strictly normal neurological examination and enjoy normal development [5, 57]. To the best of our knowledge, however, no case study on the long-term postnatal development of children diagnosed in utero with septal agenesis has ever been published. Some of the children diagnosed with isolated septal agenesis suffered from delayed acquisitions [57] or neurogenic hypernatraemia [55]. Some patients show an anterior pituitary deficiency.

Patients diagnosed with isolated septo-optic dysplasia show varying developments and have ocular impairment [57]. Approximately two-thirds of patients suffer from hypothalamic dysfunction [60]. Pituitary insufficiency, precocious puberty and diabetes insipidus may also be observed [61].

Septal agenesis shares its prognosis with the abnormalities associated with it.

References

1. Grogono JL (1968) Children with agenesis of corpus callosum. Dev Med Child Neurol 10:613–616
2. Jeret JS, Serur D, Wisniewski K, Fish C (1985) Frequency of agenesis of corpus callosum in the developmentally disabled population as determined by computerized tomography. Pediatr Neurosci 12:101–105
3. Couture A, Droullé P, Didier F (1994) Les malformations cérébrales. In: Couture A, Veyrac C, Baud C (eds) Echographie cérébrale du fœtus au nouveau-né. Sauramps Médical, Montpellier, pp 267–370
4. Destrieux C, Velut S, Kakou M (1998) I. Anatomie. A. Développement du corps calleux. Neurochirurgie 44 [Suppl 1]: 11–16
5. Barkovich AJ (2000) Congenital malformations of the brain and skull in pediatric neuroimaging. Lippincott Williams & Wilkins, pp 251–381
6. Sarnat HB (2001) Congenital malformations of the nervous system. A. Neuropathologic perspective. Neuroimaging Clin N Am 11:57–77
7. Gelot A, Lewin F, Moraine C, Pompidou A (1998) Agénésies du corps calleux : étude neuropathologique et hypothèses physiopathologiques. Neurochirurgie 44 [Suppl 1]:74–78
8. Paupe A, Bidat L, Sonigo P, Lenclen R, Molho M, Ville Y (2002) Prenatal diagnosis of hypoplasia of the corpus callosum in association with non-ketotic hyperglycinemia. Ultrasound Obstet Gynecol 20:616–619
9. Malinger G, Zakut H (1993) The corpus callosum: normal fetal development as shown by transvaginal sonography. AJR 161:1041–1043
10. Maheut-Lourmière J, Paillet C(1998) Agénésie et hypoplasie. A. Diagnostic prénatal des anomalies du corps calleux par les ultrasons: le point de vue de l'échographiste. Neurochirurgie 44 [Suppl 1]:85–92
11. Chouchane M, Benouachkou-Debuche V, Giroud M, Durand C, Gouyon JB (1999) Les agénésies du corps calleux : aspects étiologiques, cliniques, moyens de diagnostic et pronostic. Arch Pédiatr 6:1306–1311
12. Pilu G, Sandri F, Perolo A, Pittalis MC, Grisolia G, Cocchi G, Foschini MP, Salvioli GP, Bovicelli L (1993) Sonography of fetal agenesis of the corpus callosum: a survey of 35 cases. Ultrasound Obstet Gynecol 3:318–329
13. D'Ercole C, Girard N, Cravello L, Boubli L, Potier A, Raybaud C, Blanc B (1998) Prenatal diagnosis of fetal corpus callosum agenesis by ultrasound and magnetic resonance imaging. Prenat Diagn 18:247–253
14. Rapp B, Perrotin F, Marret H, Sembely-Taveau C, Lansac J, Body G (2002) Intérêt de l'IRM cérébrale fœtale pour le diagnostic et le pronostic prénatal des agénésies du corps calleux. J Gynecol Obstet Biol Reprod 31:173–182
15. Brisse H, Sebag G, Fallet C, Elmaleh M, Garel C, Rossler L, Vuillard E, Oury JF, Hassan M (1998) IRM anténatale des agénésies calleuses. Etude de 20 cas avec corrélations neuropathologiques. J Radiol 79:659–666
16. Girard N, Raybaud C, D'Ercole C, Boubli L, Chau C, Cahen S, Potier A, Gamerre M (1993) In vivo MRI of the fetal brain. Neuroradiology 35:431–436
17. Yuh WTC, Nguyen HD, Fisher DJ, Tali ET, Gao F, Simonson TM, Kao SCS, Weiner CP (1994) MR of fetal central nervous system abnormalities. AJNR Am J Neuroradiol 15:459–464

18. Resta M, Spagnolo P, Dicuonzo F, Palma M, Florio C, Greco P, D'Addario V, Vimercati A, Selvaggi L, Caruso G, Clemente R (1994) La risonanza magnetica del feto. Parte I: Tecnica d'esame ed anatomia normale dell'encefalo. Rivista di Neuroradiologia 7:53–65

19. Levine D, Barnes PD, Madsen JR, Li W, Edelman RR (1997) Fetal central nervous system anomalies: MR imaging augments sonographic diagnosis. Radiology 204:635–642

20. Gupta JK, Lilford RJ (1995) Assessment and management of fetal agenesis of the corpus callosum. Prenat Diagn 15:301–312

21. Parrish ML, Roessman U, Levinshon MW (1979) Agenesis of the corpus callosum: a study of the frequency of associated malformations. Ann Neurol 6:349–354

22. Talmant C, Yvinec M, Nomballais MF, Aubron F, David A, Rival JM, Wetzel M et les membres du Collège Français d'Echographie Foetale (1995) Agénésie du corps calleux : pronostic. Médecine Fœtale et Echographie Fœtale en Gynécologie 24:10–18

23. Mestdagh P, Daire JL, Elmaleh M, Garel C, Claude I, Robert Y, Hassan M, Sebag G (2002) Quantitative growth of the brainstem: a semiautomated MR study in fetuses. J Neuroradiol 29:1S225–1S233

24. Garel C, Chantrel E, Sebag G, Brisse H, Elmaleh M, Hassan M (2000) Le Développement du cerveau fœtal. Atlas IRM et biométrie. Sauramps Médical, Montpellier

25. Garel C, Chantrel E, Brisse H, Elmaleh M, Luton D, Oury JF, Sebag G, Hassan M (2001) Fetal cerebral cortex: normal gestational landmarks identified using prenatal MR Imaging. AJNR Am J Neuroradiol 22:184–189

26. Byrd SE, Radkowski MA, Flannery A, Mc Lone DG (1990) The clinical and radiological evaluation of the corpus callosum. Eur J Radiol 10:65–73

27. Doffe L, Adamsbaum C, Rolland Y, Robain O, Ponsot G, Kalifa G (1996) Agénésie du corps calleux et kyste interhémisphérique paramédian. J Radiol 77:427–430

28. Uematsu Y, Kubo K, Nishibayashi T, Ozaki F, Nakai K, Itakura T (2000) Interhemispheric neuroepithelial cyst associated with agenesis of the corpus callosum. Pediatr Neurosurg 33:31–36

29. Barkovich AJ, Simon EM, Walsh CA (2001) Callosal agenesis with cyst. A better understanding and new classification. Neurology 56:220–227

30. Lacey DJ (1985) Agenesis of the corpus callosum. Clinical features in 40 children. Am J Dis Child 139:953–955

31. Marszal E, Jamroz E, Pilch J, Kluczewska E, Jablecka-Deja H, Krawczyk R (2000) Agenesis of corpus callosum: clinical description and etiology. J Child Neurol 15:401–405

32. Goodyear PWA, Bannister CM, Russell S, Rimmer S (2001) Outcome in prenatally diagnosed fetal agenesis of the corpus callosum. Fetal Diagn Ther 16:139–145

33. Descamps P, Lewin F, Body G, Moutard ML, et les membres du Club Francophone de Médecine Fœtale (1998) Agénésie et hypoplasie. B. Prise en charge obstétricale des agénésies du corps calleux. Neurochirurgie 44 [Suppl 1]:93–95

34. Moutard ML, Lewin F, Baron JM, Kieffer V, Descamps P et les membres du Club Francophone de Médecine Fœtale. Agénésie et hypoplasie. C. Pronostic des agénésies isolées du corps calleux. Neurochirurgie 44 [Suppl 1]:96–98

35. Droullé P, André M (1995) Pronostic de l'agénésie calleuse. Med Fœtale Echogr Gynecol 24:22–25

36. Vergani P, Ghidini A, Strobelt N, Locatelli A, Mariani S, Bertaleo C, Cavallone M (1994) Prognostic indicators in the prenatal diagnosis of agenesis of corpus callosum. Am J Obstet Gynecol 170:753–758

37. Griebel ML, Williams JP, Russel SS, Spence GT, Glasier CM (1995) Clinical and developmental findings in children with giant interhemispheric cysts and dysgenesis of the corpus callosum. Pediatr Neurol 13:119–124

38. Rypens F, Sonigo P, Aubry MC, Delezoide AL, Cessot F, Brunelle F (1996) Prenatal MR diagnosis of a thick corpus callosum. AJNR Am J Neuroradiol 17:1918–1920

39. Bork MD, Smeltzer JS, Egan JF, Rodis JF, DiMario FJ Jr, Campbell WA (1996) Prenatal diagnosis of intracranial lipoma associated with agenesis of the corpus callosum. Obstet Gynecol 87:845–848

40. Ickowitz V, Eurin D, Rypens F, Sonigo P, Simon I, David P, Brunelle F, Avni FE (2001) Prenatal diagnosis and postnatal follow-up of pericallosal lipoma: report of seven new cases. AJNR Am J Neuroradiol 22:767–772

41. François P (1998) Lipome du corps calleux. Neurochirurgie 44 [Suppl 1]:125–126

42. Bullen PJ, Rankin JM, Robson SC (2001) Investigation of the epidemiology and prenatal diagnosis of holoprosencephaly in the North of England. Am J Obstet Gynecol 184:1256–1262

43. Matsunaga E, Shiota K (1977) Holoprosencephaly in human embryos: epidemiologic studies of 150 cases. Teratology 16:261–272

44. Oba H, Barkovich AJ (1995) Holoprosencephaly: an analysis of callosal formation and its relation to development of the interhemispheric fissure. AJNR Am J Neuroradiol 16:453–460

45. Parant O, Sarramon MF, Delisle MB, Fournié A (1997) Diagnostic anténatal de l'holoprosencéphalie. A propos d'une série de 12 cas. J Gynecol Obstet Biol Reprod 26:687–696

46. Delezoide AL, Narcy F, Larroche JC (1990) Cerebral midline developmental anomalies: spectrum and associated features. Genet Couns 1:197–210

47. Lai TH, Chang CH, Yu CH, Kuo PL, Chang FM (2000) Prenatal diagnosis of alobar holoprosencephaly by two-dimensional and three-dimensional ultrasound. Prenat Diagn 20:400–403

48. Barkovich AJ, Quint DJ (1993) Middle interhemispheric fusion: an unusual variant of holoprosencephaly. AJNR Am J Neuroradiol 14:431–440

49. Marcorelles P, Loget P, Fallet-Bianco C, Roume J, Encha-Razavi F, Delezoide AL (2002) Unusual variant of holoprosencephaly in monosomy 13q. Pediatr Dev Pathol 5:170–178

50. Odent S, Bona C, Le Marec B (1996) Holoprosencéphalie : chromosomique, syndromique ou isolée ? In: Briard ML, Dumez Y, Nioul-Fekete C (eds) 15e Séminaire de diagnostic prénatal et de médecine fœtale (Hôpital des Enfants Malades). Paris, pp 59–62

51. Odent S, Le Marec B, Munnich A, Le Merrer M, Bona-Pellié C. Segregation analysis in nonsyndromic holoprosencephaly. Am J Med Genet 1998 ; 77:139–143.

52. Odent S, Attié-Bitach T, Blayau M, Mathieu M, Augé J, Delezo AL, Le Gall JY, Le Marec B, Munnich A, David V, Vekemans M (1999) Expression of the sonic hedgehog SHH) gene during early human development and phenotypic expression of new mutations causing holoprosencephaly. Hum Mol Genet 8:1683–1689

53. Peebles DM (1998) Holoprosencephaly. Prenat Diagn 18: 477–480
54. Toma P, Costa A, Magnano GM, Cariati M, Lituania M (1990) Holoprosencephaly: prenatal diagnosis by sonography and magnetic resonance imaging. Prenat Diagn 10: 429–436
55. Garel C, Léger J, Legrand I, Stempfle N, Maiza D, Czernichow P, Hassan M (1995) Aspect IRM des hypernatrémies neurogènes. Rev Im Med 7:29–32
56. Barkovich AJ, Norman D (1989) Absence of the septum pellucidum: a useful sign in the diagnosis of congenital brain malformations. AJR 152:353–360
57. Brodsky MC, Glasier CM (1993) Optic nerve hypoplasia. Clinical significance of associated central nervous system abnormalities on magnetic resonance imaging. Arch Ophtalmol 111:66–74

58. Thomas PQ, Dattani MT, Brickman JM, McNay D, Warne G, Zacharin M, Cameron F, Hurst J, Woods K, Dunger D, Stanhope R, Forrest S, Robinson IC, Beddington RS (2001) Heterozygous HESX1 mutations associated with isolated congenital pituitary hypoplasia and septo-optic dysplasia. Hum Mol Genet 10:39–45
59. Brickman JM, Clements M, Tyrell R, McNay D, Woods K, Warner J, Stewart A, Beddington RS, Dattani M (2001) Molecular effects of novel mutations in Hesx1/HESX1 associated with human pituitary disorders. Development 128:5189–5199
60. Barkovich AJ, Fram EK, Norman D (1989) Septo-optic dysplasia: MR imaging. Radiology 171:189–192
61. Willnow S, Kiess W, Butenandt O, Dörr HG, Enders A, Strasser-Vogel B, Egger J, Schwarz HP (1996) Endocrine disorders in septo-optic dysplasia (de Morsier's syndrome): evaluation and follow-up of 18 patients. Eur J Pediatr 155:179–184

Abnormalities of Proliferation, Neuronal Migration and Cortical Organization

The various pathologies described in this chapter are all related to the organization of the cerebral cortex. Their causes are varied: genetic, infectious, metabolic, toxic, ischaemic, traumatic, etc., but whatever the causal mechanism, the consequences (which essentially depend on the stage at which the insult took place and its locus) are quite similar. Indeed, in common practice, one is often confronted with pathologies, which, for lack of anamnestic or biological data pointing to one of the causes cited above, may as well be primitive lesions or secondary lesions arisen very early in fetal life. It is thus somewhat artificial to treat some of these pathologies here, since they could also be described elsewhere, and particularly in Chap. 14.

Embryology Overview and Classification

The proliferation of neuroblasts, or neuronal precursors, starts in the 7th week of pregnancy in the subependymal region around the walls of the lateral ventricles. It has been suggested that the surplus of neuroblasts is eliminated through a process of programmed cellular death. This proliferation is particularly active between 13 and 26 weeks of gestation. Between 26 and 28 weeks of gestation, the volume of the germinal zone rapidly decreases by half. After 28 weeks of gestation, this decrease becomes more progressive. Some immature cells remain, but only around the caudothalamic groove, under the frontal horns of the lateral ventricles and around the roofs of the temporal horns. The neuronal precursors then give rise to the glial cells, astrocytes and oligodendrocytes.

Neuronal migration starts during the 8th week of pregnancy. It is maximal between 12 and 24 weeks of gestation and occurs in successive waves, forming the six layers of the cortex present as early as 20 weeks of gestation. The neurons destined to form the most superficial layer migrate first. The following waves then start by filling the deepest layer, and afterwards form the intermediate layers, the migration progressing to-

wards the most superficial layer. Neurons that leave the germinal matrix to fill the cerebral cortex are guided by the radial glial fibres (neuroglial units), which extend from the ventricular wall to the surface of the cortex. Another important group of neurons migrates tangentially within the germinal zone before starting on the classic pathway along the radial glial fibres. Moreover, a phenomenon of tangential neuronal migration has also been described at the level of the intermediate zone (the future white matter). It has been suggested that most of the interneurons that migrate tangentially originate in the ganglionic eminence. This phase of neuronal migration generally ends around 25–26 weeks of gestation.

While this phase of migration takes place, the organization of the cortex begins. After arriving in the cortex, neurons start establishing synaptic contacts with other variably distant neurons. It seems that a deep transitory layer (the seventh layer, or subplate) plays an important role in this process. Once migration is complete, the radial glial fibres transform into astrocytes.

During neuronal migration and after its completion, gyration progresses and continues until well after birth, with the appearance of primary and then secondary and tertiary sulci.

It is self-evident that any insult occurring at each one of these stages will have consequences on ulterior events.

We suggest the following schematic classification of abnormalities of proliferation, neuronal migration and cortical organization.

Brain volume abnormalities (microcephaly and macrocephaly) and abnormalities of gyration can be individualized. The latter category comprises migratory causes (heterotopias, lissencephaly and polymicrogyria without laminar necrosis) and clastic or other causes (polymicrogyria with laminar necrosis, schizencephaly and tuberous sclerosis) [1–10].

Brain Volume Abnormalities

Microcephaly

Microcephaly is defined as a cranial diameter below the 3rd percentile. Contrary to ultrasonography, MRI can measure the encephalon (and therefore evaluate micrencephaly, i. e. an abnormal diminution of cerebral volume), and not only that of the skull.

Microcephaly can be familial (numerous modes of transmission have been described), or have an infectious (Chap. 13), metabolic (phenylketonuria) or toxic [alcohol, certain drugs (Fig. 1), carbon monoxide, etc.] origin [11].

The specific cases of microcephaly associated with other cerebral malformations (Fig. 2) are dealt with in the corresponding chapters: microcephaly of clastic origin (Chap. 14), microcephaly associated with a cerebral malformation (holoprosencephaly in Chap. 8, lissencephaly; see type 1 and type 2 lissencephaly below in this section).

In the absence of a relevant familial history, a particular context, associated intra- or extracerebral abnormalities or aneuploidy, the diagnosis is oriented to a primitive form of microcephaly, microcephaly with simplified gyral pattern.

Fig. 1 a–f. Extreme micrencephaly related to maternal toxicomania (heroin and cocaine). **a** US at 25 weeks of gestation. Major microcephaly with receding forehead. **b, c** Fetal MRI done after termination of pregnancy at 26 weeks of gestation: **b** T1-weighted midline sagittal slice. The brain stem is very thin; the cerebellum is hypoplastic. The supratentorial structures are very poorly developed. The corpus callosum is not visible. **c** T1-weighted coronal slice at the level of the thalami. No sulcus is visible on the surface of the cortex. The lateral ventricles are dilated. **d** Side view of the fetus. Small skull volume and receding forehead. **e** Coronal histological slice at the level of the thalami showing a complete absence of midline structures, abnormally thin cortex and broad ventricles and coarsely outlined thalami. **f** Histological slice of the cerebral mantle. The cortical plate is very thin. A thick band of neurons (*dotted arrow*) that have not fully migrated lies between the cortical plate and the subventricular zone. The histological examination also reveals hypoplasia of the brain stem and cerebellum, abnormalities of the radial glia and an abnormal neuronal migration in the meningeal space

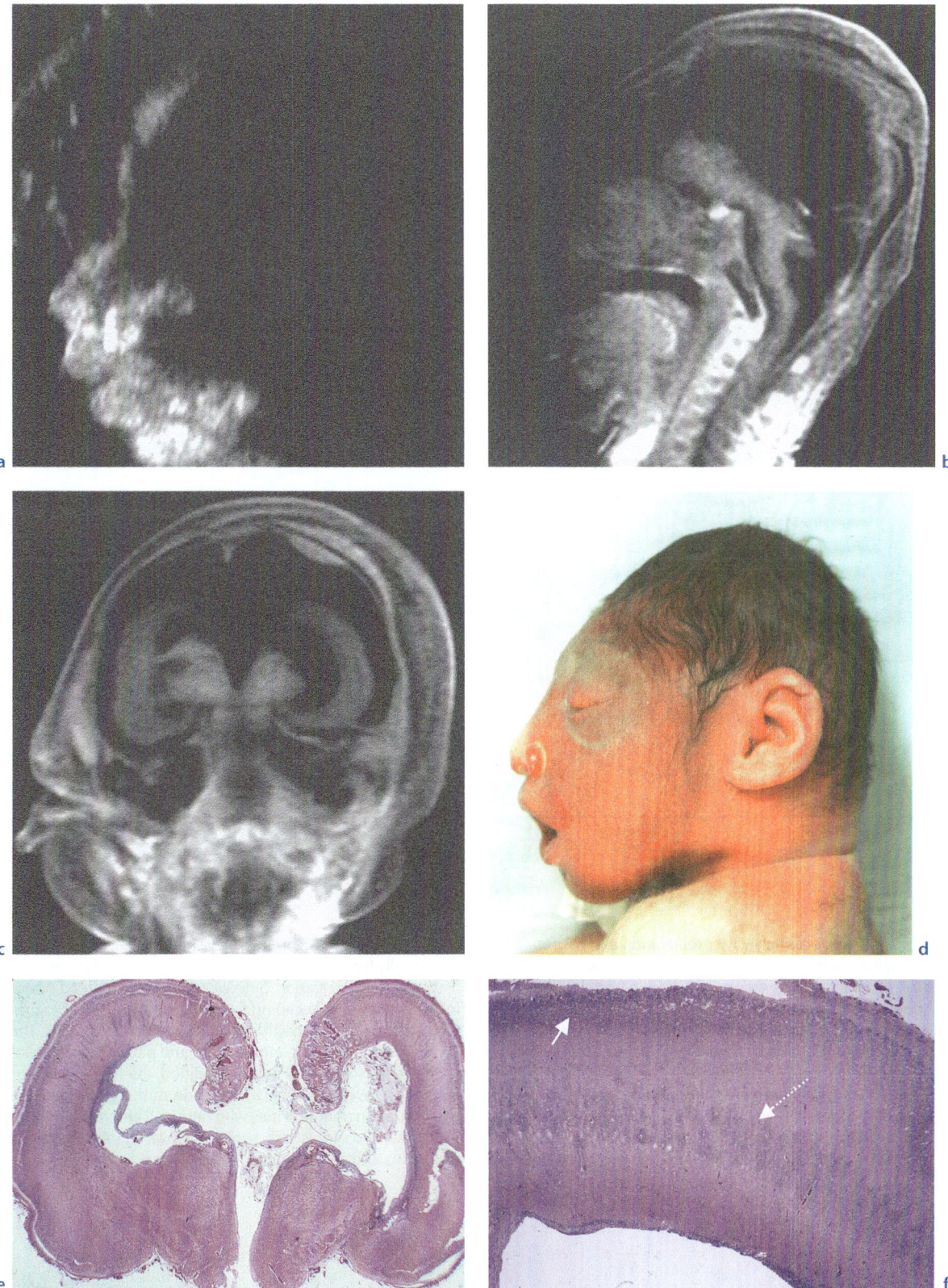

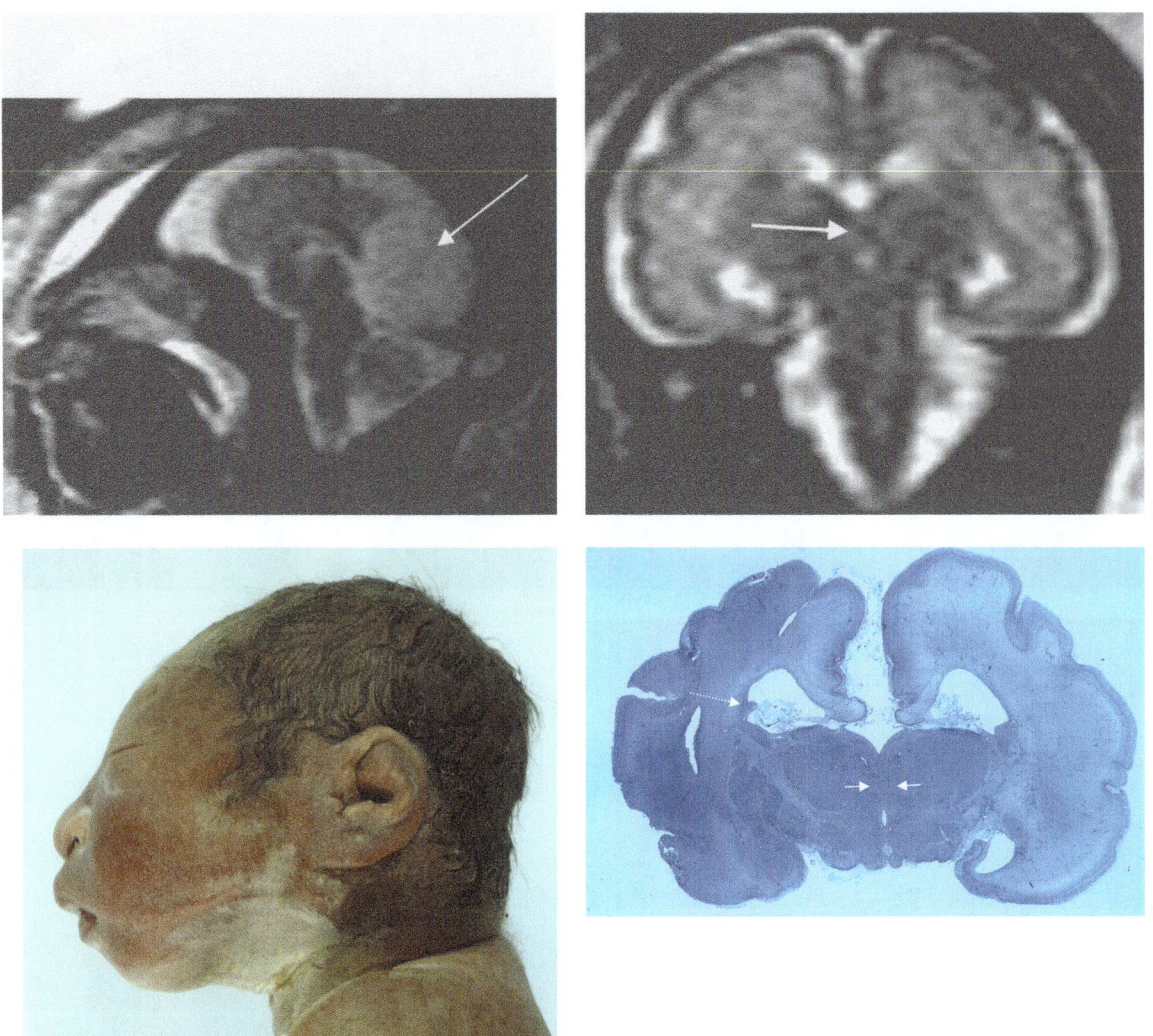

Fig. 2 a–d. Microcephaly with proliferation and migration abnormalities. Microcephaly was detected at 26 weeks of gestation, as well as a short corpus callosum and an interhemispheric cyst. **a** Fetal MR at 27 weeks of gestation. T2-weighted midline sagittal section showing microcephaly with a receding forehead, abnormally small fronto-occipital diameter and length of the corpus callosum. The rostrum and splenium seem absent. The interhemispheric cyst is clearly visible at the back (*arrow*). In histology, a continuousness between this cyst and the 3rd ventricle was depicted. **b** T2-weighted coronal slice at the level of the thalami. Gyration is practically undevel-oped. The lateral sulci are hardly visible. The thalami seem to be partially fused (*arrow*). **c** Medical termination of pregnancy at 27 weeks of gestation. Side view of the fetus' head. Major microcephaly with receding forehead. **d** Coronal histological slice at the level of the thalami (superimposable on **b**). The partial fusion of the thalami (*arrows*) and partial corpus callosum agenesis are confirmed. In addition, the histological examination revealed an early depletion of the germinal zone and migration abnormalities with neuronal heterotopias (*dotted arrow*). This fetus also showed a bilateral radiohumeral synostosis and abnormalities of the fingers

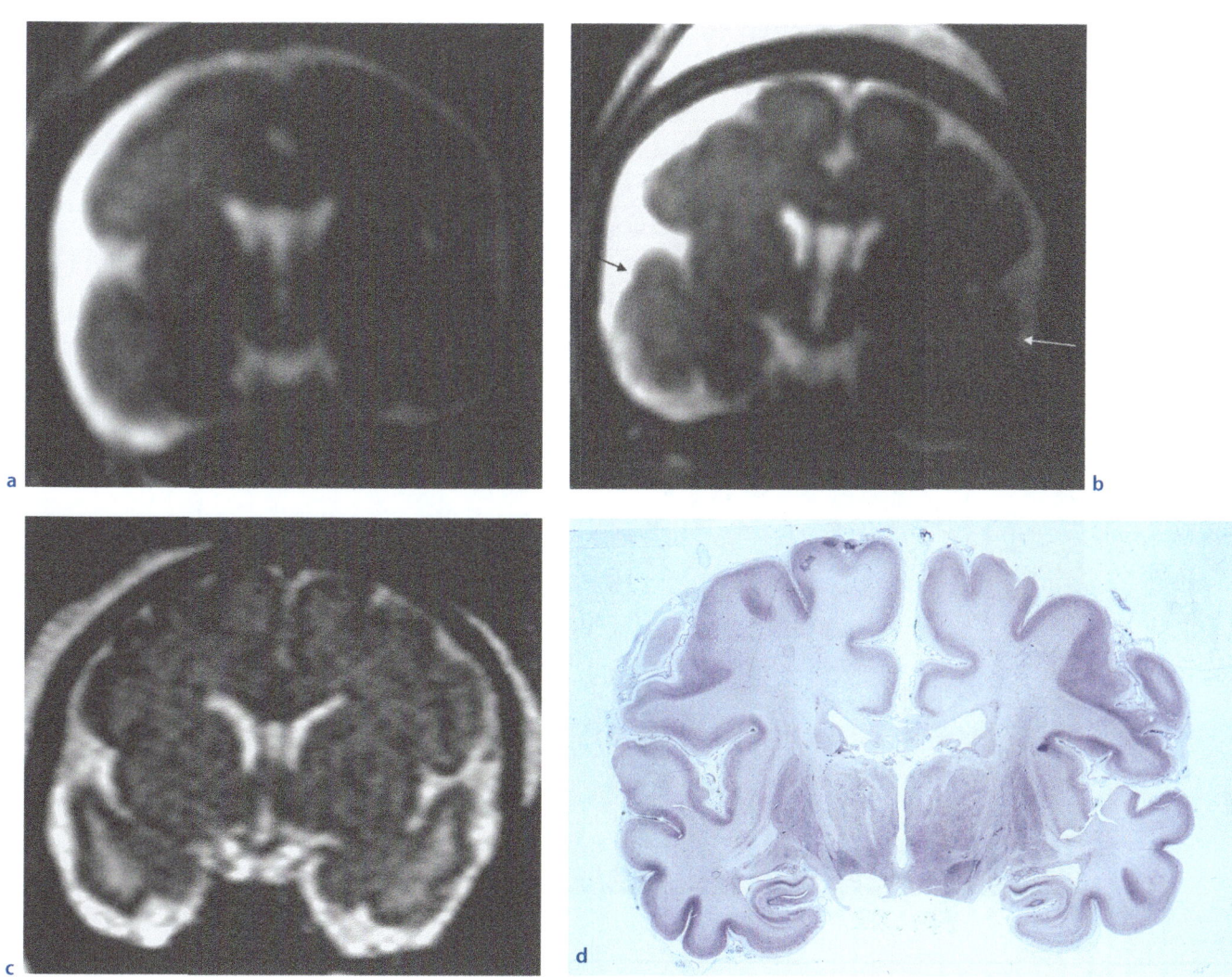

Microcephaly with Simplified Gyral Pattern

Definition, Mechanism and Prognosis

Microcephaly with simplified gyral pattern, also called microlissencephaly, corresponds to a heterogeneous group of malformations, all having in common micrencephaly, simplified gyral pattern and normal or inferior-to-normal thickness of the cortex [4]. Its mechanisms are not precisely understood, but it has been suggested that it might result from a disturbance of the proliferation of neuroblasts in the germinal zone, or from an excess of programmed cellular death [12], possibly leading to a decrease in the number of glial units and cortical neurons and a decrease in the volume of white matter.

Fig. 3 a–d. Microcephaly with simplified gyral pattern. Microcephaly was detected at 27 weeks of gestation. a, b Coronal MRI slices at the level of the third ventricle at 30 and 33 weeks of gestation. At 30 weeks gestation (a), the frontal lobes are smooth. The frontal sulci, which are usually present from 29 weeks of gestation, have not developed yet. At 33 weeks of gestation (b), the frontal sulci are present, but they are abnormally wide and shallow, compared to a control fetus at the same term (c). The anterior part of the superior temporal sulcus is only roughly sketched (*arrows*). No growth in the head circumference and the simplified gyral pattern led to termination of pregnancy at 38 weeks gestation. The neurofetopathological examination revealed that the biometric parameters were very inferior to the 3rd percentile, it also detected a reduced neuronal density. The neuronal migration, lamination and differentiation were normal. d Histological slice at the level of the 3rd ventricle and thalami. The sulci are abnormally wide and shallow for the stage. The tertiary sulci are absent

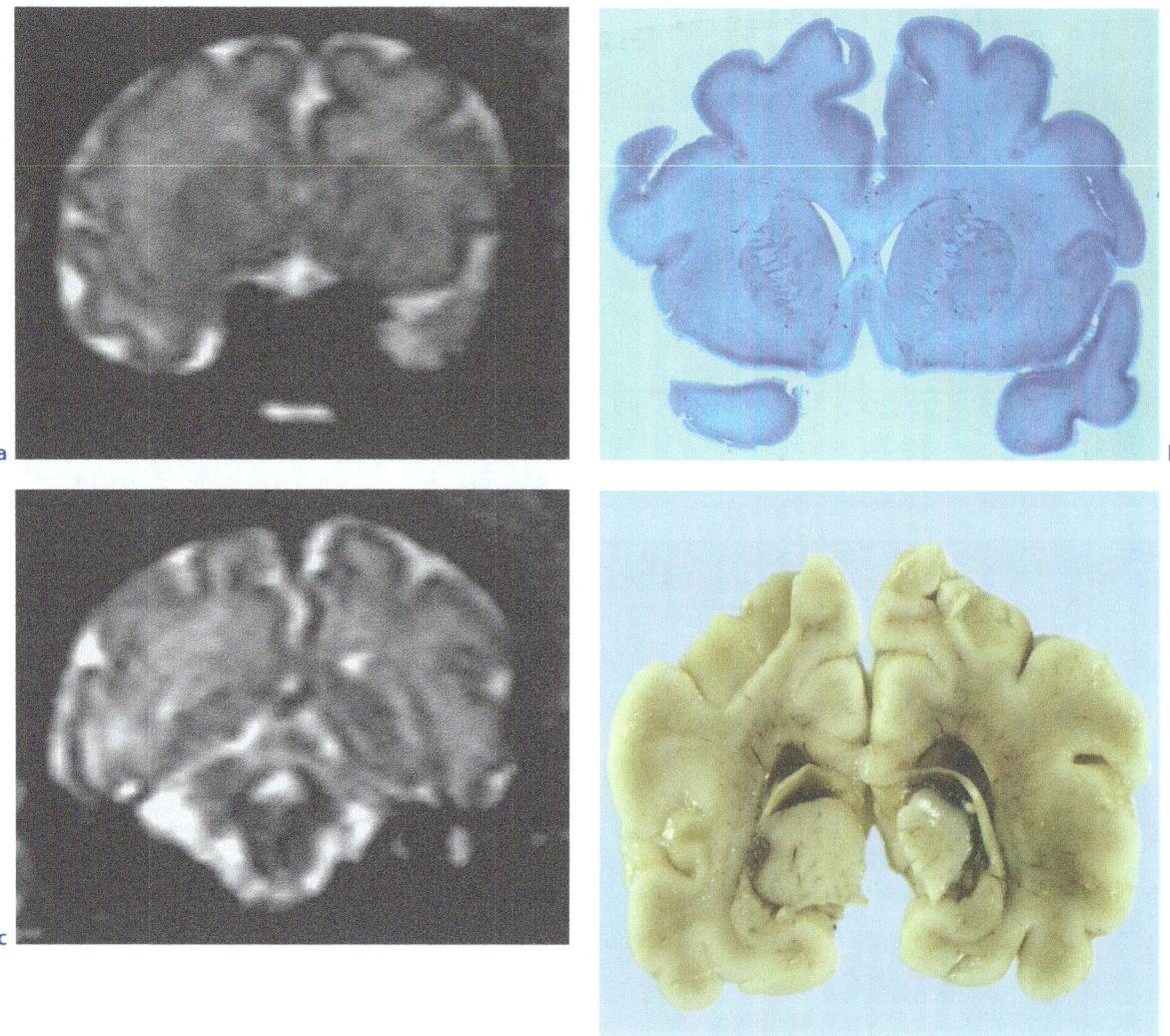

Microcephaly with simplified gyral pattern has so far been described postnatally [12–14], and a genetic origin has been suggested for some familial forms (autosomal recessive transmission) [12, 14]. Also, one case has been reported as linked with the mother's taking of carbamazepine [15]. Microlissencephaly is a heterogeneous ensemble because other signs may be associated with microcephaly such as arthrogryposis, seizures, and hip luxation. This heterogeneity probably corresponds to the large number of different mechanisms. Although the abnormalities cited above are common to all cases of microlissencephaly, the data obtained in neuroimaging examinations are variable. Postnatally, the prognosis for the reported cases was invariably negative.

To the best of our knowledge, microcephaly with simplified gyral pattern has never been reported in a

Fig. 4 a–d. Microcephaly with simplified gyral pattern. Microcephaly was detected at 26 weeks of gestation. **a, b** Anterior coronal MRI and histological slices, at respectively 35 weeks of gestation (**a**) and 36 weeks of gestation (**b**). The height of the fontal lobes is abnormally small. Sulci are scarce and abnormally wide for the stage. **c, d** Posterior coronal slices at 35 weeks of gestation in MRI (**c**), and in macroscopic view at 36 weeks of gestation (**d**). The parietal lobes are very poorly developed. Gyration is insufficiently advanced for the stage

fetus, except in our experience. In the light of the four cases we have observed so far [16], we were able to sketch a description of microlissencephaly in antenatal imaging, as it was identical in the four cases (Figs. 3, 4). In each case, the neurofetopathological examination performed following medical termination of pregnancy consolidated the physiopathological hypotheses put forward in postnatal cases: we observed no gliosis or destructive lesion. Myelination, cortical thickness and neuronal differentiation were normal, but the number of cortical neurons was very small and gyration was simplified.

Signs in Ultrasonography

In the four cases studied, microcephaly appeared relatively late, at 27 weeks of gestation for the earliest. These were severe cases of microcephaly, often less than −3 standard deviations, with a very distinct bend of the cranial perimeter line in the successive examinations and a markedly receding forehead.

Contribution of Fetal MRI

Fetal MRI plays an essential role in the diagnosis of this malformation. It can detect micrencephaly, but above all it evaluates the fetal brain gyration. This is easier when the examination takes place before 34–35 weeks of gestation, as the pericerebral space tends to narrow near the end of gestation, making it impossible to visualize the sulci properly. With MRI, the simplified gyral pattern is clear because only the primary sulci are present, and these are abnormally wide and shallow. Secondary sulci are absent, whereas they are usually developed at 34 weeks of gestation [5, 17]. The diagnosis can therefore only be made relatively late. A compromise must be found for the date of the examination, which should be performed neither too early (i. e. before the secondary sulci appear) nor too late (to evaluate gyration), hence usually between 30 and 34 weeks of gestation. Follow-up is often necessary to establish that no progress has been made in gyration between the two examinations.

Macrocephaly

Symmetrical

A distinction must be made between macrocrania, which results from an excessive growth of the skull (head circumference greater than the 97th percentile), and macrocephaly or megalencephaly, which is characterized by an excessive brain volume [11]. Measuring the biparietal diameter and head circumference enables consideration of the potential associated abnormalities of the skull shape linked with craniostenosis.

MRI has the decisive advantage over ultrasonography of distinguishing the brain (measurement of the biparietal and fronto-occipital diameters) from the pericerebral space (craniocerebral index) [5]. The significance of a widening of the pericerebral space in the fetus remains unknown. In three successive fetal MR examinations, we have observed a fetus showing a definite macrocrania with a distinct widening of the pericerebral space. This progressively came back to normal and no abnormality was detected at birth. It is indeed not certain that the concept of benign macrocrania (or external hydrocephalus) in children, which is characterized by a widening of the subarachnoid space, and often also the ventricles [18], can be transposed to the antenatal period.

Once macrocephaly is detected, the first thing to do is to look for associated intracerebral abnormalities: hydrocephalus (Chap. 11), space-occupying lesions (Chap. 10), or abnormalities of gyration, notably pachygyria (Fig. 5), and also sometimes an abnormality in the opercularization of the sylvian fissures [19].

One must also research the family history. Numerous modes of transmission have been described [11, 20] and some familial forms of macrocephaly result in mental retardation [11]. Macrocephaly may also be part of a syndromic group (notably Weaver syndrome and Proteus syndrome).

In the absence of associated cerebral abnormalities and family history, primitive macrencephaly or megalencephaly can be diagnosed. Its prognosis is still difficult, but it could lead to mental retardation [21, 22] (delayed acquisitions in 4 out of 20 children [22]). Megalencephaly is a very heterogeneous entity, which, from a neuropathology standpoint, is in some cases very close to the asymmetrical form: hemimegalencephaly.

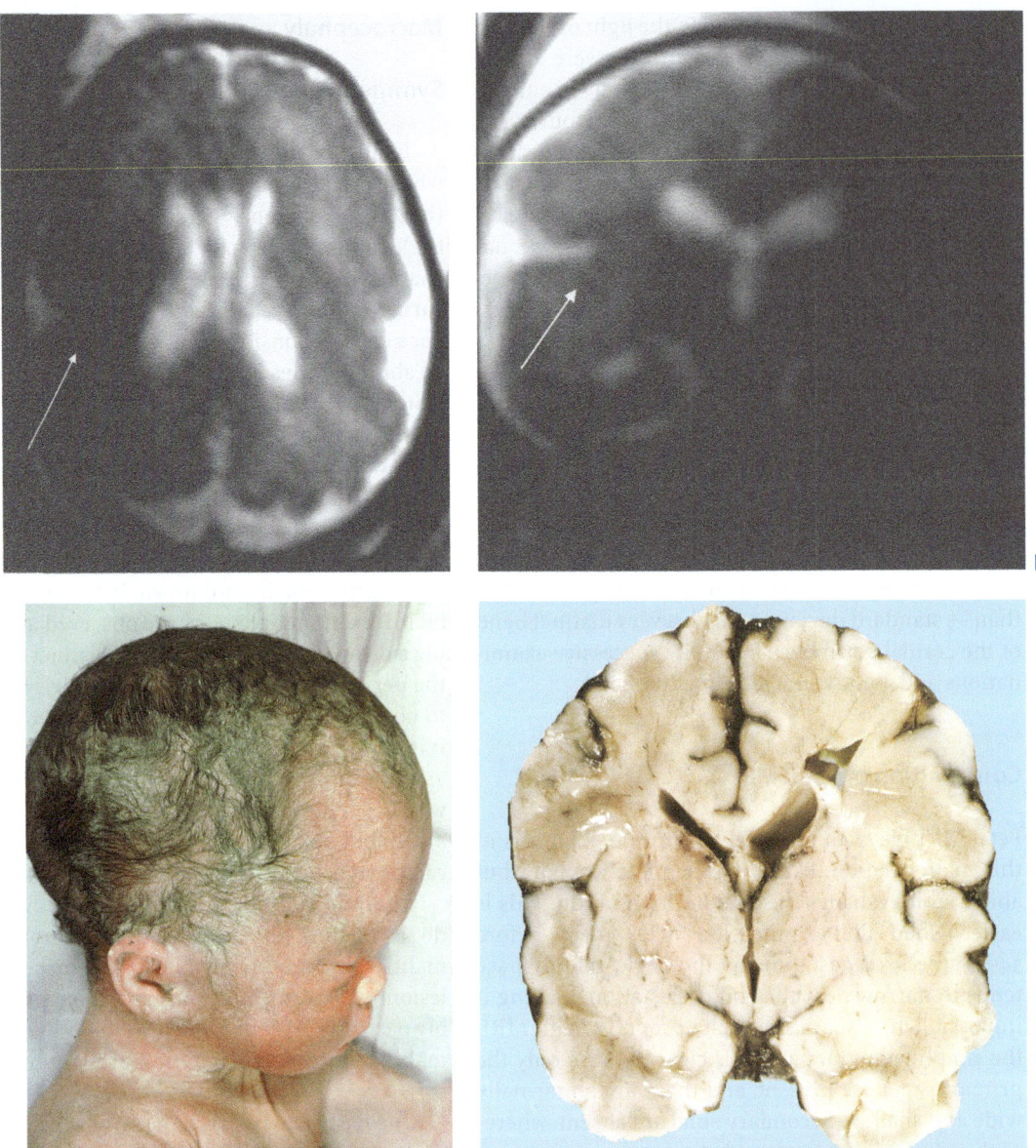

Fig. 5a–e. Megalencephaly. Fetal macrocrania with a head circumference markedly greater than the 90th percentile as early as 22 weeks gestation. **a, b** MRI done at 30 weeks of gestation. T2-weighted axial (**a**) and coronal (**b**) slices. Note the clearly visible bilateral opercular dysplasia with a thick cortical ribbon lining the sylvian fissures (*arrows*), raising suspicion of polymicrogyria. Termination of pregnancy was decided at 31 weeks of gestation. **c** Side view of the fetus's head. Typical pattern of macrocephaly. The brain's weight is greater than the 95th percentile. **d** Macroscopic coronal slice at the level of the 3rd ventricle and the mamillary bodies. The cortical ribbon around the sylvian fissures is abnormally irregular, with a pachygyric pattern. **e** Coronal histological slice. Magnification, at the same level, of a sylvian fissure. Diffuse polymicrogyria

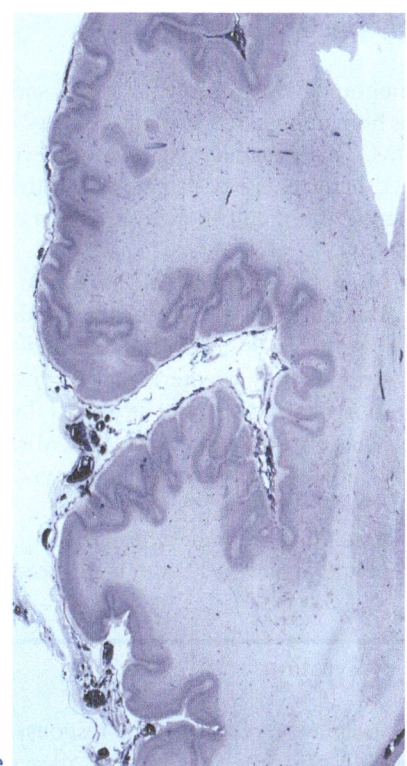

e

Asymmetrical: Hemimegalencephaly

Definition, Mechanism and Prognosis

Hemimegalencephaly (HME) corresponds to the excessive growth of a part of or an entire cerebral hemisphere. In the affected hemisphere, zones of pachygyria can be observed, or even lissencephaly, as well as zones of polymicrogyria, heterotopia and white matter gliosis [23, 24]. The brain stem and cerebellum may also be affected [24].

HME can be isolated, although in most cases it is associated in a syndromic group with corporeal hemihypertrophy (epidermal nevus syndrome, Proteus syndrome, Klippel-Trenaunay-Weber syndrome, Ito hypomelanosis) [1, 24]. In some less frequent cases, this malformation can be associated with tuberous sclerosis [25]. Neuropathological examinations show similarities between the two entities.

Indeed, the large balloon cells in HME look very similar to the abnormal cells observed in the cortical tubers of patients suffering from tuberous sclerosis. These two types of cells are, however, distinct in immunohistochemistry and in electronic microscopy [26]. Patients with HME also show cytoarchitectural abnormalities of the neurons. Histological data tend

to suggest that HME is caused by abnormalities of the neuroblasts and radial glial cells. The abnormalities in migration and cortical organization would in such cases be only secondary to the abnormal proliferation.

HME is a sporadic malformation. It is also a cerebral symmetry defect. The several genes involved in that symmetry (*Zic-3*, *Pitx-2*, *Lefty-1*, *Lefty-2*) could play a role in the pathogenesis of HME [24].

Children with HME usually show macrocrania and severe developmental retardation with hemiplegia and early seizures.

To the best of our knowledge, only one case of HME documented in the antenatal period has been reported in the literature [27].

In light of the two cases of Klippel-Trenaunay-Weber syndrome with HME (Fig. 6) we have observed and the imaging symptomatology described in postnatal cases [1, 23, 28, 29], we were able to evaluate the contributions of ultrasound and MRI examinations to the antenatal diagnosis of this malformation.

Signs in Ultrasonography

The attention is drawn to an asymmetry in the size of the hemispheres. The degree of this asymmetry is variable in itself and from one region to another. The lateral ventricle of the bigger hemisphere is usually dilated, although not in every case. The possible indented outline of the lateral ventricle supposedly is the mark of associated heterotopias (see "Subependymal Heterotopias" in this chapter. It is probably more difficult to observe abnormalities of white matter echogenicity (hyperechogenicity) in antenatal examinations, unless there are clear hamartomatous lesions (Fig. 6). Gyration abnormalities are also difficult to identify, especially in focal polymicrogyria or pachygyria. However, a defective opercularization of the sylvian fissure may be observed. Ultrasonography must naturally be used in a systematic search for an associated corporeal hemihypertrophy and for the potential hamartomatous lesions on the rest of the body, which could lead to including HME in a syndromic group.

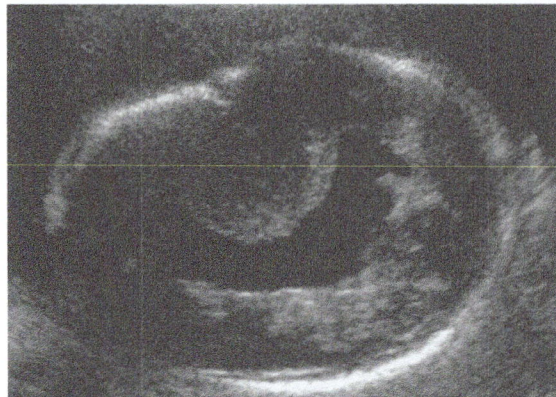

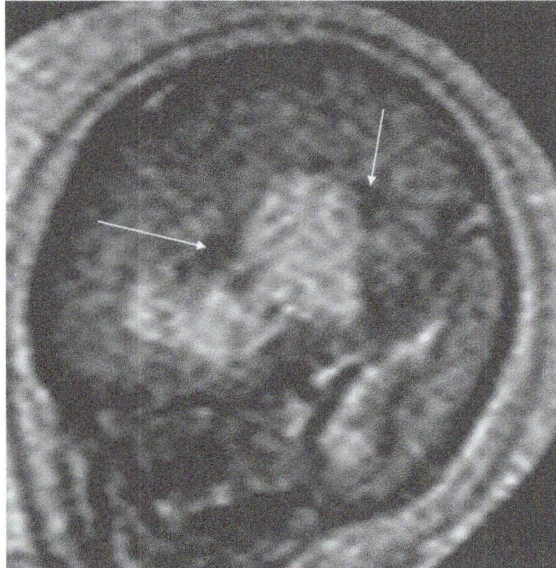

Fig. 6 a, b. Hemimegalencephaly. Fetus at 24 weeks of gestation. **a** The US examination reveals macrocephaly and the dilatation of a lateral ventricle with a hypertrophia of the homolateral hemisphere. The ventricular wall was irregular and hyperechoic. There are also multicystic lesions of the abdominal wall and inferior limbs. **b** Fetal MRI. T2-weighted coronal slice. MR confirms the asymmetry of the hemispheres, the dilatation of the right ventricle and T2-hypointense lesions on the ventricular wall (*arrows*). On neurofetopathological examination, these turned out to be angiomatous lesions associated with hemimegalencephaly. The fetus also showed a Klippel-Trenaunay-Weber syndrome

Contribution of Fetal MRI

Unlike ultrasonography, MRI systematically and clearly visualizes both hemispheres, whatever the position of the fetus. This advantage may be decisive when the affected hemisphere is also closest to the probe and is therefore difficult to analyse in ultrasonography.

The real brain biometry assessed in MRI better authenticates the asymmetry in the size of the hemispheres. The morphological abnormalities of the dilated ventricle (straightening of the frontal horns, which point superiorly and anteriorly) as well as the potential heterotopias are best analysed in MRI. MRI also provides finer analyses of the cortex and gyration.

The white matter gliosis on the affected hemisphere appears in hypersignal on T2-weighted slices.

Abnormalities of Gyration

These abnormalities may be very local, and responsible for aberrant sulci (Fig. 7). They are not always linked with migratory or clastic disorders and their prognosis is not certain.

Migratory Causes

Nodular Heterotopias: Subependymal Heterotopias

Definition, Mechanism and Prognosis

Subependymal heterotopias are formed by neurons whose migration was prematurely stopped, causing them to accumulate along the ventricular walls. These heterotopias can be focal or diffuse, uni- or bilateral. They may be isolated or associated with other malformations (corpus callosum agenesis, encephalocoele) or metabolic disorders (Zellweger syndrome, neonatal adrenoleucodystrophy).

Subependymal heterotopias are either sporadic or hereditary, with either a (probably autosomal) non X-linked or a dominant X-linked mode of transmission. Autosomal recessive forms of subependymal heterotopias have been reported.

In the latter form, the abnormality of migration results from the mutation of the *FLN1* (*Xq28*) gene, which codes for the filamin 1 phosphoprotein. Filamin 1 instigates the reorganization of actin neces-

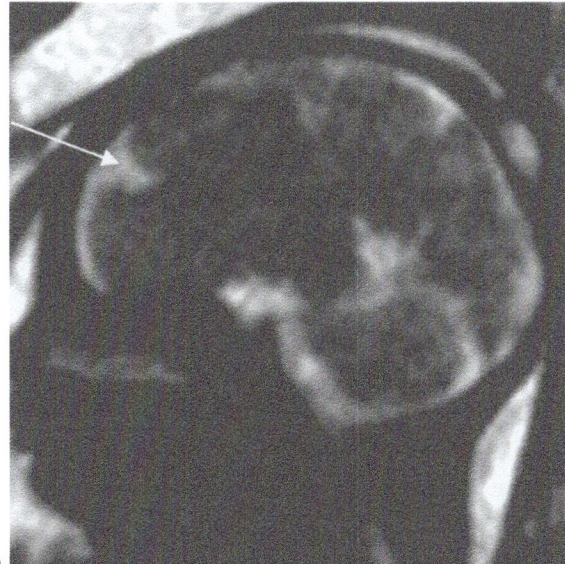

a

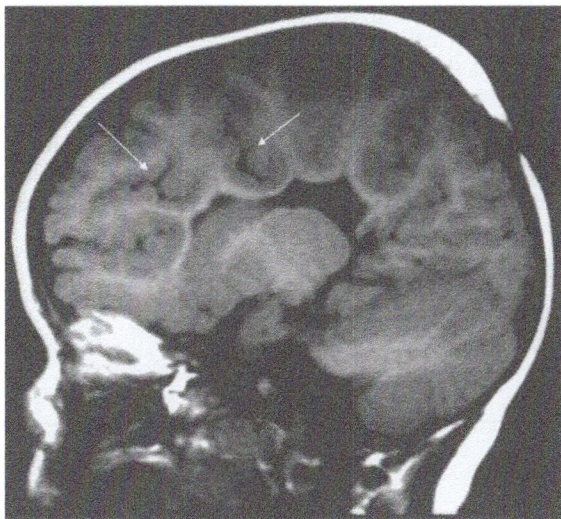

b

Fig. 7a,b. Aberrant frontal sulci. **a** Fetal MRI performed at 31 weeks of gestation following the detection of an occipital meningocoele. Many abnormal frontal sulci are visible on this slice, including notably a very wide one at the front (*arrow*). **b** Postnatal MRI at 11 months (the meningocoele was cured). The abnormal frontal sulci are still present (*arrows*). After 8 years, the clinical examination is normal

sary to the motion of migrating neurons. Without it, neuroblasts cannot migrate along the radial glial unit. This form of heterotopia is always diffuse and bilateral. Female patients have two types of neuroblasts: some migrate normally (normal *FLN1*) while others remain in the subependymal region (muted *FLN1*). Male patients have no normal *FLN1*; the disorder is therefore often lethal early in pregnancy, as filamin 1 plays an essential role in haemostasis and in the development of blood vessels. Other cerebral malformations (corpus callosum agenesis, cerebellar hypoplasia) are also frequently observed, in male and female patients alike.

Some have suggested a mechanism for subependymal heterotopias other than the interruption of migration. These may indeed also result from an abnormal proliferation of neuroblasts in the periventricular region, or from a disorder of the apoptosis of neuroblasts in the germinal zone. The neurons in the heterotopic nodules have few connections with each other and with the overlying cortex. This could be linked to the immaturity of the gamma-aminobutyric acid inhibitor neurons in the nodules, and would explain the seizures observed in these patients [3, 9, 24, 30–34].

Signs in Ultrasonography

Heterotopias are nearly identical in appearance in antenatal and in neonatal images (Fig. 8) [30, 35].

Three types of abnormalities can attract the sonographer's attention:

- The exterior outline of the lateral ventricles is indented and irregular.
- There is a hyperechoic periventricular band, usually less echoic than the choroid plexuses. It corresponds to a juxtaposition of small nodules.
- The nodules may sometimes be large (up to 20 mm in diameter) and hyperechoic, and protrude into the ventricular lumen.

In this last case, the nodules may be difficult to distinguish from a subependymal haemorrhage (if there are only one or two), or from subependymal nodules of a tuberous sclerosis. Megacisterna magna is the most frequent anomaly that has been reported in association with bilateral subependymal heterotopias [36].

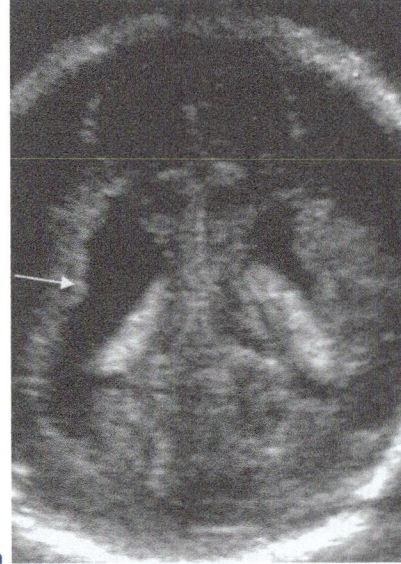

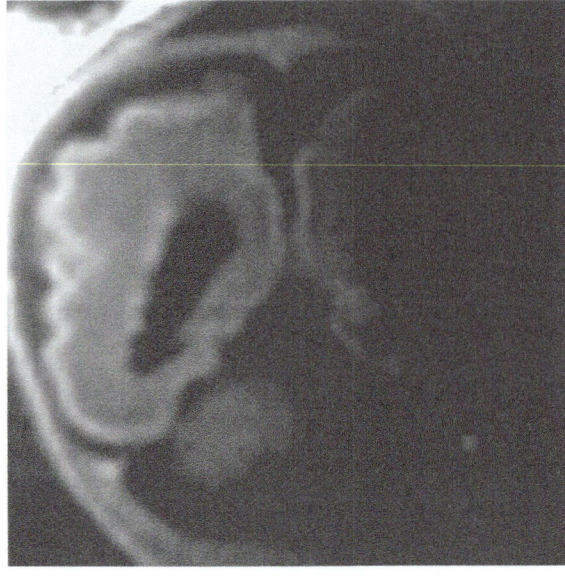

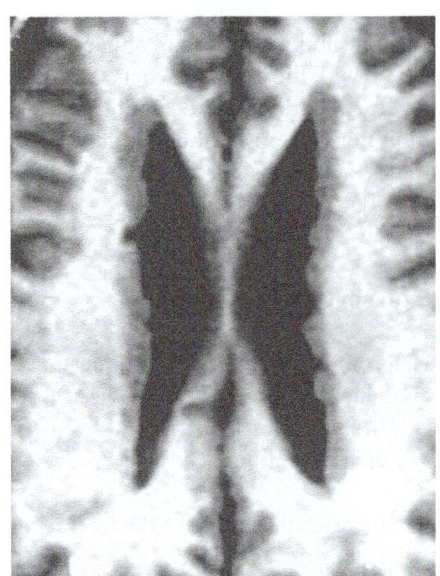

Fig. 8 a–c. Subependymal heterotopias. A mild ventricular dilatation was detected at 22 weeks of gestation. At 30 weeks of gestation, the dilatation had worsened. **a** Ultrasonography, posterior coronal slice. The ventricle outlines are indented. A hyperechoic band can be observed on their periphery (*arrow*). **b** MRI, T1-weighted coronal slice. MRI also shows the bumpy irregularity of the ventricles' surface. A band in hypersignal lines the ventricular walls. **c** Cerebral MRI of the mother. Axial slice in inversion recovery. Numerous heterotopias form indentations on the surface of the ventricular walls. The mother is asymptomatic

Contribution of Fetal MRI

MRI confirms the indented outline of the ventricles, which is better visualized than in US, since the axial slice at the level of the vertex (on which the indentations are often clearly visible) is always accessible. It should also be noted that in the four cases of subependymal heterotopias we have personally observed in fetal MRI, the ventricular dilatation in US was very mild (atria at 10–12 mm), and MRI gave the right diagnosis in only one case (Fig. 8). The subependymal nodules are isointense to the cortex, T1 hyperintense and T2 hypointense compared to the white matter.

They must not be mistaken for the germinal zone, which involutes after 26–28 weeks of gestation. An irregularity of the ventricular wall is an essential sign of heterotopia. The germinal zone does not protrude into the ventricular lumen. MRI distinguishes subependymal heterotopias from haemorrhages, since subependymal haemorrhages are sometimes associated with an intraventricular haemorrhage, ventricular dilatation, variability of the haemorrhage signal, and signs of magnetic susceptibility on the relevant sequences (gradient echo on T2*-weighted echo-planar sequences).

MRI (and ultrasonography) is used to look for potential cerebral malformations associated with heterotopias (cerebellum, corpus callosum). MRI also makes it possible to study the aetiology of heterotopias: the presence of heterotopias in the mother is a reliable sign of an X-linked dominant form (Fig. 8) [3, 36].

Prognosis

The hemizygous male patients usually die in the embryonic phase. When they do not, the neurological and intellectual disorders are often much more serious than in women.

Epilepsy is frequent in patients showing subependymal nodular heterotopias. In the isolated forms, the clinical symptomatology is in most cases discrete; the motor functions and development are normal. Moreover, in female patients, epilepsy may be accompanied by a coagulopathy and persistence of the ductus arteriosus.

When other cerebral malformations or a metabolic disease are associated with subependymal nodular heterotopias, the prognosis of the latter follows that of the former.

Subcortical Heterotopias

Definition, Mechanism and Prognosis

Subcortical heterotopias are a radiological concept. They correspond to more or less voluminous ectopic masses of neurons in the white matter somewhere in a part of a cerebral hemisphere. The affected hemisphere is often smaller than the other. The overlying cortex is thin with shallow sulci. A mass effect on the interhemispheric fissure and the adjacent lateral ventricle is possible. In some patients, there appears to be blood flow within the heterotopia. Dysgenesis of the corpus callosum is found in 70 % of cases.

Subcortical heterotopias are less frequent than subependymal heterotopias. They are often sporadic, which tends to indicate a somatic mutation rather than a the germ line mutation. They could result from a prematurely interrupted neuronal migration.

A different physiopathological explanation is suggested by studies on an animal model. Indeed, some rats have a second germinal zone in the intermediate zone of the developing brain, from which neuroblasts migrate in the periphery to the cortex and in depth towards the lateral ventricle. Subcortical heterotopias might lead to an interruption of the migration of neurons from the subependymal germinal zone and of those that migrate towards the ventricle from the second germinal zone. It is thought that capillary vessels develop inside the heterotopia along the perivascular spaces that communicate with the subarachnoid space.

The presence, or absence, of this second germinal zone in humans has, however, yet to be documented [1, 30, 31].

Antenatal Imaging

We have found only one antenatal description of a subcortical heterotopia in the literature [37]. It was detected at 22 weeks of gestation as a hemispheric formation of intermediate echogenicity, generating a mass effect on the interhemispheric fissure that increased in size in the course of pregnancy, with no associated abnormalities, which could also suggest a space-occupying lesion. The postnatal MR examination performed on the 1st day, in which the mass was isointense to the cortex, suggested this diagnosis. It was later confirmed by the biopsy.

In these cases, MRI is probably more efficient than ultrasonography because of its better contrast resolution. The analysis of the overlying cortex is also finer in MRI.

Prognosis

The motor and intellectual disorders the patients showing such heterotopias suffer from depend on the size of the lesion and its mass effect on the adjacent cortex. In the extensive unilateral forms, cases of hemiplegia have been described.

Very small lesions do not affect normal development.

Intracortical Heterotopias

Migration has stopped in the deepest layer of the cortex. This is notably seen in the cerebro-hepato-renal syndrome (Zellweger syndrome) of autosomal recessive transmission and linked with a peroxisomal disorder. Heterotopias are also found in the cerebellum [9]. It seems that such heterotopias have never been described in the antenatal period.

Molecular and/or Meningeal Heterotopias

In cases of molecular and/or meningeal heterotopia, there is an excess of migration in the superficial molecular layer of the cortex (layer 1) or in the meningeal space. This can be observed notably in connection with cocaine intoxication (Fig. 1). Other infectious (cytomegalovirus, toxoplasmosis) or toxic (alcohol) environments and ionizing radiations have also been implicated in the genesis of migratory disorders. In most cases, the question of their mechanism remains unsolved [9].

Subcortical Band Heterotopia: Double Cortex Syndrome

Definition and Mechanism

A layer of neurons with a clear outline lying inside the white matter characterizes this abnormality, also called the double cortex. This layer corresponds to the premature interruption of the migration of these neurons. The overlying cortex is of normal thickness, with shallow sulci; it may, however, also be more or less agyric. Band heterotopia can be complete or partial; in the latter case it predominantly affects the frontal lobes. Some patients may show a second band heterotopia in the temporal lobes.

This abnormality is determined by the *DCX* gene, also known as *XLIS* (long arm of the X chromosome), coding for double cortin. This protein stabilizes the microtubules by linking with them. Microtubules are intracellular components that play an essential role in cellular division, intracellular transport, morphogenesis and neuronal migration. Numerous mutations of the *DCX* gene have been described. The great majority (>90%) of patients showing subcortical band heterotopias are female. In these women, it is assumed that the band heterotopia corresponds to neurons where the mutant *DCX* gene is active, whereas the overlying cortex is formed by neurons with an active normal *DCX* gene. No correlation between genotype and phenotype was observed in these women; this was ascribed to a variable inactivation of the X chromosome. Gonadal or somatic mosaicism and interactions with other genes have also been suggested. Some rare cases of males with a band heterotopia and a mutant *DCX* gene without somatic mosaicism suggest that some neurons migrate despite their abnormal double cortin.

In most cases, however, males show a complete lissencephaly linked with a premature interruption of neuronal migration. The involvement is most serious in the frontal lobes. These patients' mothers all have subcortical band heterotopias.

Approximately 10% of patients show a typical band heterotopia, but no mutation of the *DCX* gene. Here, the aetiology remains unknown [1, 9, 24, 30, 31, 38–41].

Antenatal Imaging

We have not found a single antenatal diagnosis of this form of heterotopia in the literature. We have personally observed one case in a fetus sent to MRI after a mild bilateral ventricular dilatation was detected in US. The antenatal diagnosis could only be made retrospectively in the light of the postnatal imaging data (Fig. 9).

In ultrasonography, one should seek an inhomogeneity of the cerebral parenchyma, in which the band heterotopia is more echoic than the adjacent white matter. MRI is certainly more sensitive: it shows a T1-hyperintense band in the cerebral parenchyma and provides a good analysis of the cortical sulci.

Prognosis

The thicker the band heterotopia and the more shallow the cortical sulci, the worse the prognosis of subcortical band heterotopia. Epilepsy, cognitive and developmental disorders of variable seriousness are observed. Some patients have few noticeable clinical manifestations.

The prognosis of lissencephaly in males with this malformation is as negative as that of other types of lissencephaly.

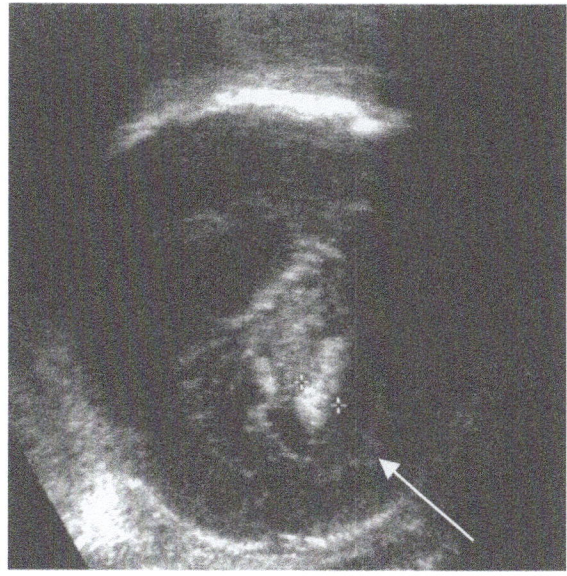

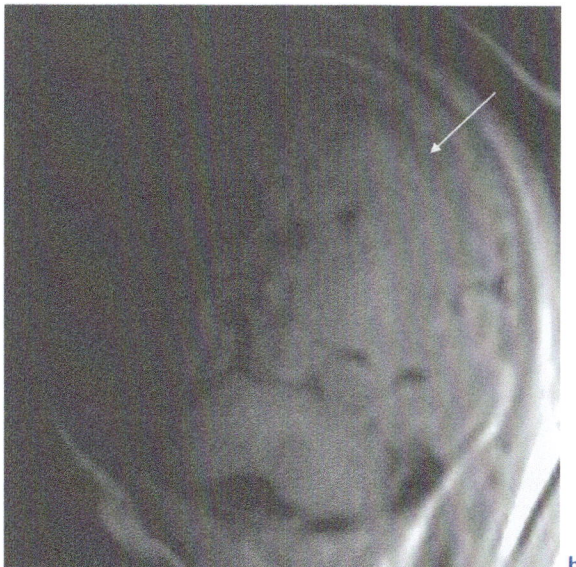

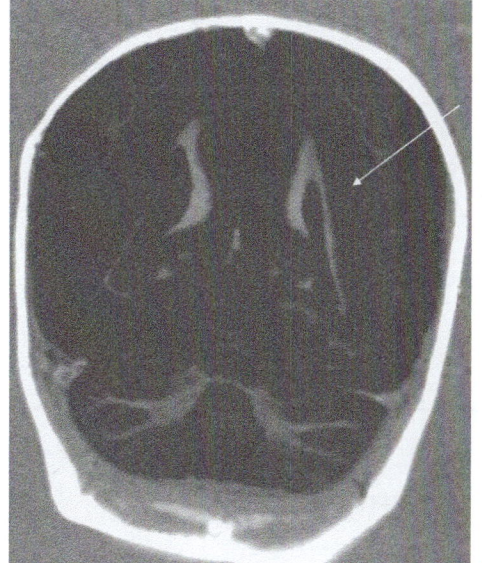

Fig. 9a–c. Band heterotopia. Fetus at 36 weeks of gestation. **a** US examination detects a mild bilateral ventricular dilatation. On this coronal slice, we retrospectively detected a hyperechoic band at a distance from the lateral ventricle (*arrow*). **b** Fetal MRI. T1-weighted coronal slice (done with a 0, 5-T MRI). We note the heterogeneousness of the cerebral parenchyma; it is hypointense inside with a hyperintense periphery (*arrow*). **c** Postnatal MRI. Coronal inversion recovery slice. The band heterotopia is clearly visible (*arrow*) in the hyposignal inside the hyperintense white matter. At 20 months, a slight balance disorder is noted

Type I Lissencephaly

Definition and Mechanism

Agyria is defined as the complete absence of sulci; it is a synonym of complete lissencephaly. Pachygyria is defined as a low number of shallow sulci with an abnormally thick cortex (incomplete lissencephaly).

Type I lissencephaly (Fig. 10) is characterized in histology by a four-layer cortex. The thick deepest layer is made up of neurons whose migration has stopped. This interruption of the migration supposedly occurred between 12 and 16 weeks of gestation.

This type of lissencephaly has been observed in patients showing mutations of the *DCX* and *LIS1* genes. The *DCX* (or *XLIS*) gene codes for double cortin. Males show lissencephaly with an anteroposterior gradient (the involvement is most serious at the level of the frontal lobes) (see "Subcortical Band Heterotopias" in this chapter). The *LIS1* gene is located on chromosome *17p13.3*. It codes for the LIS1 protein (PAF acetylhydrolase), which, like double cortin, has a stabilizing effect on the microtubules. Deletions of the *LIS1* gene are found in all patients with Miller-Dieker syndrome, which associates lissencephaly with a very typical facies. This lissencephaly obeys a

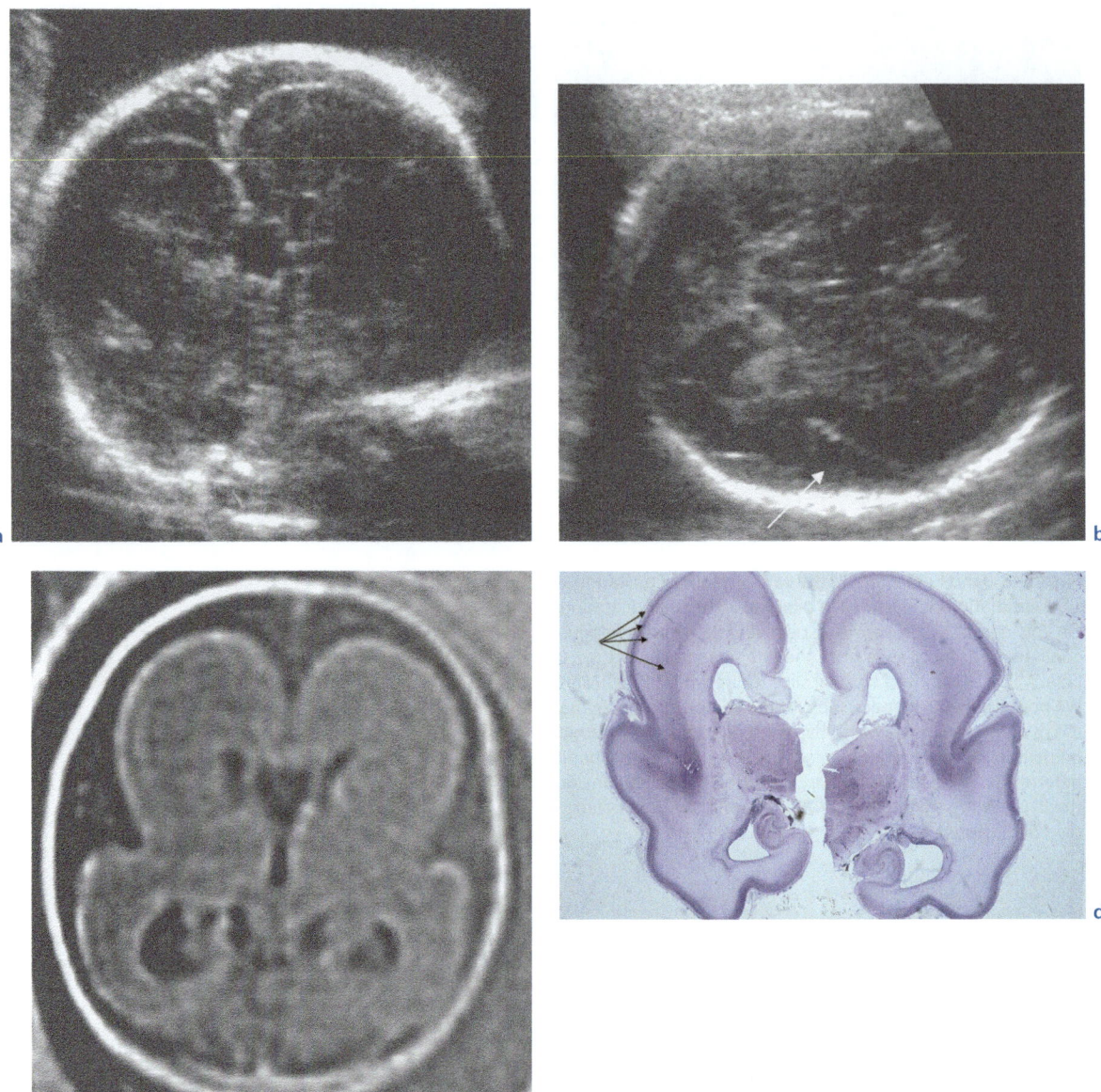

posteroanterior gradient; the most serious lesions are indeed parieto-occipital. Some cerebral abnormalities observed in Miller-Dieker syndrome might also be secondary to an excess of glutamatergic transmission.

Such deletions and mutations are found in approximately 64% of patients with type I lissencephaly. Roughly 20% of patients have normal *LIS1* and *DCX* genes, but other genes are involved in neuronal migration and may cause or contribute to lissencephaly [1, 4, 9, 24, 39, 42–44].

Fig. 10a–d. Type I lissencephaly. **a, b** Coronal (**a**) and axial (**b**) US slices taken at 35 weeks of gestation. The brain surface is abnormally smooth. The lateral ventricles are dilated and no opercularization of the sylvian fissures is visible (*arrow*). **c** Axial MRI slice at the same stage. Not one sulcus is visible. The sylvian fissures are not opercularized. The brain has a characteristic figure-eight shape. **d** Coronal histological slice at 35 weeks of gestation + 5 days. Both hemispheres are completely smooth, the ventricles are dilated, the sylvian fissure is absent. The cortex is organized in four layers (*arrows*)

Signs in Ultrasonography

In our own experience (four cases), and in the articles [3, 42, 45] reporting an antenatal diagnosis of lissencephaly (in which, moreover, the type is not always stated), the ultrasonographic sign most likely to attract attention is ventricular dilatation.

This may be associated with microcephaly, corpus callosum dysgenesis or with an abnormality of the posterior fossa (Dandy-Walker malformation, cerebellum hypoplasia). In light of what is observed postnatally [35], one should, at a sufficiently late stage, look for the absence of normally present sulci [5]; but we know ultrasonography is not entirely reliable regarding the visualization of sulci in the antenatal period. The lack of opercularization of the sylvian fissures (always clearly seen) can also be seen. The lateral sulci are abnormally wide and vertical.

Contribution of Fetal MRI

MRI is very efficient in this kind of diagnosis. Indeed, MRI provides a better analysis of fetal gyration than US, and this whatever the position of the head, on condition of course, that the examination is done at a stage where the principal primary sulci are normally present [5, 10, 17]. A smooth cerebral surface and wide sylvian fissures naturally hold no pathological value at 22 weeks of gestation.

In type I lissencephaly, the brain is described as figure-eight-shaped due to bilateral opercular dysplasia. The thick deepest cortical layer can be visualized in MRI (Fig. 10). Sometimes, lissencephaly is only partial and zones of normal cortex and zones of pachygyric or even agyric cortex alternate.

The potentially associated abnormalities of the corpus callosum, brain stem and cerebellum are also better seen in MRI [45, 46].

Prognosis

Whatever the gene involved, children suffering from classic lissencephaly almost always present an overall developmental retardation and experience seizures.

The age at which these symptoms arise and their severity depend on the extent to which the cortex is affected.

Type II Lissencephaly

Definition, Mechanism and Prognosis

Also known as cobblestone lissencephaly, type II lissencephaly (Fig. 11) is the most common form of lissencephaly. It corresponds to vascular–mesenchymal abnormalities associated with abnormalities of neuronal positioning. It is observed in a number of syndromes: Walker-Warburg syndrome, Fukuyama congenital muscular dystrophy and COM (cerebro-oculo-muscular) syndrome. These syndromes result from a deficiency of a protein group that plays a fundamental role in muscular contraction, but also in central nervous system development (hence the frequent presence of other abnormalities of the brain stem, cerebellum and white matter). The best known among these proteins is merosin, the deficiency of which is implicated in Fukuyama dystrophy. It intervenes in the migration of oligodendrocyte precursors, hence the myelination abnormalities observed in these patients. Other proteins probably play a role in the formation of glial and retinal limiting membranes and, consequently, in the final stage of migration and cortical organization. In these patients, the cortex has a chaotic aspect; the layers are not clearly individualized. The neurons inside are disoriented and are not where they should be. Histology reveals that groups of neurons are separated by fibroglial vascular tissue that stretches through the cortex, from the white matter to the subarachnoid space. Mutations in the *O*-mannosyltransferase gene *POMT1* give rise to the Walker-Warburg syndrome.

The Walker-Warburg, or HARD±E syndrome associates hydrocephaly, severe hypotonia linked to muscular dystrophy, ocular malformations, malformations of the posterior fossa and sometimes an encephalocoele. Most patients suffer from an absence of psychomotor development and die in the 1st year of life [1, 4, 24, 42, 43, 47].

Signs in Ultrasonography

Among all the syndromes associated with type II lissencephaly, Walker-Warburg syndrome is the most frequently observed in antenatal sonography [48–53] in the Western world. Its main signs are ventricular dilatation, abnormalities of the posterior fossa (Dandy-Walker malformation), ocular abnormalities (cataract, retinal dysplasia), and the presence of an encephalocoele.

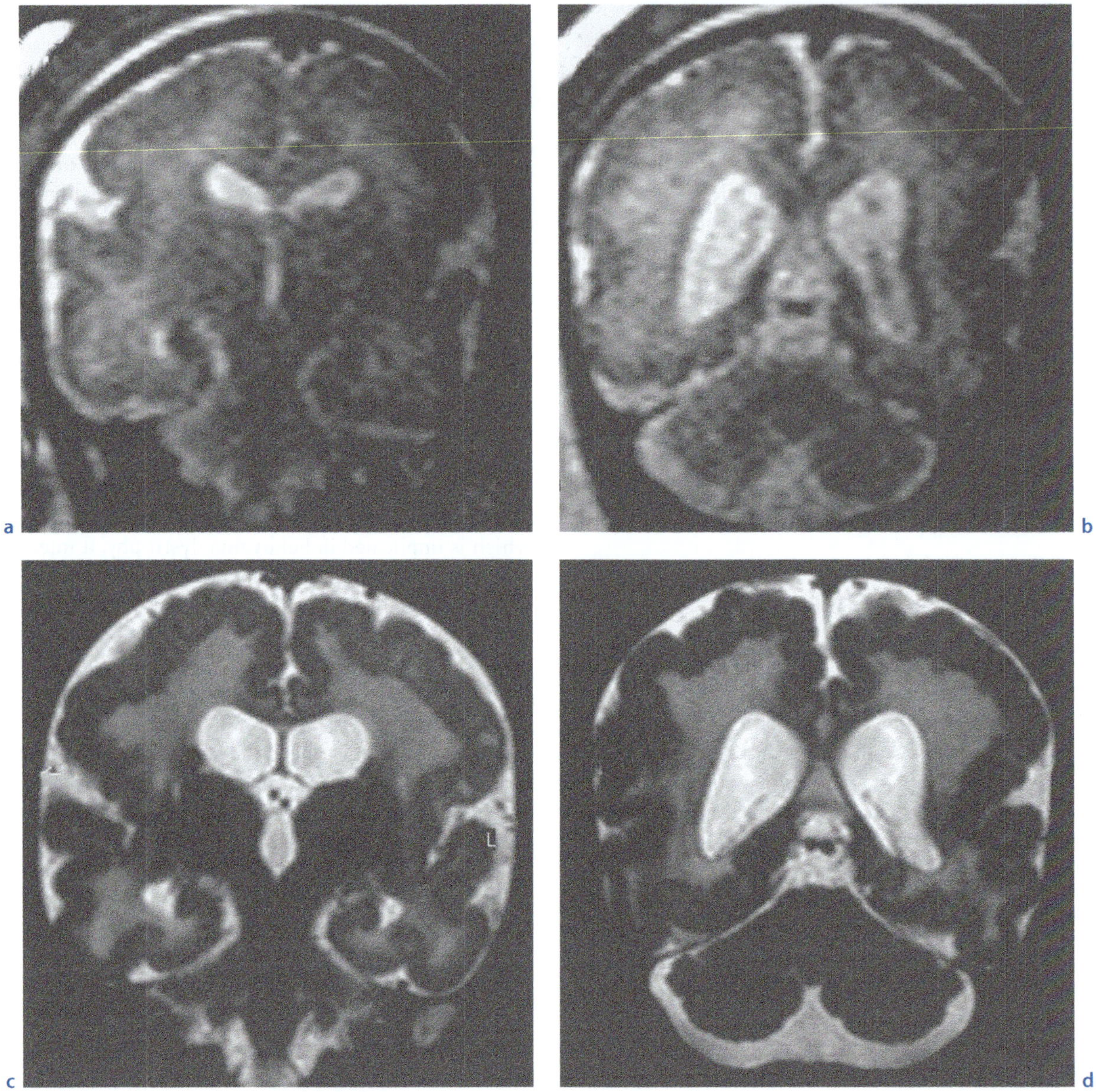

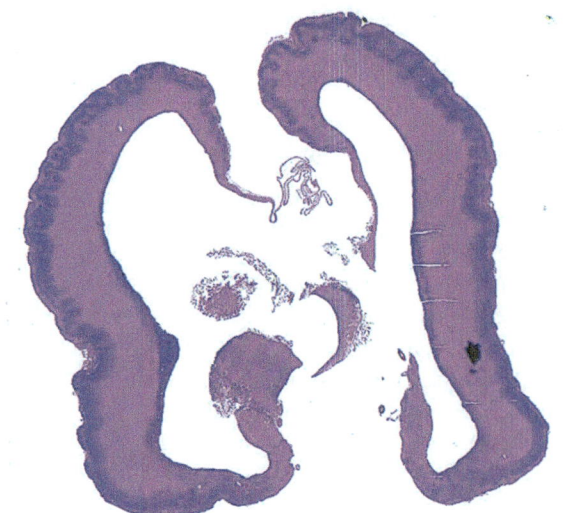

Fig. 11 a–e. Type II lissencephaly: Walker-Warburg syndrome. The sonographic examination at 35 weeks of gestation revealed a mild dilatation of the atria (10 mm) and raised suspicion of vermian hypoplasia. **a, b** Fetal MRI taken at 35 weeks of gestation. T2-weighted coronal slices. The atria are dilated (14 and 15 mm). We also note a lack of opercularization of both sylvian fissures and a pattern of extensive pachygyria. Indeed, the sulci usually visible at this stage are not present (frontal and inferior temporal sulci, sulci on the inferior aspect of the hemispheres), the cortex is abnormally thick and the border between the cortex and white matter looks regular. Subtentorial biometric data are below the 10th percentile. **c, d** Postnatal MRI (refusal of termination of pregnancy). T2-weighted coronal slices. The aspect is entirely superimposable to the one observed in the antenatal MRI. **e** Fetopathological examination of a fetus from the same sibship. Posterior coronal histological slice showing the major ventricular dilatation and the meningeal cortical dysplasia characteristic of type II lissencephaly

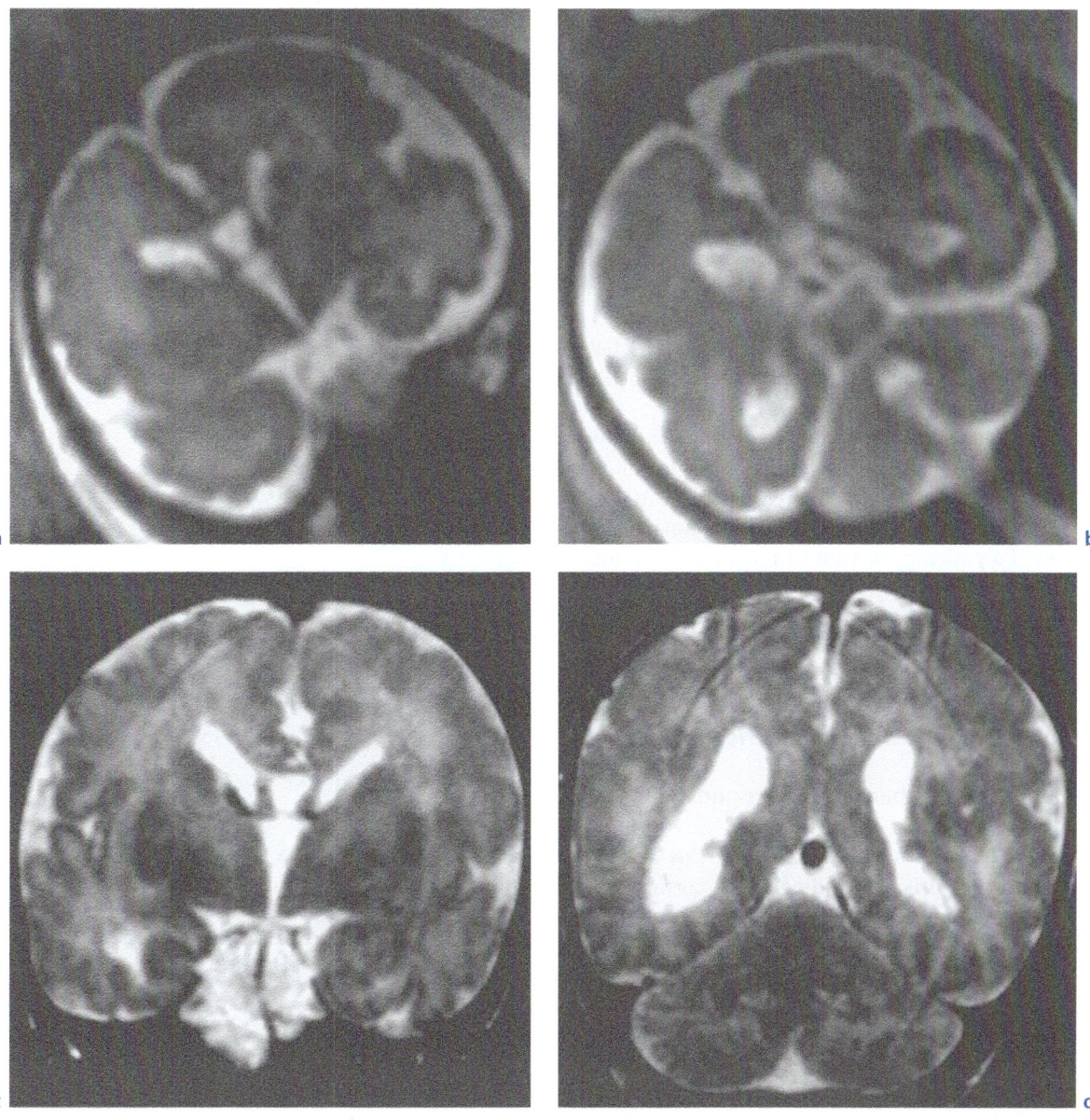

Contribution of Fetal MRI

The main asset of MRI [54–55] is its better analysis of the posterior fossa (brain stem and cerebellum hypoplasia) and of gyration, which are not clearly visible in sonography [5, 10, 17] (Fig. 11).

Polymicrogyria Without Laminar Necrosis

Atypical polymicrogyria is a heterogeneous group of migration abnormalities that all have in common a secondary overfolding of the cortical ribbon without laminar necrosis. It is related to a causal factor occur-

Fig. 12 a–d. Polymicrogyria in a Zellweger syndrome. **a, b** Antenatal MRI performed at 35 weeks of gestation following the detection on US of ventricular dilatation. T2-weighted coronal slices. MRI reveals a bilateral opercular dysplasia and extended polymicrogyria. The frontal and temporal sulci are not clearly individualized. **c, d** Postnatal MRI on the 5th day of life. T2-weighted coronal slices (movement artefacts). Polymicrogyria is particularly visible around the left sylvian fissure and in the frontal lobes. The cortex seems abnormally thick and the cortex–white matter junction line is irregular. Moreover, this child showed a bilateral germinolysis (not shown), renal cysts and facial dysmorphy with major hypotonia

ring well before 15–20 weeks of gestation. Carbon monoxide intoxication, for example, may give rise to polymicrogyria without laminar necrosis if it occurs between 12 and 17 weeks of gestation, and to polymicrogyria with laminar necrosis between 18 and 24 weeks of gestation. Polymicrogyria without laminar necrosis may therefore be a consequence of an early insult in the second trimester.

The presence of associated heterotopias is another argument pointing to a causal event occurring before 20 weeks of gestation.

This type of polymicrogyria is observed in Zellweger syndrome (Fig. 12), glutaric acidaemia type II and mitochondrial cytopathies.

It is of course impossible to distinguish between the different types of polymicrogyria in antenatal MRI. The pattern here is therefore similar to the one described for polymicrogyria with laminar necrosis (see "Polymicrogyria with Laminar Necrosis" below) [56].

Clastic and Other Causes

Polymicrogyria with Laminar Necrosis

Definition, Mechanism and Prognosis

Polymicrogyria with laminar necrosis associates laminar necrosis, overfolding of the cortical ribbon and a fusion of the molecular layers of two adjacent sulci. In most cases, laminar necrosis affects layer V. It was suggested that this abnormality originates in a causal mechanism occurring between 20 and 27 weeks of gestation. During this period, the supragranular layers are immature, and thus more exposed to hypoxia and to hypoperfusion. This abnormality could therefore be experimentally produced by injecting a glutamatergic agent into the forming cortex, thus inducing an excitotoxic cascade. When the insult occurs around 18–20 weeks of gestation, migration abnormalities may be associated with polymicrogyria, since at this stage the neurons bound for the most superficial layers of the neocortex have not yet migrated.

The aetiologies of this type of microgyria are diverse: congenital cytomegalovirus (CMV) infection, toxoplasmosis, syphilis and maternal shocks.

Some patients also show syndromes with focal, bilateral and symmetrical polymicrogyria located either in the perisylvian cortex (Foix-Chavany-Mary syndrome) or in the frontoparietal or paramedian

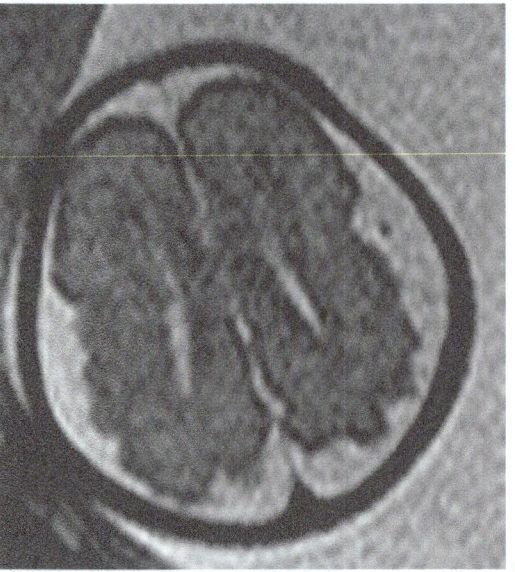

a

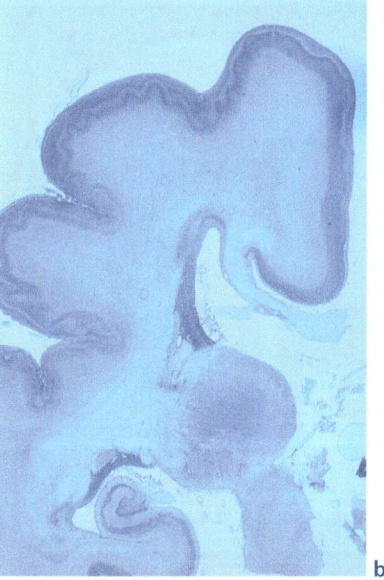

b

Fig. 13a, b. Polymicrogyria with laminar necrosis. Fetus at 29 weeks of gestation with a group of malformations, among which a partial corpus callosum agenesis (CCA) and a supratentorial biometry far below the 10th percentile. **a** T2-weighted axial slice. The lateral ventricles are parallel due to partial CCA. Polymicrogyria manifests itself in the overfolding of the cortical ribbon clearly visible at the posterior frontal and parietal levels. **b** Coronal histological slice of the right hemisphere showing the midcortical laminar necrosis

parieto-occipital cortex. Some familial forms of these syndromes have been reported.

When the perisylvian region is affected, patients show a pseudobulbar syndrome at birth characterized by dysphagy, epilepsy, mental retardation and sometimes arthrogryposis.

Moreover, both focal and diffuse bilateral polymicrogyria have been documented, the latter with seizures, hypotonia and mental retardation.

Some syndromes of bilateral polymicrogyria have been mapped to specific genetic loci. Unilateral polymicrogyria has been reported in relation with *PAX6* mutation [56–58].

Antenatal Imaging

To the best of our knowledge, there has been no report of an antenatal diagnosis of polymicrogyria in ultrasonography, which is hardly surprising considering the poor visibility of the cortex's surface in US. In fetal MRI, however, polymicrogyria is visible (we have observed five cases), with the usual restriction regarding gyration abnormalities, i. e. that the examination should be done before 34 weeks of gestation, when the pericerebral space is still wide enough to clearly visualize the cerebral cortex (Fig. 13). Polymicrogyria may be located anywhere, although it is more frequent in the perisylvian regions. It may be difficult to distinguish from pachygyria. Using thin high-resolution slices in postnatal MRI provides a good view of the junction between white and grey matter. The junction line is smooth in pachygyria and irregular in polymicrogyria [1]. Naturally, these abnormalities are not always detectable in fetal MRI, because of its lower spatial resolution.

MRI also detects opercular dysplasia (Figs. 10–12).

Schizencephaly

Definition and Mechanism

Schizencephaly is characterized by an abnormal cleft between the lateral ventricle and the cortex's surface, edged with polymicrogyric dysplastic grey matter without normal lamination. The cleft can be uni- or bilateral, symmetrical or asymmetrical. In many cases, it is located on both sides of the central sulcus. Its lips are either closed or open.

The aetiology of schizencephaly remains unclear. Two types of mechanisms have been suggested. One consists of mutations of the *EMX2* homeobox gene, which is expressed in the germinal matrix, and has been implicated in some familial cases. It seems that this genetic abnormality particularly affects the perisylvian regions. The other mechanism is of an environmental nature, the original insult occurring in the second trimester of pregnancy. The insult may be viral (notably CMV infection; see Chap. 13), or an exposure to organic solvents, a haemorrhage with fetal hypotension, or a vascular occlusion (see Chap. 14) [60]. Polymicrogyria and schizencephaly might in some cases have very similar aetiopathogenic mechanisms.

It is within the scope of this ischaemic theory that schizencephaly may be associated with an absence of septum pellucidum (see Chap. 8). One-third of the children with schizencephaly also suffer from hypoplasia of the optical nerves [1, 24, 59, 60].

Signs in Ultrasonography

So far, only open-lip schizencephalies have been diagnosed in utero. A few antenatal diagnoses (by US and MRI) of schizencephaly have been reported and analysed [60–62]. Ventricular dilatation is found in 70 % of cases. Schizencephaly is characterized by what seems like a rupture of the ventricular wall, and an abnormal communication between the ventricular lumen and the subarachnoid space [35]. The cortical ribbon extends along the two edges of the cleft. Cortical atrophy may also play a part in ventricular dilatation. In ultrasonography, one should look for a potentially associated absence of septum pellucidum and also for a corpus callosum dysgenesis or an abnormality of the posterior fossa.

Contribution of Fetal MRI

Fetal MRI allows a good analysis of the hemisphere affected by schizencephaly, but also of the other hemisphere, in which one should look for a bilateral cleft and for a mirror image of the affected hemisphere, including cortical dysplasia. Slices should be made in several planes, as one may fail to notice the schizencephaly when it is parallel to the planigraphic plane.

MRI also offers a clearer view of the cortex lining the cleft [60]; it is often dysplastic, with abnormal sulci (polymicrogyria and grey matter heterotopias lining the cleft). Furthermore, MRI distinguishes open-lip schizencephaly from other fluid-filled formations such as porencephaly and arachnoid cysts and makes it possible to look for associated abnormalities of the posterior fossa and corpus callosum.

Prognosis

The prognosis depends on the size and location of the cleft and also on whether it is uni- or bilateral. It is negative in wide open-lip bilateral schizencephaly (mental retardation, delayed speech). It is better in unilateral forms, since cerebral plasticity allows a reorganization of the cognitive functions in the contralateral hemisphere. Hypotonia and seizures may also be observed. When schizencephaly is located in the frontal lobes, there is a greater incidence of motor dysfunctions [60].

Tuberous Sclerosis Complex

Definition, Mechanism and Prognosis

Tuberous sclerosis complex (TSC) is an autosomal dominant phakomatosis characterized by a lesion that combines a migratory disorder and a space-occupying lesion. Birth incidence is approximately 1/6,000 or 10,000 [63]. Two distinct genes involved in TSC (*TSC1* [*9q34*], *TSC2* [*16p13–3*]) have been identified; mutations or deletions of these genes have been observed in some patients with TSC. However, the genetic heterogeneity of TSC and the great variety of mutations currently preclude any possibility of diagnosing this pathology antenatally. The cerebral abnormalities observed in TSC cases are assumed to result from an abnormal expression of the *TSC1* and *TSC2* genes in the germinal zone cells. This is said to give rise to abnormalities of differentiation, development and migration of the neuroblasts, hence the presence of dysplastic cells in the subependymal regions (periventricular nodules), in the cortex (cortical tubers) and along the path taken by the neurons that migrate between the two regions (diffuse infiltrates of white matter) [64, 65].

The balloon cells observed in TSC are very similar to those encountered in hemimegalencephaly, although they differ on an immunohistochemical level and in electronic microscopy [26].

Signs in Ultrasonography

In the absence of a family history of TSC, ultrasonography of the fetal brain rarely shows signs leading to a suspicion of TSC. Indeed, whereas postnatal neuroimaging reveals abnormalities in over 95% of patients with TSC [65], most antenatal sonographies are normal due to the low sensitivity of the examination in this field. Subependymal nodules are hyperechoic; they are difficult to distinguish from subependymal haemorrhages or heterotopias. They are rarely calcified before 1 year after birth [65]. The cortical tubers are described as hyperechoic foci in postnatal and antenatal imaging. Infiltrates of white matter are not visible in US.

The most easily identifiable lesions in antenatal US are the voluminous subependymal nodules or giant cell tumours, which are usually located near the Monro foramina or elsewhere on the surface of the ependyma [27, 66]. In some rare cases, a hemimegalencephaly is associated with TSC [27].

In fact, the antenatal sonographic sign that most commonly leads to suggesting a diagnosis of TSC is the discovery of intracardiac masses reminiscent of rhabdomyomas.

Rhabdomyomas are the most common aetiology of intracardiac masses (58%); they are found in 50%–80% of patients with TSC [67]. They are not usually seen until the third trimester, and they tend to regress spontaneously [66, 67]. In a series of eight fetuses with such cardiac tumours, five showed abnormalities in cerebral imaging that suggested TSC [68].

Contribution of Fetal MRI

Apart from one diagnosis of probable hemimegalencephaly reported at 26 weeks of gestation (no postnatal MRI was done) in a fetus whose father and two siblings suffered from TSC (and cardiac rhabdomyomas) [27], only subependymal nodules have been described in fetal MRI (two cases [64], four cases [68], and five cases of our own). For all these fetuses, the cerebral US was normal, and MR examinations were made following the detection of intracardiac masses. The sensitivity of MRI seems to be much better than that of US in the detection of subependymal nodules. It remains, however, very low, as was shown by the correlation made with postnatal MR data (in our own experience) or with neurofetopathological examinations, which demonstrated that many subependymal nodules had not been detected in antenatal MRI [63,

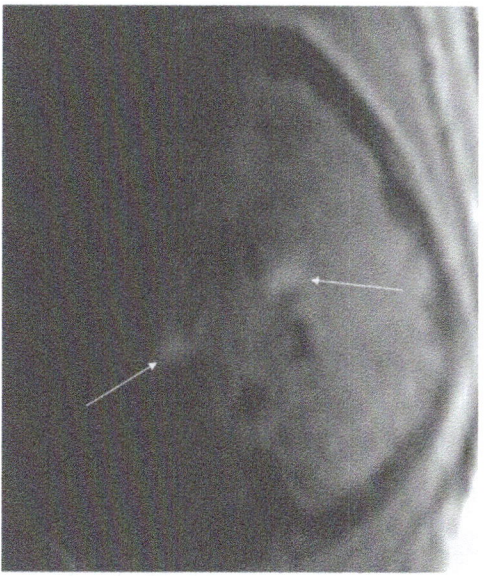

Fig. 14. Tuberous sclerosis. Fetus at 32 weeks of gestation. MRI was done following the discovery in US of numerous intracardiac tumours reminiscent of rhabdomyomas. The cerebral ultrasonography was normal. T1-weighted axial slice. The two subependymal nodules visible on this slice are hyperintense (*arrows*)

68]. Therefore, antenatal MRI cannot rule out this diagnosis.

The subependymal nodules are T1 hyperintense and T2 hypointense (Fig. 14). This T1 hyperintensity contrasts with the marked hypointensity of the fetus's nonmyelinated white matter.

The cortical hamartomas described in postnatal as T1 hyperintense, T2 hypointense lesions [65] can also be observed in fetal MRI. The observation of diffuse infiltration of white matter has not been reported yet.

References

1. Barkovich AJ (2000) Congenital malformations of the brain and skull in pediatric neuroimaging. Lippincott Williams & Wilkins, Philadelphia pp 251–381
2. Chong BW, Babcook CJ, Salamat MS, Nemzek W, Kroeker D, Ellis WG (1996) A magnetic resonance template for normal neuronal migration in the fetus. Neurosurgery 39:110–116
3. Mitchell LA, Simon EM, Filly RA, Barkovich AJ (2000) Antenatal diagnosis of subependymal heterotopia. AJNR Am J Neuroradiol 21:296–300
4. Barkovich AJ, Kuzniecky RI, Dobyns WB, Jackson GD, Becker LE, Evrard P (1996) A classification scheme for malformations of cortical development. Neuropediatrics 27:59–63
5. Garel C, Chantrel E, Sebag G, Brisse H, Elmaleh M, Hassan M (2000) Le développement du cerveau fœtal : atlas IRM et biométrie. Ed Sauramps Médical, Montpellier
6. Sidman RL, Rakic P (1973) Neuronal migration with special reference to developing human: a review. Brain Res 62:1–35
7. Jammes JL, Gilles FH (1983) Telencephalic development: matrix volume and isocortex and allocortex areas. In: Gilles FH, Leviton A, Dooling EC (eds) The developing human brain. John Wright-PSG, Boston, pp 87–93
8. Brisse H, Fallet C, Sebag G, Nessmann C, Blot P, Hassan M (1997) Supratentorial parenchyma in the developing fetal brain: in vivo MR study with histologic comparison AJNR Am J Neuroradiol 18:1491–1497
9. Gressens P (2000) Mechanisms and disturbances of neuronal migration. Ped Res 48:725–730
10. Adamsbaum C, Gelot A, André C, Baron JM (2001) Atlas d'IRM du cerveau fœtal. Masson
11. Perelman R (1990) Pathologie du tissu nerveux. In: Perelman R (ed) Pathologie du système nerveux et des muscles. Psychiatrie-Maloine, Paris, pp 181–472
12. Barkovich AJ, Ferriero DM, Barr RM, Gressens P, Dobyns WB, Truwit CL, Evrard P (1998) Microlissencephaly: a heterogeneous malformation of cortical development. Neuropediatrics 29:113–119
13. Sztriha L, Al-Gazali L, Varady E, Nork M, Varughese M (1998) Microlissencephaly. Pediatr Neurol 18:362–365
14. Sztriha L, Al-Gazali, Varady E, Goebel HH, Nork M (1999) Autosomal recessive micrencephaly with simplified gyral pattern, abnormal myelination and arthrogryposis. Neuropediatrics 30:141–145
15. Hashimoto LN, Bass WT, Green GA, Werner AL, Reagan TJ (1999) Radial microbrain form of micrencephaly: possible association with carbamazepine. J Neuroimaging 9:243–245
16. Garel C, Brisse H, Hornoy P, Lamer S, Fallet C, Vuillard E, Hassan M (1998) Fetal MRI in microlissencephaly. Pediatr Radiol 28:367
17. Garel C, Chantrel E, Brisse H, Elmaleh M, Luton D, Oury JF, Sebag G, Hassan M (2001) Fetal cerebral cortex: normal gestational landmarks identified using prenatal MR imaging. AJNR Am J Neuroradiol 22:184–189
18. Alper G, Ekinci G, Yilmaz Y, Arikan C, Telyar G, Erzen C (1999) Magnetic resonance imaging characteristics of benign macrocephaly in children. J Child Neurol 14:678–682
19. Göhlich-Ratmann G, Baethmann M, Lorenz P, Gärtner J, Goebel HH, Engelbrecht V, Christen HJ, Lenard HG, Voit T (1998) Megalencephaly, mega corpus callosum and complete lack of motor development: a previously undescribed syndrome. Am J Med Genet 79:161–167

20. Bodensteiner JB, Chung EO (1993) Macrocrania and megal-encephaly in the neonate. Seminars in Neurology. 13:84–91
21. Petersson S, Pedersen NL, Schalling M, Lavebratt C (1999) Primary megalencephaly at birth and low intelligence level. Neurology 53:1254–1259
22. Sandler AD, Knudsen MW, Brown TT, Christian RM (1997) Neurodevelopmental dysfunction among nonreferred children with idiopathic megalencephaly. J Pediatr 131:320–324
23. Barkovich AJ, Chuang SH (1990) Unilateral megalencephaly: correlation of MR imaging and pathologic characteristics. AJNR 11:523–531
24. Sarnat HB (2001) Congenital malformations of the nervous system. A neuropathologic perspective. Neuroimaging Clin N Am 11:57–77
25. Griffiths PD, Gardner SA, Smith M, Rittey C, Powell T (1998) Hemimegalencephaly and focal megalencephaly in tuberous sclerosis complex. AJNR Am J Neuroradiol 19:1935–1938
26. Arai Y, Edwards V, Becker LE (1999) A comparison of cell phenotypes in hemimegalencephaly and tuberous sclerosis. Acta Neuropathol 98:407–413
27. Brackley KJ, Farndon PA, Weaver JB, Dow DJ, Chapman S, Kilby MD (1999) Prenatal diagnosis of tuberous sclerosis with intracerebral signs at 14 weeks' gestation. Prenat Diagn 19:575–579
28. Lam AH, Villanueva AC, de Silva M (1992) Hemimegalencephaly. Cranial sonographic findings. J Ultrasound Med 11:241–244
29. Fariello G, Malena S, Lucigrai G, Toma P (1993) Hemimegalencephaly: early sonographic pattern. Pediatr Radiol 23:151–152
30. Barkovich AJ, Kuzniecky RI (2000) Gray matter heterotopia. Neurology 55:1603–1608
31. Barkovich AJ (2000) Morphologic characteristics of subcortical heterotopia: MR imaging study. AJNR Am J Neuroradiol 21:290–295
32. Fox JW, Lamperti ED, Eksioglu YZ, Hong SE, Feng Y, Graham DA, Scheffer IE, Dobyns WB, Hirsch BA, Radtke RA, Berkovic SF, Huttenlocher PR, Walsh CA (1998) Mutations in filamin 1 prevent migration of cerebral cortical neurons in human periventricular heterotopia. Neuron 21:1315–1325
33. Sheen VL, Topcu M, Berkovic S, Yalnizoglu D, Blatt I, Bodell A, Hill RS, Ganesh VS, Cherry TJ, Shugart YY, Walsh CA (2003) Autosomal recessive form of periventricular heterotopia. Neurology 60:1108–1112
34. Sheen VL, Feng Y, Graham D, Takafuta T, Shapiro SS, Walsh CA. Filamin A and Filamin B are co-expressed within neurons during periods of neuronal migration and can physically interact. Hum Mol Genet 11:2845–2854
35. Pellicer A, Cabanas F, Perez-Higueras A, Garcia-Alix A, Quero J (1995) Neural migration disorders studied by cerebral ultrasound and colour Doppler flow imaging. Arch Dis Child 73F51–F61
36. Bargallo N, Puerto B, de Juan C, Martinez-Crespo JM, Lourdes Olondo M (2002) Hereditary subependymal heterotopia associated with megacisterna magna: antenatal diagnosis with magnetic resonance imaging. Ultrasound Obstet Gynecol 20:86–89
37. Onyeije CI, Sherer DM, Jarosz CJ, Divon MY (1998) Prenatal sonographic findings associated with sporadic subcortical nodular heterotopia. Obstet Gynecol 91:799–801
38. Walsh CA, Goffinet AM (2000) Potential mechanisms of mutations that affect neuronal migration in man and mouse. Cur Opin Genet Dev 10:270–274

39. Leventer RJ, Pilz DT, Matsumoto N, Ledbetter DH, Dobyns WB (2000) Lissencephaly and subcortical band heterotopia: molecular basis and diagnosis. Mol Med Today 6:277–284
40. Aigner L, Uyanik G, Couillard-Despres S, Ploetz S, Wolff G, Morris-Rosendahl D, Martin P, Eckel U, Spranger S, Otte J, Woerle H, Holthausen H, Apheshiotis N, Fluegel D, Winkler J (2003) Somatic mosaicism and variable penetrance in double cortin-associated migration disorders. Neurology 60:329–332
41. D'Agostino MD, Bernasconi A, Das S, Bastos A, Valerio RM, Palmini A, Costa da Costa J, Scheffer IE, Berkovic S, Guerrini R, Dravet C, Ono J, Gigli G, Federico A, Booth F, Bernardi B, Volpi L, Tassinari CA, Guggenheim MA, Ledbetter DH, Gleeson JG, Lopes-Cendes I, Vossler DG, Malaspina E, Franzoni E, Sartori RJ, Mitchell MH, Mercho S, Dubeau F, Andermann F, Dobyns WB, Andermann E (2002) Subcortical band heterotopia (SBH) in males: clinical, imaging and genetic findings in comparison with females. Brain 125:2507–2522
42. Sergi C, Zoubaa S, Schiesser M (2000) Norman-Roberts syndrome: prenatal diagnosis and autopsy findings. Prenat Diagn 20:505–509
43. Dobyns WB, Truwit CL (1995) Lissencephaly and other malformations of cortical development:1995 update. Neuropediatrics 26:132–147
44. Kato M, Dobyns WB (2003) Lissencephaly and the molecular basis of neuronal migration. Hum Mol Genet 12 [Suppl 1]: R89–R96
45. Greco P, Resta M, Vimercati A, Dicuonzo F, Loverro G, Vicino M, Selvaggi L (1998) Antenatal diagnosis of isolated lissencephaly by ultrasound and magnetic resonance imaging. Ultrasound Obstet Gynecol 12:276–279
46. Okamura K, Murotsuki J, Sakai T, Matsumoto K, Shirane R, Yajima A (1993) Prenatal diagnosis of lissencephaly by magnetic resonance image. Fetal Diagn Ther 8:56–59
47. Beltran-Valero de Bernabe D, Currier S, Steinbrecher A, Celli J, Van Beusekom E, Van der Zwaag B, Kayserili H, Merlini L, Chitayat D, Dobyns WB, Cormand B, Lehesjoki AE, Cruces J, Voit T, Walsh CA, Van Bokhoven H, Brunner HG (2002) Mutations in the O-mannosyltransferase gene POMT1 give rise to the severe neuronal migration disorder Walker-Warburg syndrome. Am J Hum Genet 71:1033–1043
48. Beinder EJ, Pfeiffer RA, Bornemann A, Wenkel H (1997) Second-trimester diagnosis of fetal cataract in a fetus with Walker-Warburg syndrome. Fetal Diagn Ther 12:197–199
49. Van Zalen-Sprock RM, van Vugt JM, van Geijn HP (1996) First-trimester sonographic detection of neurodevelopmental abnormalities in some single-gene disorders. Prenat Diagn 16:199–202
50. Chitayat D, Toi A, Babul R, Levin A, Michaud J, Summers A, Rutka J, Blaser S, Becker LE (1995) Prenatal diagnosis of retinal nonattachment in the Walker-Warburg syndrome. Am J Med Genet 56:351–358
51. Holzgreve W, Feil R, Louwen F, Miny P (1993) Prenatal diagnosis and management of fetal hydrocephaly and lissencephaly. Childs Nerv Syst 9:408–412
52. Vohra N, Ghidini A, Alvarez M, Lockwood C (1993) Walker-Warburg syndrome: prenatal ultrasound findings. Prenat Diagn 13:575–579
53. Gasser B, Lindner V, Dreyfus M, Feidt X, Leissner P, Treisser A, Stoll C (1998) Prenatal diagnosis of Walker-Warburg syndrome in three sibs. Am J Med Genet 76:107–110

54. Huppert BJ, Brandt KR, Ramin KD, King BF (1999) Single-shot fast spin-echo MR imaging of the fetus: a pictorial essay. Radiographics 19:S215–S227

55. Kojima K, Suzuki Y, Seki K, Yamamoto T, Sato T, Tanaka T, Suzumori K (2002) Prenatal diagnosis of lissencephaly (type II) by ultrasound and fast magnetic resonance imaging. Fetal Diagn Ther 17:34–36

56. Gressens P, Barkovich AJ, Evrard P (2003) Polymicrogyria: role of the excitotoxic damage. In: Barth PG (ed) Disorders of neuronal migration, MacKeith, London, pp 170–181

57. Mitchell TN, Free SL, Williamson KA, Stevens JM, Churchill AJ, Hanson IM, Shorvon SD, Moore AT, van Heyningen V, Sisodiya SM (2003) Polymicrogyria and absence of pineal gland due to PAX6 mutation. Ann Neurol 53:658–663

58. Chang BS, Piao X, Bodell A, Basel-Vanagaite L, Straussberg R, Dobyns WB, Qasrawi B, Winter RM, Micheil Innes A, Voit T, Ellen Grant P, Barkovich AJ, Walsh CA (2003) Bilateral frontoparietal polymicrogyria: clinical and radiological features in 10 families with linkage to chromosome 16. Ann Neurol 53:596–606

59. Lyon G, Evrard P (2000) Infirmité motrice cérébrale. In: In: Lyon G, Evrard P (eds) Neuropédiatrie. Masson, Paris, pp 57–72

60. Denis D, Maugey-Laulom B, Carles D, Pedespan JM, Brun M, Chateil JF (2001) Prenatal diagnosis of schizencephaly by fetal magnetic resonance imaging. Fetal Diagn Ther 16:354–359

61. Lituania M, Passamonti U, Cordone MS, Magnano GM, Toma P (1989) Schizencephaly: prenatal diagnosis by computed sonography and magnetic resonance imaging. Prenat Diagn 9:649–655

62. Senat MV, Bernard JP, Schwärzler P, Britten J, Ville Y (1999) Prenatal diagnosis and follow-up of 14 cases of unilateral ventriculomegaly. Ultrasound Obstet Gynecol 14:327–332

63. Levine D, Barnes P, Korf B, Edelman R (2000) Tuberous sclerosis in the fetus: second-trimester diagnosis of subependymal tubers with ultrafast MR imaging. AJR Am J Roentgenol 175:1067–1069

64. Jan W, Lacey NA, Langford KS, Bewley SJ, Maxwell DJ (2003) The antenatal diagnosis of migration disorders: a series of four cases. Clin Radiol 58:247–256

65. Barkovich AJ (2000) The phakomatoses In: Barkovich AJ (ed) Pediatric Neuroimaging. Lippincott Williams & Wilkins, Baltimore, pp 383–442

66. Sgro M, Barozzino T, Toi A, Johnson J, Sermer M, Chitayat D (1999) Prenatal detection of cerebral lesions in a fetus with tuberous sclerosis. Ultrasound Obstet Gynecol 14:356–359

67. Axt-Fliedner R, Qush H, Hendrik HJ, Ertan K, Lindinger A, Mäusle R, Remberger K, Schmidt W (2001) Prenatal diagnosis of cerebral lesions and multiple intracardiac rhabdomyomas in a fetus with tuberous sclerosis. J Ultrasound Med 20:63–67

68. Sonigo P, Elmaleh A, Fermont L, Delezoide AL, Mirlesse V, Brunelle F (1996) Prenatal MRI diagnosis of fetal cerebral tuberous sclerosis. Pediatr Radiol 26:1–4

Intracranial Space-Occupying Lesions

Intracerebral Tissue Space-Occupying Lesions

Congenital cerebral tumours are extremely rare; they are defined as the tumours observed in the antenatal period or in the first 2 months of life. They account for 0.5%–1.5% of cerebral tumours in children [1–5]. The occurrence rate is approximately 0.34 per million live births [6, 7].

Given the rarity of this pathology, most of the cases reported in antenatal US are unique. In light of these cases and a small series of seven cases [8], we were able to attempt to describe the ultrasonographic symptomatology of this pathology. Furthermore, some tumours have also been studied in fetal MRI [1, 3, 8–10]; we can thus try to evaluate the contribution of MRI to the diagnosis of this pathology.

The most frequent congenital cerebral tumours are teratomas, which account for around half of all these tumours [1, 2, 6, 7, 11–13]. Gliomas are the second most common tumours (approximately 25%) [1, 2, 7]. The remaining 25% correspond to tumours observed only very exceptionally in antenatal examinations: astrocytoma [1], glioblastoma multiforme [7, 8], neuroblastoma [4], primitive neuroectodermal tumour (PNET) [4, 8, 14, 15], gangliocytoma [16], meningeal sarcoma, craniopharyngioma, capillary haemangioblastoma [17], hypothalamic hamartoma and choroid plexus papilloma [7, 18]. It seems that no case of ependymoma or ependymoblastoma has been described in the literature [12].

Furthermore, in cerebral tumours occurring in the 1st year of life, medulloblastomas and teratomas are much more frequent in the Far East, whereas astrocytomas are less common there than in the rest of the world [9].

Ultrasonographic Patterns of Cerebral Tumours

There can of course be no question here of describing a specific symptomatology for each histological type, but rather to provide a few elements peculiar to certain tumours.

These tumours frequently take root in the supratentorial space and more rarely in the posterior fossa [14]. Some tumours located in the skull [19] in the meninges [20] may have an intracranial extension. The diagnosis is generally assessed after 20 weeks of gestation, rarely before (one case at 18 weeks of gestation [8]), and usually before 33–34 weeks of gestation (one case at 37 weeks of gestation [6]).

They are in most cases associated with macrocrania, hydrocephalus, and with hydramnios probably linked with a swallowing disorder [6, 8]. Some very vascularized tumours may be responsible for heart failure, in connection with intratumoral arteriovenous shunts [21]. Associated cardiac and urinary malformations and cleft palate have been described in almost 14% of the children with congenital cerebral tumours.

The majority of these tumours are so voluminous at the time they are detected (at least 6–7 cm in diameter) that the surrounding cerebral structures are often affected beyond recognition (Fig. 1). The tumour is not always easily located [4]; this is all the more difficult because some initially subtentorial tumours may invade the supratentorial space [14].

Teratomas generally have a mixed, solid and cystic component [3, 8–13, 21]. When this cystic component predominates, it may be difficult to distinguish from an arachnoid cyst, or indeed from any other cystic lesion [8]. Calcifications may be observed [6, 8, 12], as well as an intense hypervascularization [8, 12]. These calcifications are, however, not characteristic, as they are observed in other histological types (notably PNET [4]).

In the few cases reported, glioblastomas were described as diffusely and intensely hyperechoic tumours that could be mistaken for voluminous haemorrhages [2, 7, 8]. Often, these tumours are located in the supratentorial space, although it can sometimes be near impossible to locate them with any precision.

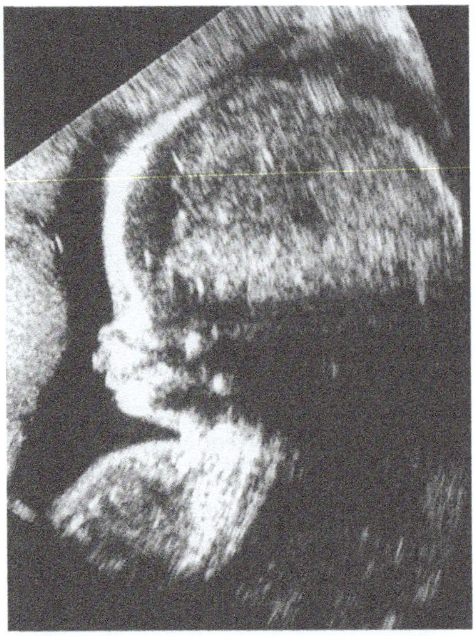

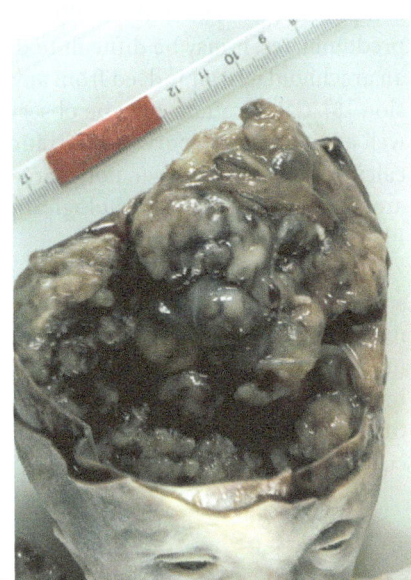

Fig. 1 a–e. Intracranial teratoma. Detection at 25.5 weeks of gestation on US examination of a macrocrania related to an intracranial space-occupying lesion of heterogeneous echogenicity associated with a labiopalatine cleft and hypertelorism. **a, b** Ultrasonography. Midline sagittal slice (**a**) and axial slice (**b**). **c, d** MRI performed at 26 weeks of gestation. T2-weighted coronal (**c**) and axial (**d**) slices. Apart from the occipital horns (*arrows*), no cerebral structure is identifiable in the supratentorial space (the posterior fossa, not shown here, is normal). Voluminous mixed space-occupying lesion with both cyst and tissue areas. Termination of pregnancy at 26 weeks of gestation. **e** View of the tumoral mass after opening of the skull. No cerebral structure is recognizable. The mass is polylobar. The histological examination confirms the teratoma pattern

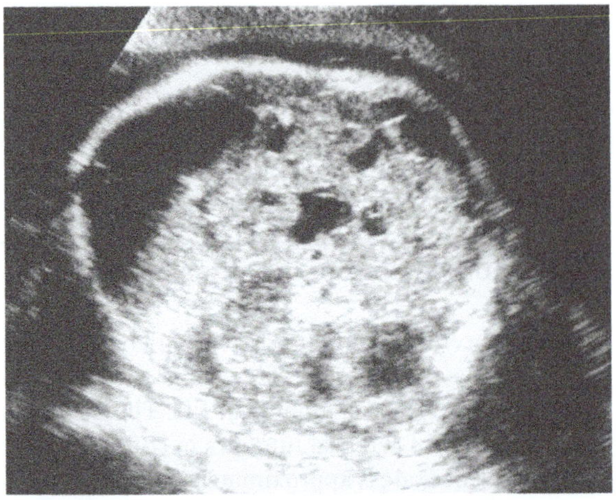

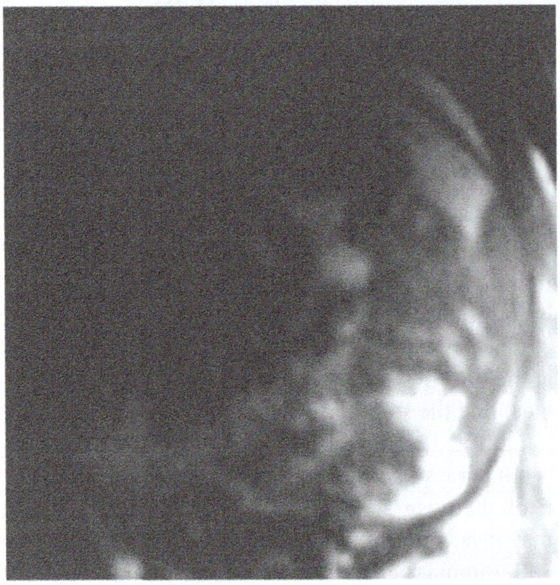

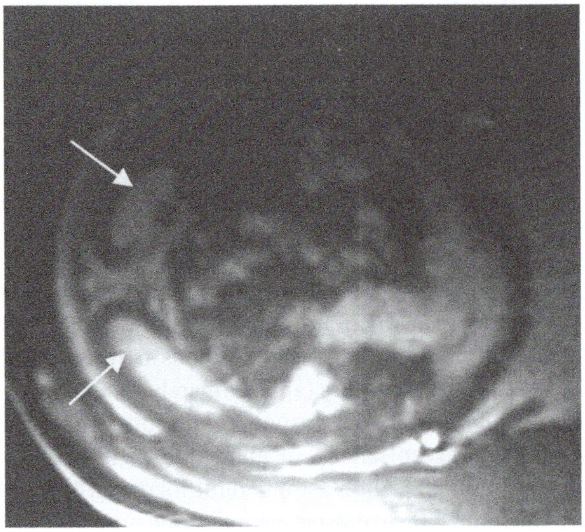

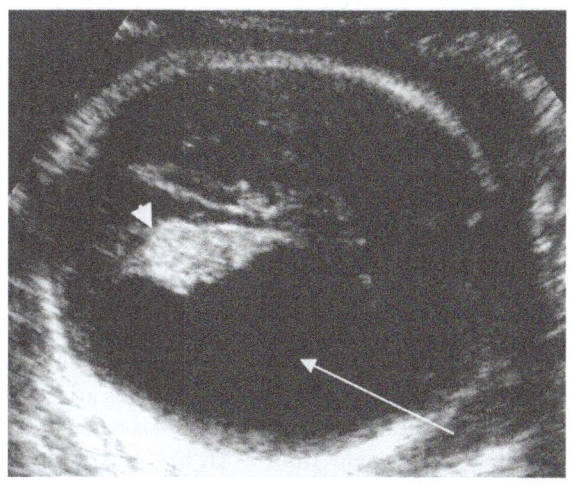

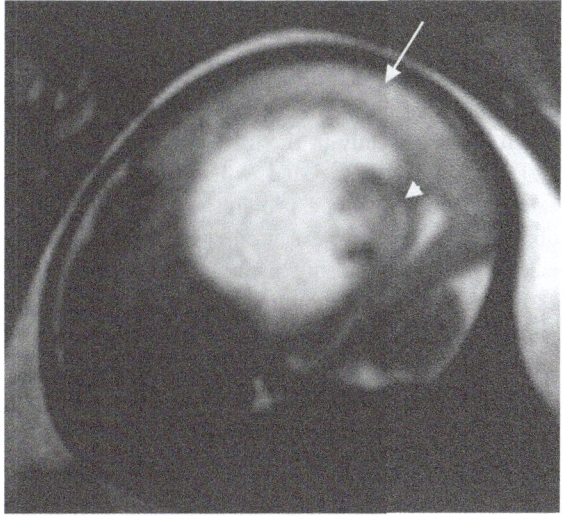

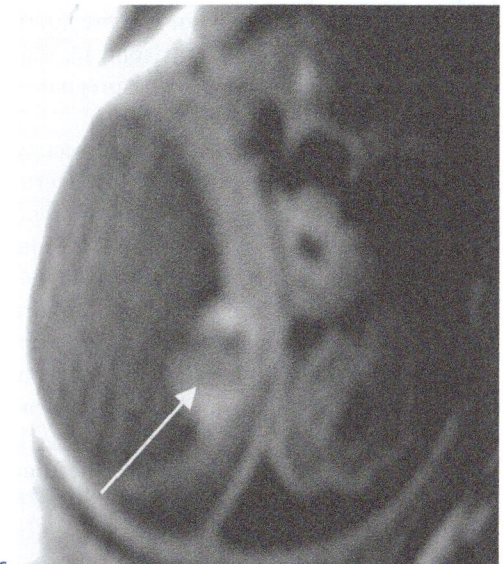

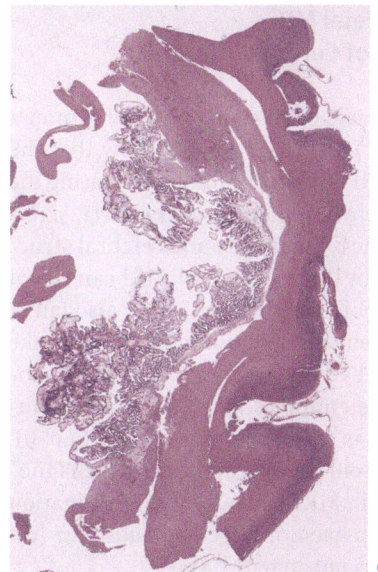

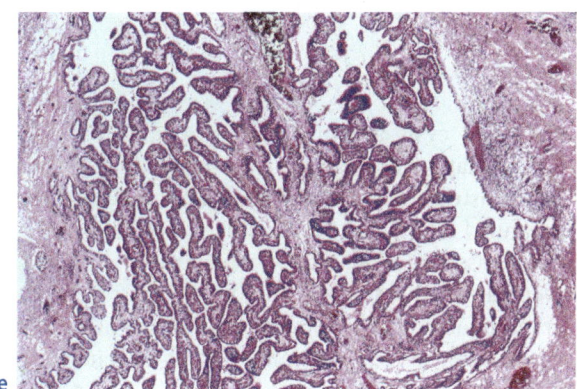

Fig. 2a–e. Choroid plexus papilloma. **a** US performed at 32 weeks of gestation. Axial slice at the level of the lateral ventricles. The voluminous cystic structure (*arrow*) had originally been interpreted as an arachnoid cyst. The adjacent oval-shaped hyperechoic structure (*arrowhead*) corresponds to a voluminous choroid plexus. **b** MRI taken at 32 weeks of gestation. T2-weighted parasagittal slice. The choroid plexus is heterogeneous, voluminous and in hyposignal (*arrowhead*). The cerebral parenchyma lining the dilated ventricle is abnormally hyperintense (*arrow*). **c** T1-weighted axial slice at the level of the occipital lobes. The left choroid plexus is heterogeneous, hypointense in the centre and hyperintense in the periphery (*arrow*). Termination of pregnancy at 33.5 weeks of gestation. The neurofetopathological examination confirms the marked dilatation of the left lateral ventricle, which is in contact with a tumour-looking greyish tissue scattered with haemorrhagic suffusions. The cerebral parenchyma lining the occipital horn (not shown) is the seat of ischaemic changes. **d, e** Coronal histological slices of the left occipital lobe at the level of the tumour. The histological pattern is that of a differentiated choroid plexus papilloma (**e**)

Choroid plexus papillomas have a much better prognosis, comparable to that of low-grade astrocytomas [2]. These generally benign tumours are located in the choroid plexus of a lateral ventricle (and much less frequently in the third or fourth ventricle [12]); they are associated with a hydrocephalus caused either by a hyperproduction of CSF or by an obstruction. They appear as a hyperechoic mass, adjacent to the choroid plexus in an atrium, generally associated with ventricular dilatation (Fig. 2) and a widening of the pericerebral space [12]. Doppler velocimetry locates the feeding arteries, but it does not show any vascularization inside the tumoral mass [12]. The main complication of these tumours is haemorrhage [22].

Contribution of Fetal MRI to the Diagnosis of Cerebral Tumours

The few reported cases of antenatal cerebral tumours studied in US and in MRI [1, 3, 8–10] show that the contribution of MRI is relatively limited. Locating the mass more precisely is sometimes possible [1, 3, 10], as is recognizing the remaining sound cerebral structures not involved by the tumour [10]. MRI can reveal intratumoral haemorrhages [8], but it may also fail to recognize very haemorrhagic tumours and mistake them for isolated haemorrhages [1]. However, subcortical nodular heterotopias may have a pseudotumoral appearance in ultrasonography (seeChap. 9). In one case of choroid plexus papilloma, the diagnosis was suggested in MRI when the US examination hesitated between a haemorrhage and a tumour (diagnostic arguments not stated) [18].

Prognosis

The prognosis of congenital cerebral tumours is very poor. Of the 21 fetuses whose cases were studied in the different articles cited in this chapter [1–11, 14, 16] two died in utero and eight in the immediate neonatal period; seven pregnancies were terminated. Three children suffered from severe developmental retardation. The only subject who had a normal development at 2 years, after a cystoperitoneal shunt was placed, was the one whose antenatal diagnosis of cystic teratoma was corrected in postnatal MRI. It was in fact an arachnoid cyst [8].

Cystic Intracranial Space-Occupying Lesions

The detection in antenatal US of a cystic (anechoic) intracranial space-occupying lesion is followed by a study of its size, location, contents and outline. One must determine whether the cyst is single or multiple, whether there is some vascularization inside this space-occupying lesion and whether there are any associated cerebral or extracerebral malformations.

The most frequently observed cystic space-occupying lesion, the choroid plexus cyst, is immediately recognizable. It is lined with ependyma and generally located at the level of the atria. Problems arise not so much regarding its diagnosis, which is made in US and does not benefit from MRI, but regarding its prognosis. The persistence of such a cyst after 28 weeks of gestation calls for the preparation of a karyotype, notably to look for trisomy 18. Many choroid plexus cysts disappear during pregnancy in the successive US examinations [23].

The other principal cystic space-occupying lesions encountered are arachnoid cysts, arteriovenous malformations of the vein of Galen, porencephalic cysts, open-lip types of schizencephaly, interhemispheric cysts and posterior fossa cysts [24–26]. In the last four entities, associated cerebral abnormalities generally lead to the diagnosis. These are detailed in the corresponding chapters: porencephaly in Chap. 14, schizencephaly in Chap. 9, interhemispheric cysts in Chap. 8 and posterior fossa cysts in Chap. 12. To these should be added the tumours in which the cystic component predominates (notably teratomas), which may be difficult to distinguish from arachnoid cysts.

Arachnoid Cysts

Arachnoid cysts account for approximately 1% of nontraumatic intracranial space-occupying lesions in the postnatal neuroradiological and neurosurgical literature [26]. With the exception of interhemispheric cysts associated with CCA, which belong to a distinct class of disease, arachnoid cysts are rarely observed in antenatal examinations. Most publications on the subject are based either on case reports or rather small series.

Description

Congenital arachnoid cysts develop from a splitting of the arachnoid membrane, their walls are made up of arachnoid cells [24–30]. The cells lining the cyst have organelles and an enzymatic activity specialized in a secretory function; they can therefore secrete CSF, which accumulates inside the cyst [28]. The cysts are independent of the ventricular system [27], but they may communicate with the subarachnoid space [29, 31].

Congenital cysts must be distinguished from those arachnoid cysts secondary to an infection, haemorrhage or trauma [24, 27, 28, 30, 31].

Location and Sex

Most arachnoid cysts are supratentorial (approximately 90%) [26], most frequently in the sylvian fissures and in the inferior and anterior parts of the temporal fossa (50%–65%) [32]. Arachnoid cysts can also be observed in the suprasellar region (5%–10%), the quadrigeminal cistern (5%–10%) or at the convexity (5%) [26].

These figures were taken from the postnatal literature. Actually, in a recent antenatal series [33], temporal cysts were exceptional (1.8%), cysts of the tentorial notch were not rare (15%) and cysts of the posterior fossa accounted for 22% of cases. The authors suggest that temporal cysts, which are frequent in the postnatal period, are probably not congenital, and that cysts of the tentorial notch, which are less frequently observed in children than in fetuses, may sometimes disappear postnatally. We have personally observed two cases of temporal cysts diagnosed postnatally in children whose mothers had undergone fetal MRI examination for ventricular dilatation. Even a posteriori, we could not tell whether the cyst was present in the antenatal period because of the significant physiological widening of the fetus's temporal pericerebral space. This might in any case constitute an alternative explanation for the difference in frequency observed between antenatal and postnatal studies.

Several antenatal studies (notably [31]) have noted a clear male predominance among the fetuses with arachnoid cysts. This male predominance is at the limit of significance in another study [33], in which the authors ascribe it to the fact that some traumas more frequent in male patients lead to the fortuitous discovery of cysts after birth, or to their clinical decompensation.

Stage of Discovery

Most arachnoid cysts reported in the literature were detected after 20 weeks of gestation. The detection of a cyst of the posterior fossa at 18 weeks of gestation [34] and five cases diagnosed before 20 weeks of gestation in a series of 15 arachnoid cysts [31] must, however, be cited. In a large series of 54 intracranial cysts [33], 55% had been diagnosed between 20 and 30 weeks of gestation and 45% after 30 weeks of gestation. According to the authors, this can be ascribed to the late development of some lesions, and notably arachnoid cysts consecutive to an inflammation or a haemorrhage.

Ultrasonographic Diagnosis

Arachnoid cysts are described as homogeneous anechoic structures with a distinct, thin wall [24, 26, 27, 31, 34]. In some rather rare occurrences, there may be lobulations [31] or intracystic septa [24]. No vascularization is shown with Doppler imaging.

In some cases, the fact that a cyst is extracerebral and distinct from the ventricular system is not clearly seen in US examinations [24].

False images of intracranial cysts have been reported many times [35, 36]. They were ascribed to ultrasonographic artefacts; hence the necessity of taking slices in many different planes.

Hydrocephaly and macrocrania are frequently encountered in the neonatal period [30]. These signs are, however, not always present, depending on the location of the cyst. There may also be a mass effect on the adjacent ventricular structures or the midline [27, 29], or ventriculomegaly by compression of the aqueduct [25], particularly for the cysts located in the suprasellar or quadrigeminal cisterns [26] or in the tentorial notch [33]. In an antenatal series of 54 arachnoid cysts [33], only 16.6% of fetuses had ventricular dilatation. There did not seem to be a correlation between the volume of the cyst and the size of the ventricles. Other authors [24] have made the opposite observation; they found that ventriculomegaly was always associated with voluminous cysts.

Arachnoid cysts can be multiple, notably on the midline [26]. The discovery of an interhemispheric cyst associated with corpus callosum agenesis raises the question of the cyst's nature. It seems indeed that many interhemispheric cysts are not proper arachnoid cysts in this context, but rather more like expansions of the dilated third ventricle, and that actual interhemispheric arachnoid cysts are rare [26].

Ultrasonography also makes it possible to evaluate the malformations potentially associated with the arachnoid cyst: Fallot's tetralogy, sacrococcygeal tumour, septal agenesis, syndactylism and arteriovenous malformation [27]. In the postnatal literature, we noted a high occurrence rate of arachnoid cysts in patients with autosomal dominant polycystic kidney disease (up to 8 % of patients) [28]. It seems, however, that these findings are not transposable to the fetus, since this association has, to our knowledge, never been reported in antenatal studies. Actually, most of the cysts diagnosed in the antenatal period are isolated. Some rare karyotypic abnormalities such as unbalanced translocation [34] have been reported in the absence of associated abnormalities. On the karyotypes of 40 fetuses with isolated intracranial cysts, no abnormality was observed [33].

Contribution of Fetal MRI

The question of the role of fetal MRI has been poorly addressed in the antenatal literature, with the exception of one recent series [33]. The following considerations are based on this article and on our own experience involving 15 cases.

MRI can play a major part in the precise localization of the cyst and the determination of its relations with the adjacent cerebral structures, notably with the ventricular system (Figs. 3–5). Indeed, as we have mentioned above, these structures may be difficult to evaluate precisely in US. This is all the more difficult indeed when the cyst is voluminous, superficial or located into the posterior fossa or in the supratentorial space. The distinct issue of cysts of the posterior fossa is addressed in Chap. 12.

Fetal MRI can also help reveal the nature of the cyst, as it distinguishes between arachnoid cysts, porencephalic cysts and schizencephaly by bringing to light pericystic gliosis (T2 hyperintense), abnormal sulci or signs of haemorrhage. The presence of a tissue component associated with the cyst could be one element suggesting a teratoma.

Likewise, the detection of heterotopias and corpus callosum agenesis would suggest a glioependymal cyst rather than an arachnoid cyst.

On a macroscopic level, these cysts look identical. Only in histology can they be distinguished from one another, as the former are lined with ependyma. Glioependymal cysts are much less frequent than arachnoid cysts; they can also be located in the supratentorial space or in the posterior fossa. In this

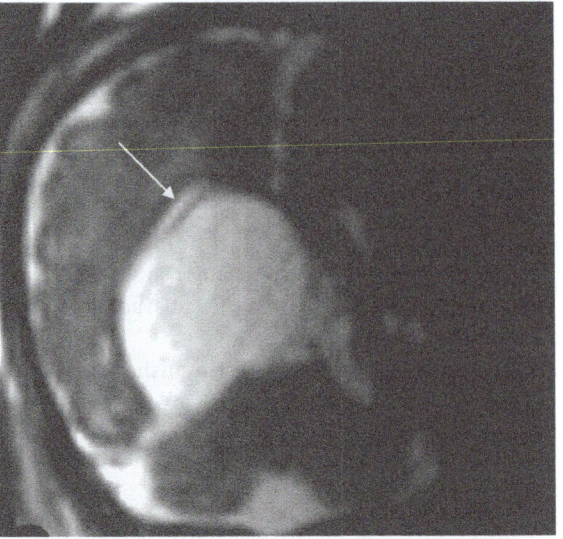

a

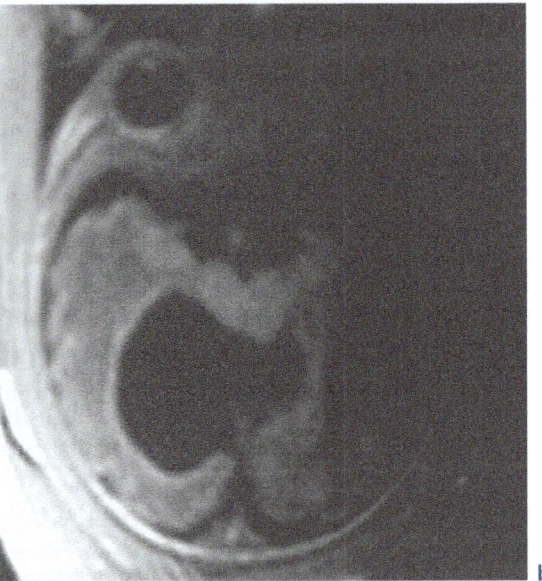

b

Fig. 3 a, b. Arachnoid cyst of the tentorial notch. Detection at 33 weeks of gestation of a right medial occipital cystic formation difficult to distinguish from the right lateral ventricle. **a, b** Fetal MRI performed at 34 weeks of gestation. T2-weighted posterior coronal slice (**a**) and T1-weighted axial slice (**b**). An apparently isolated cyst of the tentorial notch displaces the right atrium (*arrow*). Postnatal MRI confirms the antenatal data. The arachnoid cyst is stable. At 18 months, the child's psychomotor development is normal

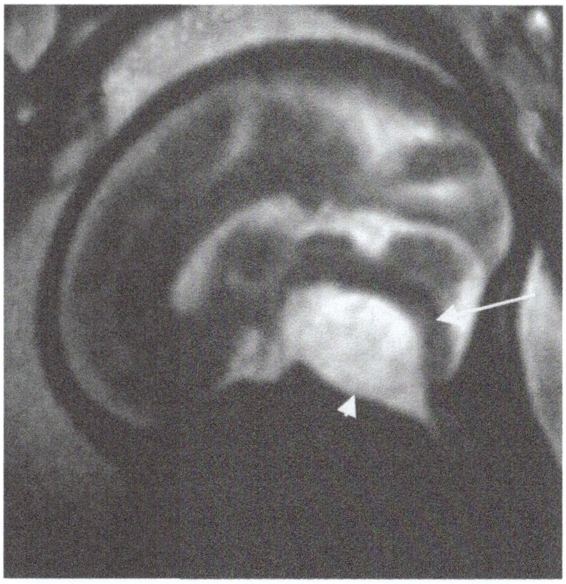

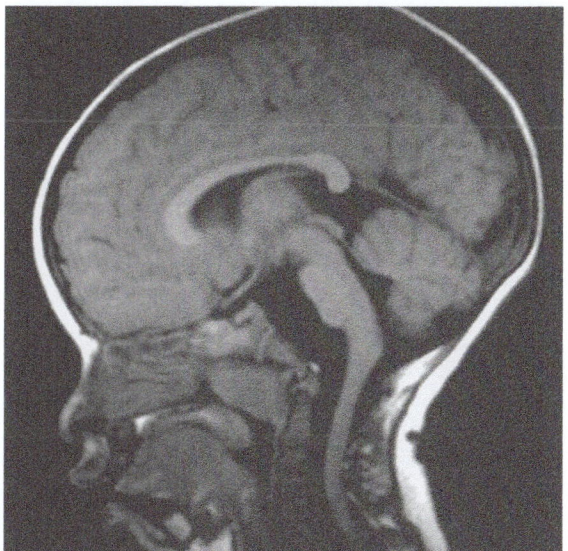

Fig. 4 a–g. Arachnoid cyst of the posterior fossa. Detection in US at 27 weeks of gestation of a cystic lesion of the posterior fossa, difficult to localize with respect to the different components of the posterior fossa. **a, b** Fetal MRI at 27.5 weeks of gestation. T2-weighted midline sagittal slice (**a**) and axial slice at the level of the posterior fossa (**b**). The hyperintense cyst (*arrowhead*) is in the retroclival region; it displaces the brain stem to the back and to the right (*arrow*); the protruding bulge of the pons has disappeared. **c, d** MRI at 8 months. T1-weighted midline sagittal slice (**c**) and T2-weighted axial slice (**d**): the mass effect on the pons is still present. **e** MRI at 18 months. T1-weighted midline sagittal slice: the cyst has decreased in size and the bulge is beginning to appear.
Fig. 4 f, g. See next page

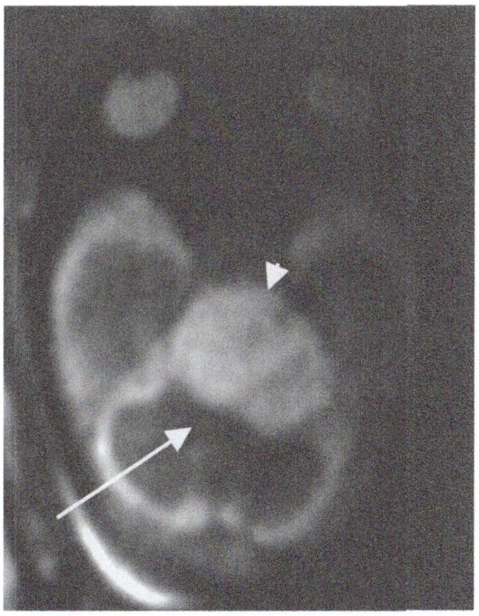

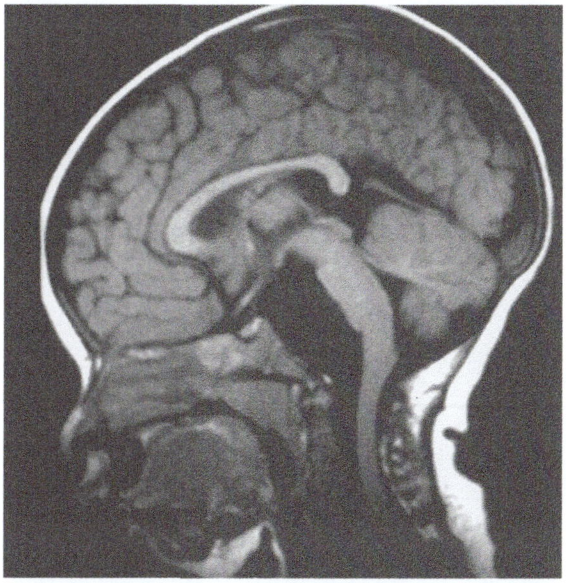

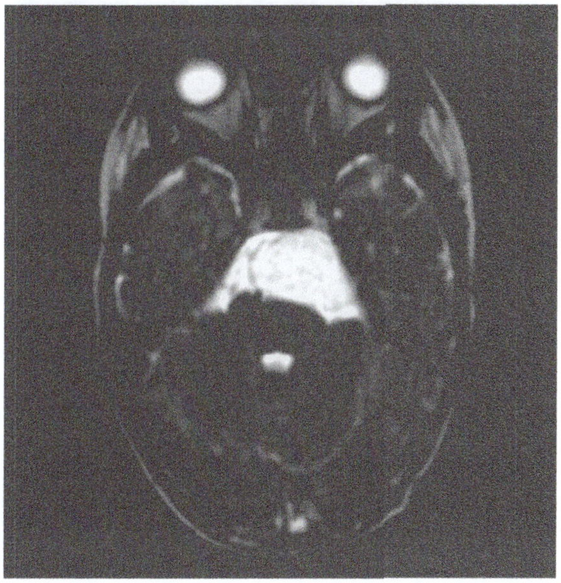

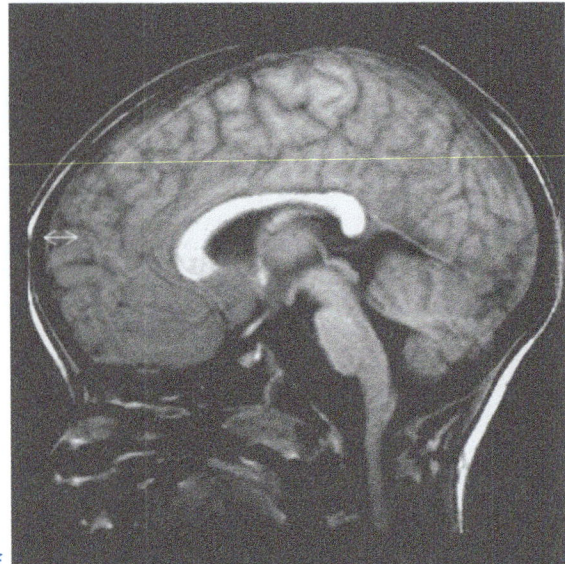

f

Fig. 5 a–f. Arachnoid cyst of the quadrigeminal cistern. Patient ▶
sent to MRI following the detection in US at 38 weeks of gestation of a cystic lesion of the midline at the junction between
the middle and the posterior parts. **a** US taken at 38 weeks of
gestation. Axial slice showing the midline cystic formation (*arrow*) at the back of the thalami (*arrowheads*). **b–d** Fetal MRI at
38 weeks of gestation. T2-weighted midline sagittal (**b**) and
posterior coronal (**c**) slices, T1-weighted axial slice (**d**). At the
back of the third ventricle, there is a cystic formation (*arrow*)
measuring 20 mm in diameter that recalls an arachnoid cyst of
the quadrigeminal cistern. **e** Postnatal MRI at 2 months. T2-
weighted midline sagittal slice confirming the antenatal data.
The cyst exerts a mass effect on the quadrigeminal plate (*arrow*) and on the corpus callosum splenium (*arrowhead*). **f** Follow-up MRI at 3 years. T2-weighted midline sagittal slice. The
cyst is distinctly smaller and the mass effect on the adjacent
structures is clearly less visible. The psychomotor development at 3 years is normal

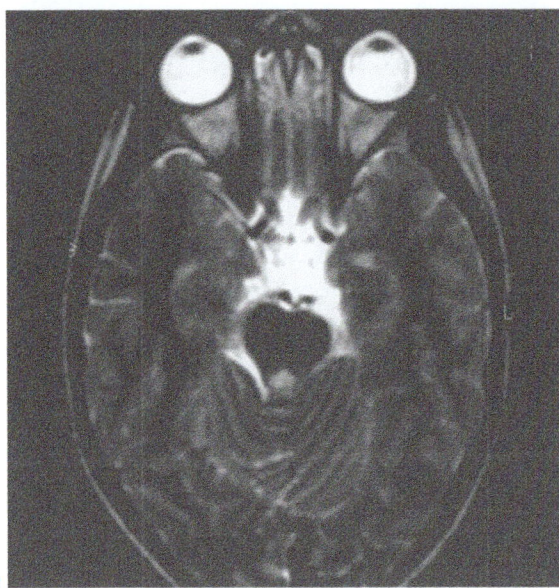

g

Fig. 4 f, g. T1-weighted midline sagittal slice (**f**) and T2-weight-
ed axial slice (**g**) at 4.5 years. A slight mass effect persists on
the pons; the cyst is distinctly smaller. The psychomotor development of the child at 6 years is normal

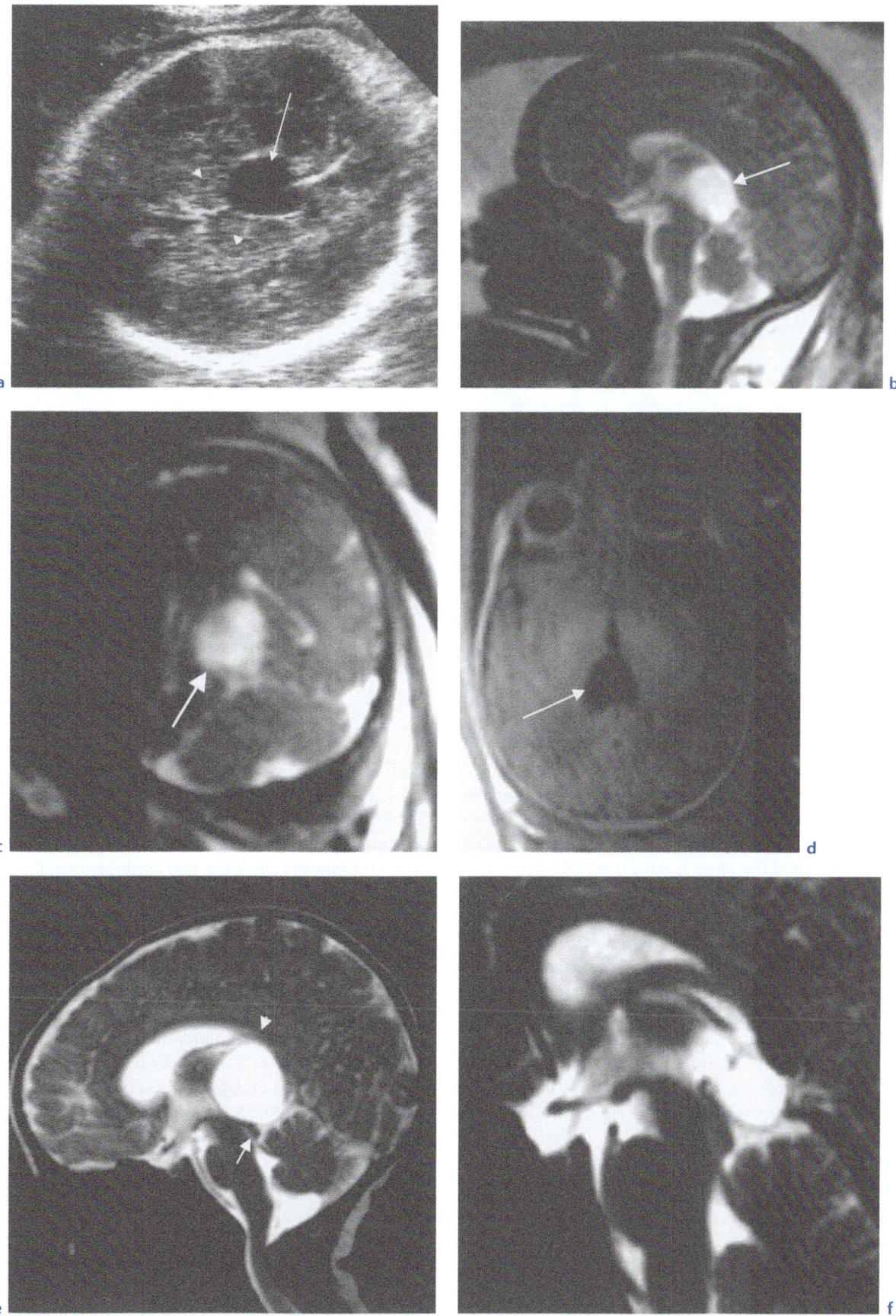

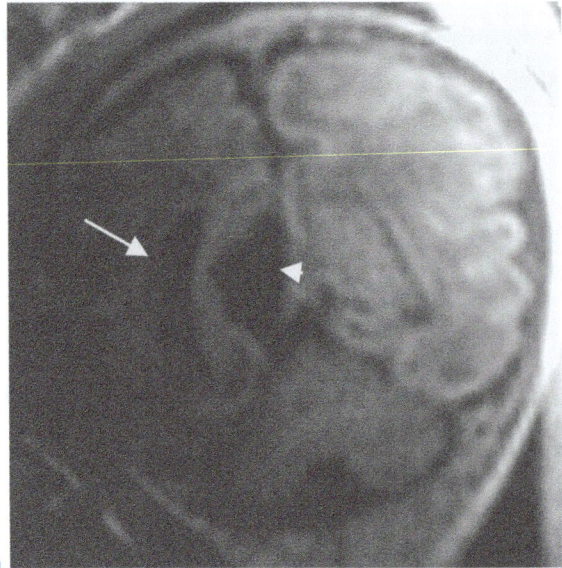

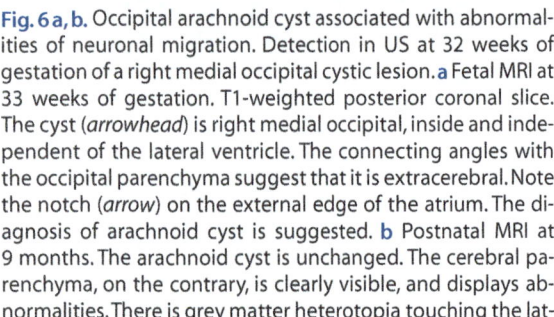

a

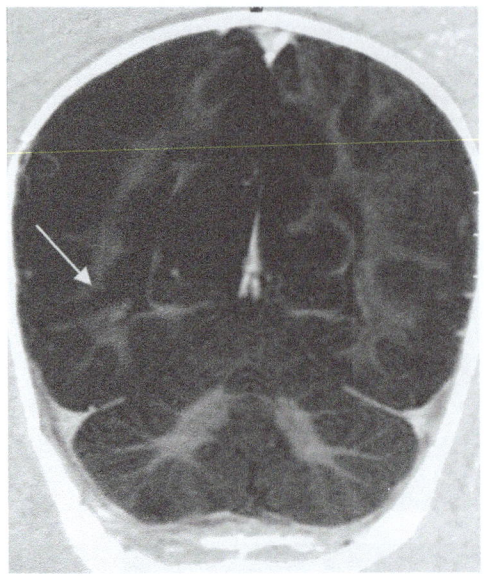

b

Fig. 6 a, b. Occipital arachnoid cyst associated with abnormalities of neuronal migration. Detection in US at 32 weeks of gestation of a right medial occipital cystic lesion. a Fetal MRI at 33 weeks of gestation. T1-weighted posterior coronal slice. The cyst (*arrowhead*) is right medial occipital, inside and independent of the lateral ventricle. The connecting angles with the occipital parenchyma suggest that it is extracerebral. Note the notch (*arrow*) on the external edge of the atrium. The diagnosis of arachnoid cyst is suggested. b Postnatal MRI at 9 months. The arachnoid cyst is unchanged. The cerebral parenchyma, on the contrary, is clearly visible, and displays abnormalities. There is grey matter heterotopia touching the lat-

eral ventricle (which probably corresponds to the notch seen in antenatal examination), with a band of grey matter stretching from the cortex to the right atrium, reminiscent of closed-lip schizencephaly (*arrow*). Another subependymal heterotopia (not shown) is present at the level of the right frontal horn. At 2.5 years, the psychomotor development is satisfactory on motor and comprehension skills, but there is a slight retardation in language acquisition. Note that here, the fetal MRI examination was done using a 0.5-T MRI unit. Thin slices taken on a 1.5-T MRI unit may have shown evidence of the abnormalities overlooked here

last occurrence, an intracerebellar location is particularly suggestive of the diagnosis [25]. Some cerebellar migration abnormalities associated with a supratentorial glioependymal cyst have been reported [25].

One could therefore assume that MRI might point to this aetiology by revealing the above-mentioned cerebral abnormalities, these being more easily diagnosed in MRI than in US. This distinction, however, is purely academic, and carries no consequences when the cyst is isolated, since nothing currently sets the prognoses of these two entities apart.

However, the resolution of fetal MRI is not limitless, and some heterotopias, some discreet cortical malformations or small abnormalities of the white matter can be overlooked [33] (Fig. 6).

Progression and Prognosis of Arachnoid Cysts

Our knowledge of the antenatal natural history of arachnoid cysts is incomplete. Some cysts have a close communication with the cerebrospinal fluid that accumulates inside the cyst, causing it to expand. This phenomenon has only been reported on a sporadic basis (one case [31], three cases of voluminous cysts [24], two other cases [29, 30]). In a large antenatal series, approximately 20 % of cysts increase in volume during pregnancy [33]. Some cysts remain unchanged throughout pregnancy and start expanding after birth. This increase in volume seems to be more frequent with interhemispheric cysts and with cysts at the base of the skull. Regression of the cyst is more often observed after birth (24 %) than before (3.7 %). It might result from a spontaneous rupture of the cyst into either the subarachnoid space or the ventricles [33].

The prognosis is directly dependent on the abnormalities associated with the cyst [33, 37]. In most cas-

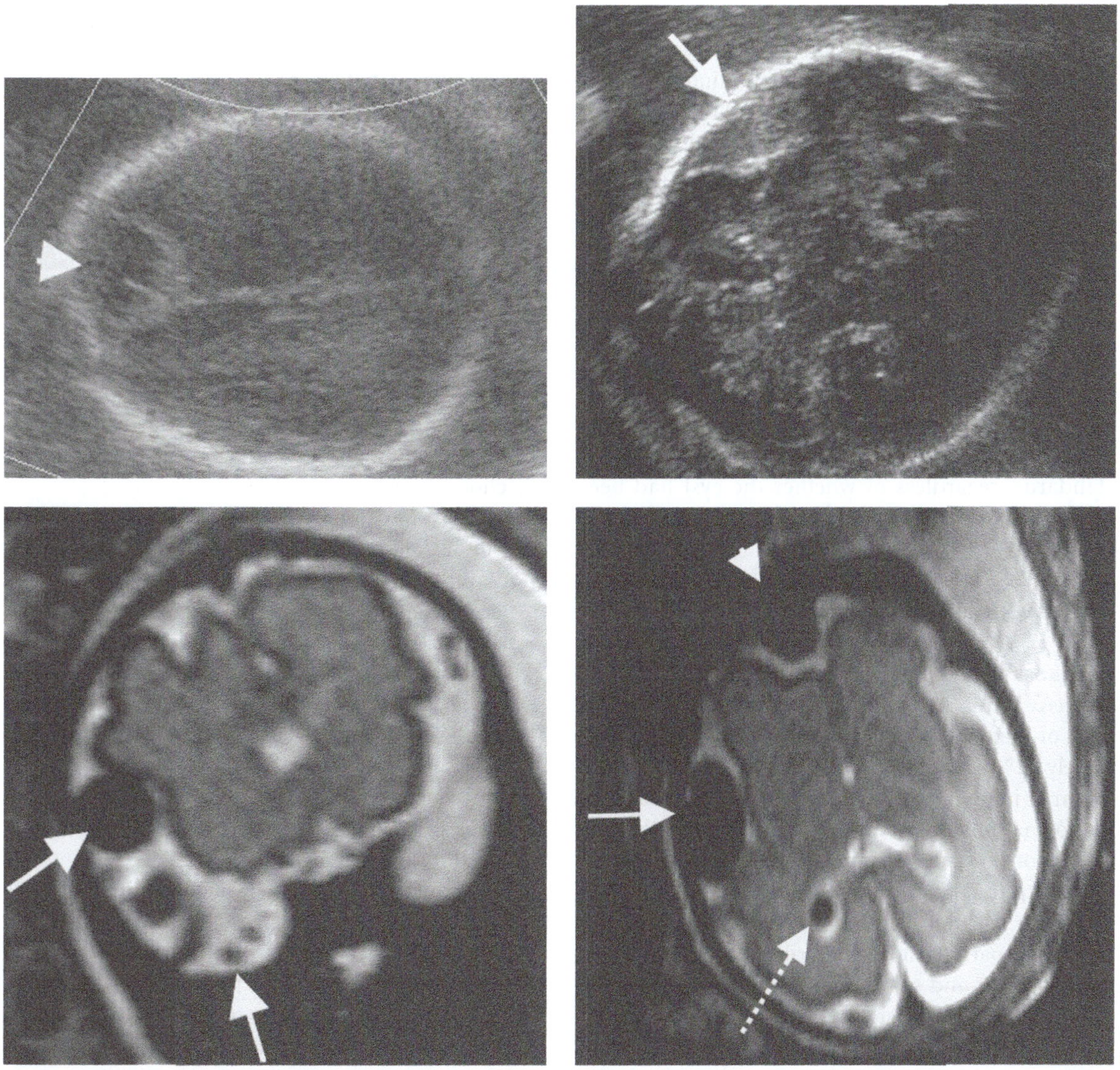

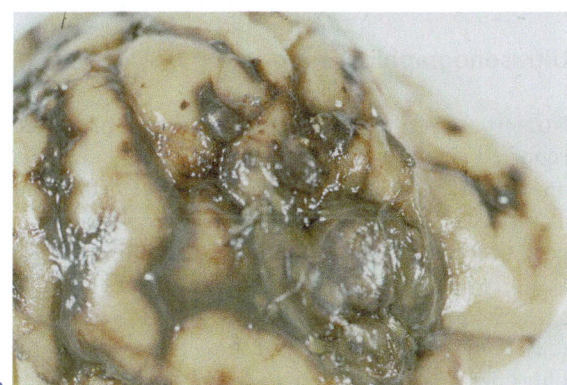

Fig. 7a–e. Pericerebral vascular malformation. **a, b** Fetus at 28 weeks of gestation. US axial slice at the level of the vertex (**a**) and temporal slice at the level of the temporal lobes (**b**). They show an extracerebral right paramedian frontal space-occupying lesion (*arrowhead*). It is heterogeneous, hyperechoic in the periphery and hypoechoic in the centre and not vascularized on Doppler examination. In addition, there is a nonvascularized hyperechoic space-occupying lesion in the right sylvian fissure (*arrow*). **c, d** Fetal MRI at 28 weeks of gestation. T2-weighted anterior coronal (**c**) and axial (**d**) slices. The vascular malformation manifests itself in the presence of dilated vessels in the pericerebral space. In the front, the superior longitudinal sinus is hyperintense and dilated (*arrowhead*). Numerous vessels (*arrows*), void of signal, are seen in the right sylvian fissure and under the right temporal lobe. Additionally, the right choroid plexus has increased in volume and appears in T2-hyposignal (and T1-hypersignal, not shown) (*dotted arrow*). The absence of satisfactory growth of the fetal brain between two successive MRI examinations, and the uncertainty concerning the frontal gyration around the malformation led to suggesting termination of pregnancy. It was terminated at 31 weeks of gestation, and the autopsy revealed a meningeal vascular malformation with haemorrhagic complications. **e** Oblique view of the right sylvian fissure. Voluminous thrombosed vessel of the sylvian fissure, suggesting a vascular malformation

es of isolated cysts, the prognosis is good. Some seizures, headaches and sometimes hemiparesis have been described in relation with voluminous cysts of the middle cerebral fossa. Intracranial hypertension, developmental retardation and abnormalities of the hypothalamo-pituitary axis can be observed in association with suprasellar cysts [28]. The placement of a cystoperitoneal shunt or a ventriculocystostomy is sometimes necessary ([27], in 28 % of children [33], [37]). It seems that temporal arachnoid cysts can be accompanied by memory and cognitive disorders, which regress in the postoperative period [38]. In a postnatal follow-up of cysts that had been diagnosed in the antenatal period [33], the children's development and intelligence quotients were comparable to standards, regardless of whether the cyst had been drained or not.

Arteriovenous Malformations

The most frequent type of arteriovenous malformation (AVM) is the aneurysmal malformation of the vein of Galen (VGAM), which represents approximately 92 % of the antenatal AVMs reported in the literature (in 1995 [39]). The other cerebral vascular malformations observed in fetuses are mostly malformations of a dural sinus [40]; pial AVMs are usually exceptional in the antenatal period [40].

These vascular malformations have a common particular pattern in US (described for VGAM in the next section) and share the same risk of fetal heart failure and vascular steal phenomena (see "Vein of Galen Aneurysmal Malformation").

In two cases of antenatal AVM reported in the literature that did not affect the vein of Galen [41, 42], the lesion was located at the frontal level. In the first case [41], the AVM was detected at 23.5 weeks of gestation; it was accompanied by heart failure and mild left ventriculomegaly.

A cystic mass with a turbulent flow was discovered in the frontal lobe. The autopsy revealed that it was a leptomeningeal mass with dilated dural sinuses and a left frontoparietal haematoma, hence probably a malformation of a dural sinus. The diagnosis of such vascular malformations very probably benefits greatly from fetal MRI, as MR images show the dilatation of the vessels in the pericerebral space. This has been the case twice in our experience (Fig. 7).

Vein of Galen Aneurysmal Malformation

Anatomical Substratum

The term "vein of Galen aneurysmal malformation" (VGAM) in the literature actually corresponds to diverse entities. A distinction should indeed be made between [40, 43, 44]:

- A VGAM corresponding to a dilatation of the median prosencephalic vein, embryological precursor of the vein of Galen. This dilatation is associated either with arteriovenous fistulas in the vein wall (mural type) or with numerous shunts communicating with the anterior part of the vein (choroid type).
- A pial AVM drained by the true, i. e. fully formed, vein of Galen. This type is rare in neonates and in infants and, it seems, exceptional in the antenatal period, these AVMs essentially developing postnatally [40]. We have observed three such cases.
- A vein of Galen varix with no associated AVM that can be observed in postnatal examination, but this type has not been reported in antenatal examinations.

Only the first type of VGAM is further described in this section.

The principal feeding arteries are the choroidal, anterior cerebral and transmesencephalic arteries [45]. Venous drainage is usually in the falcine sinus or in other embryonic sinuses. The right sinus may be absent or thrombosed. This type of AVM shows a marked male predominance [40, 45].

Ultrasonographic Diagnosis

Numerous cases of US diagnoses of VGAM have been reported in the antenatal literature [24, 39, 42–44, 46–49]. In US, VGAM is almost always detected after 28 weeks of gestation (two-thirds after 34 weeks of gestation [39]); this also applied to Lasjaunias's series [40]. Two early diagnoses have been reported at 22 weeks of gestation [44] and 24 weeks of gestation [24]. For the great majority of these fetuses, sonographies performed as early as 4 weeks [42] prior to the diagnosis were considered normal.

The VGAM is located on the midline, behind the third ventricle. It is oval-shaped, it communicates with a tubular structure behind it (corresponding to a drainage venous sinus), which gives an overall aspect classically described as a keyhole pattern. The VGAM is anechoic, and could therefore be mistaken with other cysts, notably with arachnoid cysts. The Doppler mode reveals the presence of a flow inside the VGAM. Colour Doppler shows the afferent and efferent vessels (see "Anatomical Substratum" above). Pulse Doppler shows an arterial-type flow in the afferent vessels, a venous-type flow in the efferent vessels, and a mixed, arterial and venous flow inside the VGAM. The drainage veins are generally much easier to spot than the afferent arteries. The cerebral evaluation of VGAM in US must also include a thorough study of the cerebral parenchyma, looking for ischaemic lesions, and notably for those linked with a vascular steal phenomenon, which jeopardizes the brain vascularization by diverting the blood flow towards the VGAM and therefore has a decisive influence on prognosis (see "Progression of VGAM and Prognosis" above) [46].

Macrocrania is also sometimes present [40].

In the 23 cases of the literature reported by Sepulveda et al. [39], 17 fetuses showed associated abnormalities: ventricular dilatation, cardiomegaly and dilatation of the neck vessels.

Ventricular dilatation was observed in four cases. Its mechanism remains a moot point: some ascribe it to a direct compression by the malformation on the aqueduct [39], while others suggest that since the aqueduct is in most cases permeable [40], ventricular dilatation may result from an increase in venous pressure hindering the resorption of CSF [39, 40, 45]. It could also be caused in vacuo by clastic lesions [44].

Cardiomegaly is observed in 60% of cases [39]; it is an essential element of the prognosis, as we will see below. In a series of 18 cases diagnosed with VGAM in antenatal examination [50], 17 were born with mild heart failure, although cardiomegaly had only been diagnosed in four of the fetuses. It should be remembered here that the discovery of cardiomegaly of unknown origin in a fetus must be followed by a search for an arteriovenous shunt, notably a cerebral one.

Dilatation of the neck vessels is observed in 26% of cases; to some, it is a very good sign of a cerebral AVM [39].

Other less frequent abnormalities are sometimes observed [39]: hydramnios, hepatomegaly, ascites and intrauterine growth restriction.

Contribution of Fetal MRI

A few fetal MRI observations of VGAM have been reported in either single cases or series [40, 43, 45, 49, 51–54]. The contribution of MRI is not always stated. We have personally observed five cases (Fig. 8).

As always, the advantage of MRI resides in the possibility of taking slices in the three planes of space, whatever the position of the fetus's head. Therefore, it facilitates the analysis of the vascular malformation, and the afferent arteries are also probably more clearly visible than in US [45]. On both T1- and T2-weighted slices, the vein of Galen aneurysmal dilatation, as well as the arteries and the veins, are void of signal. The acquisition of cerebral angiography sequences is possible in the antenatal period. The morphology of the dilated vein and of the drainage venous sinuses is identical to that described in US.

The main assets of MRI, however, certainly remain the better analysis of the cerebral parenchyma, and the opportunity to look for ischaemic-haemorrhagic lesions [43], which greatly influence the prognosis. These lesions may have diverse appearances, depending on their type and age: cerebral atrophy with widened subarachnoid space [45], periventricular leucomalacia lesions [46] in T1 hypersignal or hyposignal, depending on whether there are any calcifications, and in T2 hypersignal. Areas of cortical necrosis and polymicrogyria may also be observed. In fact, every type of ischaemia and haemorrhage described in Chap. 14 is possible.

MRI also provides a good analysis of the corpus callosum, which may be very thin (Fig. 8). Delayed development of the corpus callosum is observed postnatally in this type of malformation [40].

When taking an antenatal MRI of a fetus with a VGAM, it is, as a rule, more useful to look for cerebral lesions that would definitively jeopardize the child's neurological future than to establish a precise mapping of the malformation, as this can be done postnatally.

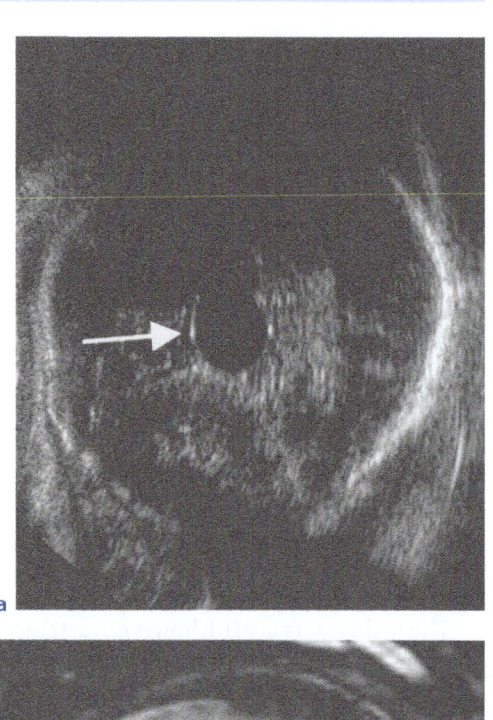

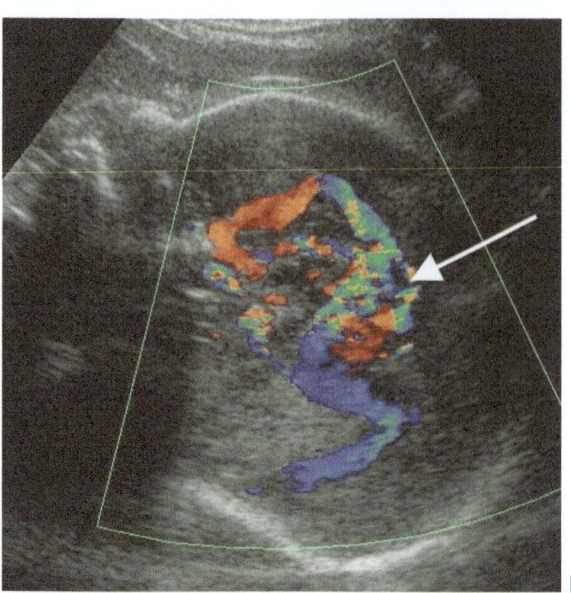

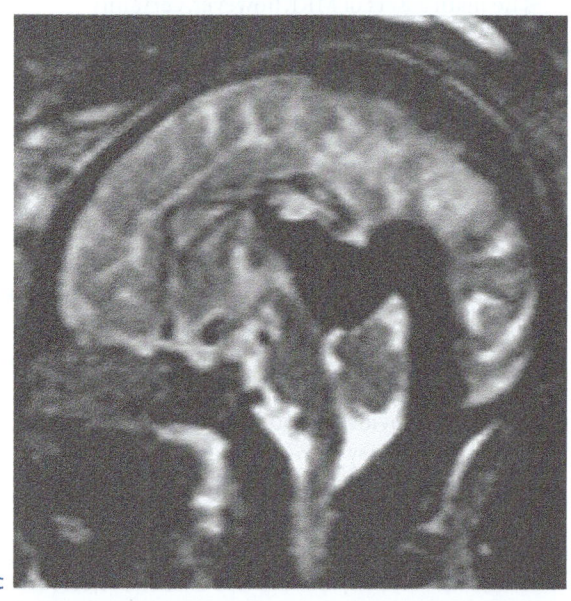

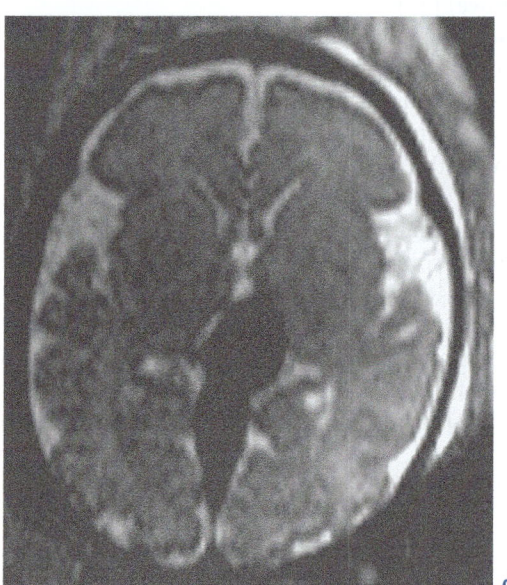

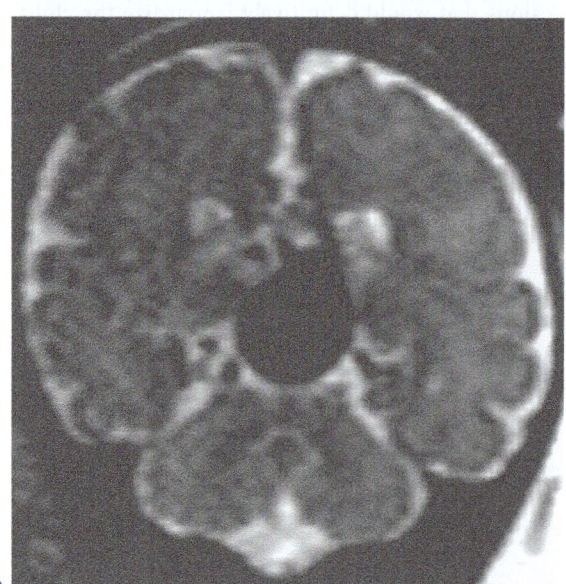

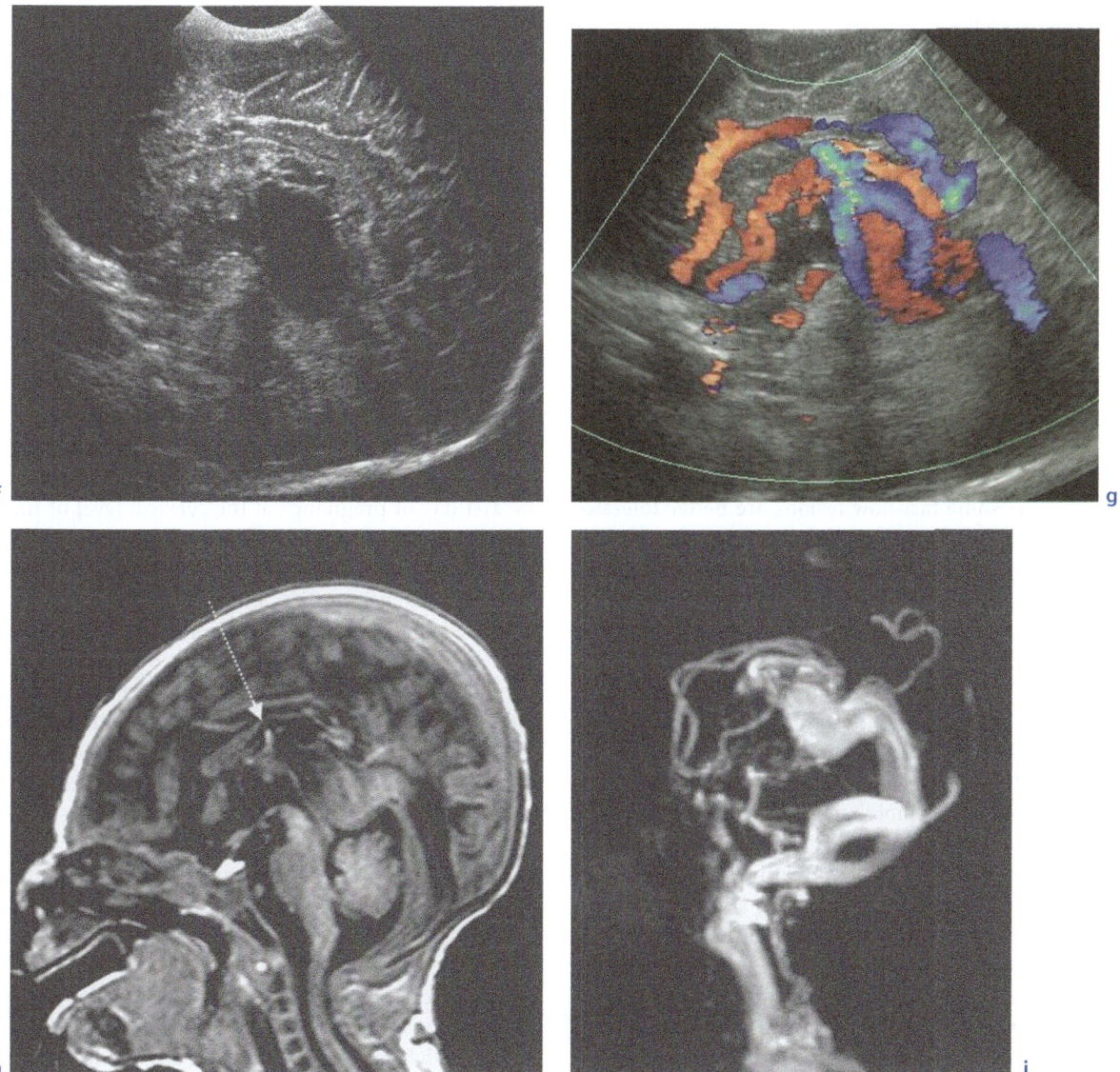

Fig. 8a–i. Vein of Galen aneurysmal malformation. **a, b** Ultrasonography at 35 weeks of gestation. Posterior coronal slice (**a**): midline oval-shaped cystic mass (*arrow*) at the back of the third ventricle. Midline sagittal slice with colour Doppler (**b**): the afferent arteries (anterior cerebral and anterior choroidal arteries) appear in red. The flow inside the malformation is turbulent (*arrow*). The venous drainage (*in blue*) is clearly visible in the falcine sinus. **c–e** Fetal MRI at 35 weeks of gestation. T2-weighted sagittal (**c**), axial (**d**) and coronal (**e**) slices. The different elements of the VGAM are void of signal. The axial slice displays the typical keyhole pattern. This fetus also showed mild cardiomegaly. Given the absence of major cardiac repercus-sions and the absence of abnormalities of the cerebral paren-chyma, the pregnancy was pursued. The child was born at 38 weeks of gestation with no sign of heart failure. **f, g** Postnatal transfontanellar US on the 2nd day of life. Midline sagittal slice without (**f**) and with Doppler (**g**), in an aspect superimposable on the antenatal sonography (**b**). **h, i** Postnatal MRI on the 4th day of life. T1-weighted midline sagittal slice (**h**) and MR angiography sequence on a sagittal slice (**i**). The corpus callosum is thin (*dotted arrow*). No abnormality of the cerebral parenchyma's signal is detected on this examination. The vascular mapping of the malformation confirms the antenatal data. Note the dilatation of the jugular veins

Progression of VGAM and Prognosis

Without postnatal treatment, the spontaneous thrombosis of the VGAM is rare (4% in Lasjaunias's series [40]), and it is not necessarily the sign of a good prognosis, as only two of the five children with a spontaneous thrombosis of the VGAM in this study enjoyed normal neurological development. One should therefore not wait for this hypothetical event to begin treatment.

In the absence of treatment, the mortality rate reaches 90%; the immediate postnatal progression is conditioned by the occurrence of heart failure [45].

It should be noted that the degree of heart failure is variable from one child to another, and that it seems to be independent of the characteristics of the shunt, as some fast-flow lesions are better tolerated than some seemingly small shunts. Therefore, the detailed analysis of the lesion cannot provide sufficient prognostic elements [40].

As seen above, VGAM may also be associated with ischaemic cerebral lesions, which can result from the following mechanisms: vascular steal phenomena, ischaemia or a decrease in cerebral perfusion linked to heart failure, venous thrombosis, or atrophy of the adjacent structures caused by compression. These lesions include haemorrhages, periventricular leucomalacia and laminar cortical necroses [45].

In the absence of early treatment, the surviving children may suffer from seizures and mental retardation. The rate of mental retardation is difficult to establish, since it takes into account cerebral lesions existing before treatment, the type and date of the treatment, and these details are not always stated. The rate is as high as 62% in some series [45]. Late endocrine manifestations such as precocious puberty and failure to thrive have also been described [40].

Cardiomegaly and the presence of antenatal ischaemic cerebral lesions are obviously arguments for a poor prognosis, whereas macrocrania is not. Diminished cerebral parameters, however, should lead to suspicion of cerebral atrophy [40].

Interestingly enough, when one compares a series of VGAM cases diagnosed in antenatal examinations [50] and other series of VGAM, the percentage of patients with irreversible cerebral lesions is relatively stable (22% vs 25%). These 22% of neonates die shortly after birth. For the remaining 78%, however, the antenatal diagnosis helps to better determine the time at which the malformation should be treated, thus improving neurological progression (88% good neurological progression in the antenatal diagnosis series vs 78% in the other series) [40].

The treatment is based on an embolization aimed at the definitive occlusion of the fistulas, while preserving the normal vascularization of the brain [40, 45]. Surgical treatment is difficult, dangerous and often incomplete [45]. Among Lasjaunias's series of 78 embolized children [40], the mortality rate was 9%.

Meningocoeles and Encephalocoeles

Definition, Description of the Malformation and Epidemiology

Meningocoeles and encephalocoeles are neural tube closure abnormalities. The closure normally starts on the 21st day of pregnancy at the cervical level of the embryo. The closure of the anterior neuropore takes place on the 24th day, and that of the posterior neuropore intervenes on the 26th day [55]. It has been suggested that these malformations may also result from a secondary lesion occurring on an initially normal neural tube [56]. The term "cephalocoele" corresponds to the protrusion of any one intracranial element through a congenital defect of the skull, whether at the base or on the vault [56]. There are two types [57, 58]:

- The meningocoele, a protrusion of meninges only
- The encephalocoele, a hernia of the cerebral parenchyma

Some authors [58] introduced an additional subtlety by distinguishing between the encephalocoele, in which the herniated cerebral parenchyma displays a gyral pattern, and the cranial meningomyocoele, in which the neural tissue of the herniated sac shows

Fig. 9a–f. Nasofrontal encephalocoele. Detection in US at ▶ 25 weeks of gestation of a mixed mass containing anechoic and echoic structures above the root of the nose, with a supranasal bone defect. **a, b** MRI taken at 26 weeks of gestation. T2-weighted axial (**a**) and sagittal (**b**) slices. Presence of a mixed hyperintense and intermediary signal mass (*arrowhead*) isointense at the cerebral parenchyma. This mass is located above the nose and communicates with the encephalon through a frontal bone defect. Termination of pregnancy at 29 weeks of gestation. **c** T2-weighted midline sagittal slice. Post-termination of pregnancy MRI showing the same elements as the MRI done before. **d** Side view of the skull showing the frontal bone defect (*arrow*). **e** Fetus's profile: above the root of the nose, a prominent epidermized formation. **f** Side view of the brain showing the pedicle that links the encephalocoele with the frontal lobe

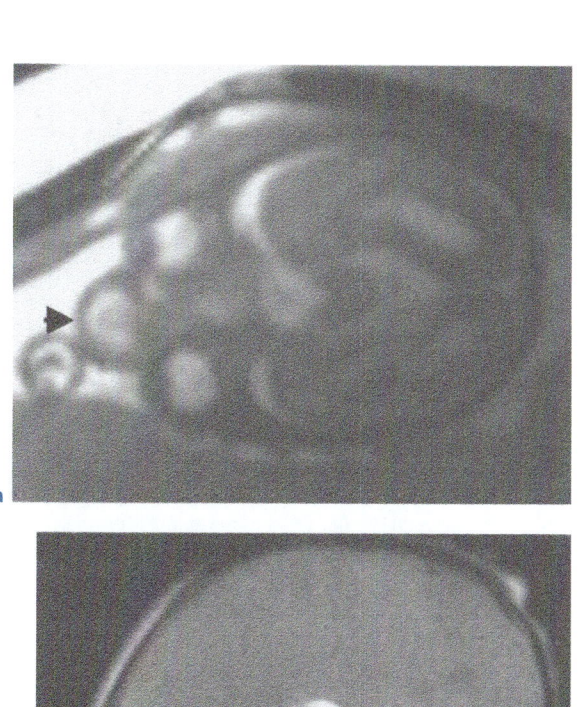

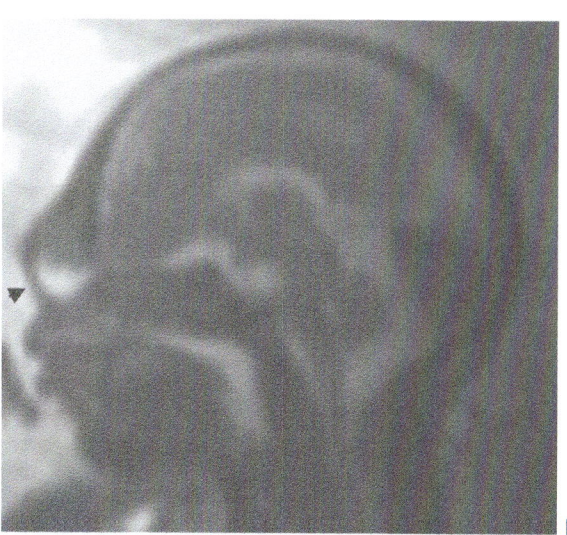

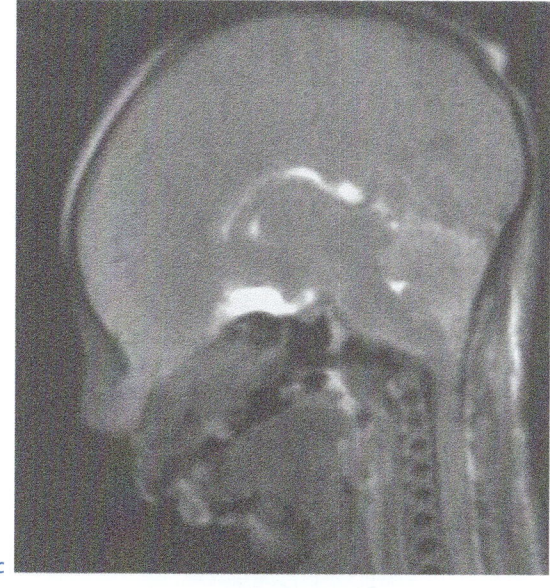

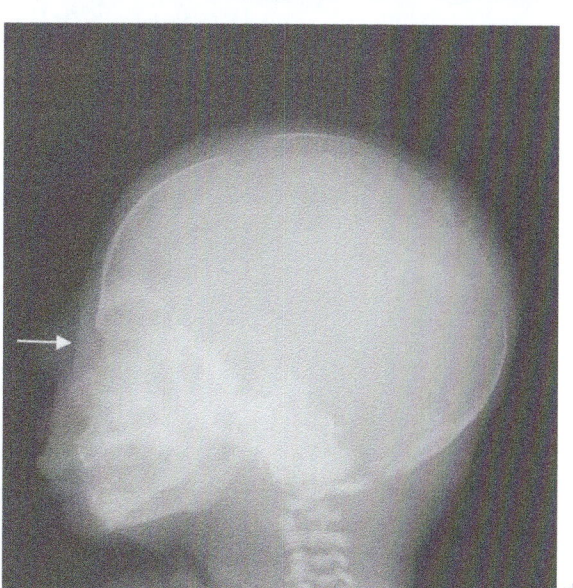

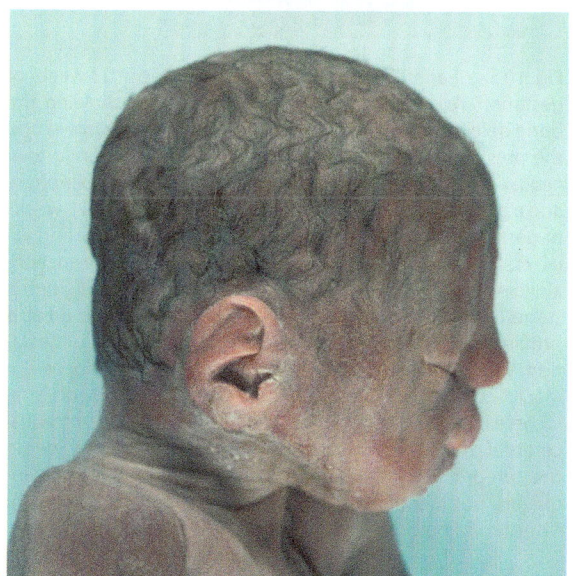

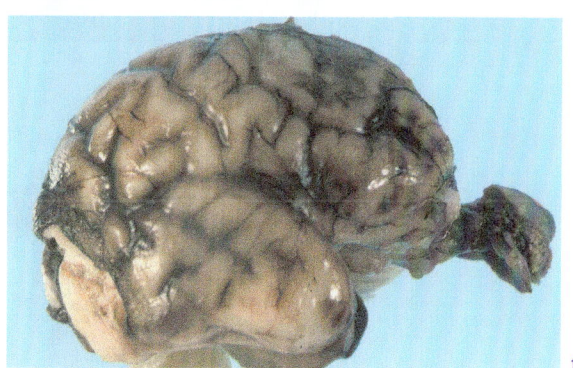

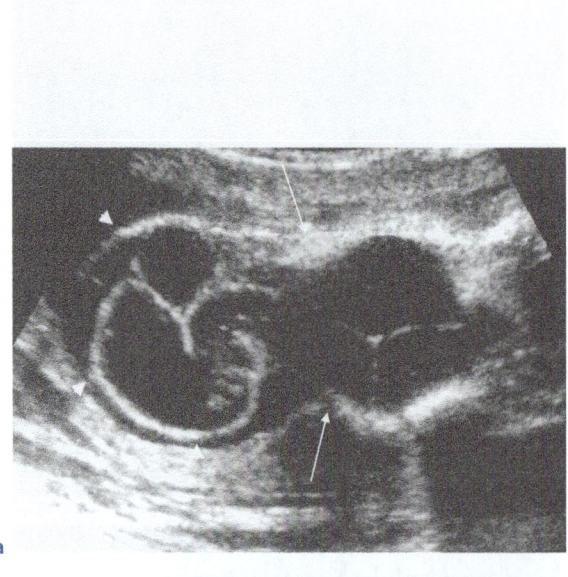

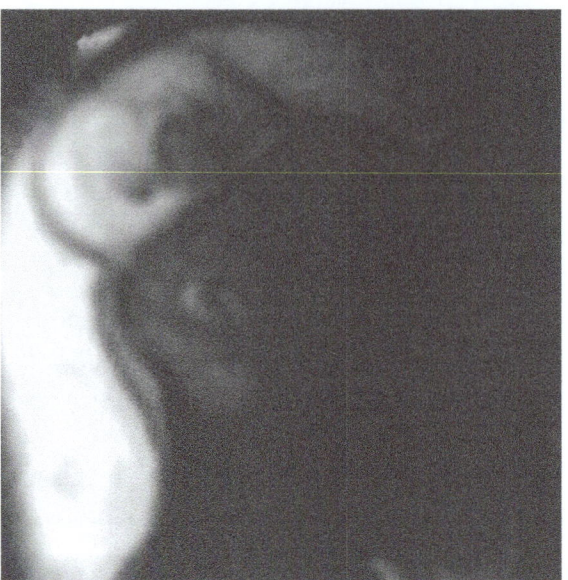

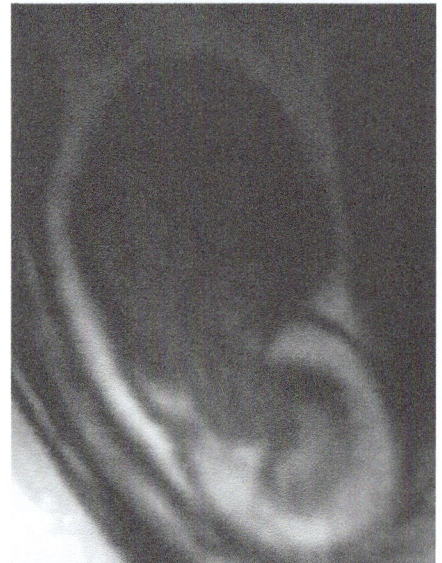

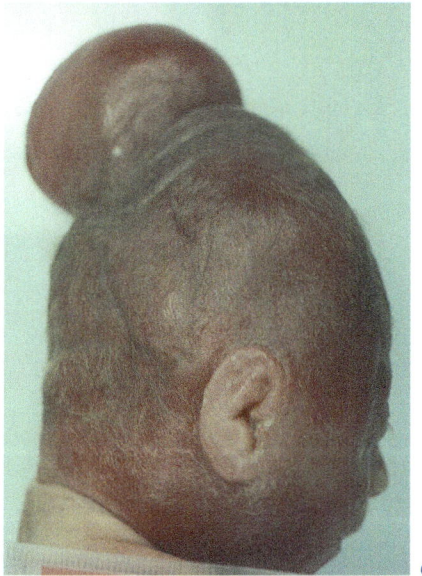

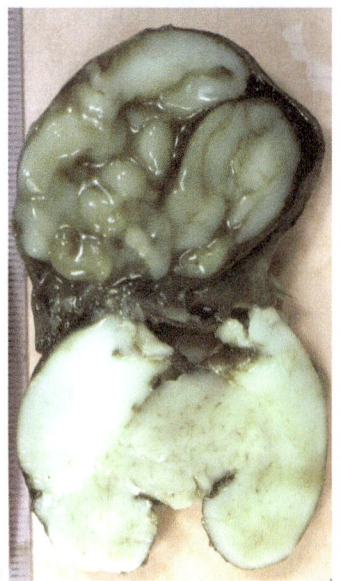

Fig. 10 a–e. Parietal encephalocoele. **a** US done at 23 weeks of gestation. Axial slice at the level of the vertex showing the bone defect of the cranial vault (delimited by the *arrows*) and the presence of a pericranial space-occupying lesion (*arrowheads*) of mixed echogenicity, with a hypoechoic periphery and a gyriform pattern in the centre. **b, c** Fetal MRI at 23 weeks of gestation: T2-weighted left paramedian sagittal (**b**) and axial (**c**) slices. The continuity between the brain and the encephalocoele is clearly visible. The pericerebral space is thin for the stage. No individual cerebral structure is identifiable. **d** Fetus profile after termination of pregnancy at 24 weeks of gestation. View of the left paramedian parietal encephalocoele. **e** Macroscopic view. Coronal slice. The contents of the encephalocoele display a gyriform structure. There is also substantial cerebral dysgenesis, with an absence of ventricular cavities in the cerebral hemispheres and fused thalami. The basal ganglia are not identifiable. The histological study shows major disorders of neuronal migration

neither a gyral pattern nor a clear link with the brain. In addition, the term "encephalocystomeningocoele" is used when the ventricles are at least partly included in the herniated sac [58]. The encephalocoele is usually covered with skin, which explains why a majority of these malformations are not accompanied by an increased alphafetoprotein level in the maternal serum [59].

These malformations are rare, and the occurrence rate of each type is difficult to assess, since the figures given in the literature concern the broader terms of "cephalocoeles" and "encephalocoeles", and therefore include different types of malformations. The frequency is estimated at approximately 0.8–3 cases per 10,000 births [57, 59–61].

Encephalocoeles represent roughly 5% of neural tube closure abnormalities [62]. There are marked variations in the spatial distribution of the encephalocoeles according to the geographic origin and ethnic group.

Indeed, in North America and Europe, the occipital encephalocoeles are the most frequent (75%–80% of cases) [60–63] and females are more often affected than males [61]. Encephalocoeles of the skull base (in which the defect is located in the frontal, ethmoidal or sphenoidal bone) are less frequent: they account for only 15% of all encephalocoeles [60]. In Asia, Africa, Australia and Latin America, these are more frequent, with a slight male predominance [61, 63] (Fig. 9).

Parietal and temporal localizations [61, 63] are possible, although very rare (Fig. 10).

Most encephalocoeles are sporadic and of unknown origin. Environmental and genetic factors – the latter being more frequent for encephalocoeles of the posterior fossa – have been blamed [57].

Ultrasonographic Diagnosis

US examination shows a pericranial, extracerebral space-occupying lesion, the location, size and echogenicity of which must be evaluated.

The location is in most cases occipital, the size is variable, from 5 mm to approximately 10 cm [64].

The contents have a fundamental influence over the prognosis. They are typically anechoic in meningocoeles and hyperechoic or mixed in encephalocoeles. They can be hyperechoic in the centre, or have a hyperechoic periphery corresponding to some cerebral parenchyma. Out of 24 cephalocoeles, 15 show some measure of gyration inside the malformation

[64]. In some cases, the encephalocoele pattern is reminiscent of a cyst inside a cyst [65].

The contents of the mass vary with time: they may initially look solid and later become cystic [64] or vice versa [63]. Apart from these extreme cases, it may be difficult to distinguish an encephalocoele from a meningocoele in sonography [63, 65].

The other pivotal sign looked for in US examination is the defect of the cranial vault (found in 88% of fetuses in a series of 26 cephalocoeles [64]). It may be difficult to visualize because of its small size, cephalic presentation or oligohydramnios [64]. Some authors [58] consider that ascertaining the presence of such a defect is very difficult because of the variability in size of the posterior fontanelle, and also because such a defect may be difficult to distinguish from a cranial suture. The presence of such a defect should allow for differentiation between a meningocoele from an epidermoid cyst [59, 60, 66]. It has also been reported that some artefacts may mimic these defects.

An absence of vascularization in Doppler imaging rules out a fast-flow vascular malformation that could be located in front of a suture, and hence be difficult to distinguish from an encephalocoele [67].

Likewise, a teratoma or a hygroma may look very similar to an encephalocoele, but neither is associated with a skull defect. Moreover, the hygroma forms an obtuse connecting angle with the cranial vault, whereas this angle is acute with encephalocoeles [65].

In US, one must also look for a lemon sign, a microcephaly and a flattened configuration to the basiocciput. Hydrocephalus is observed in 80% of occipital meningocoeles, in 65% of occipital encephalocoeles and in 15% of frontal encephalocoeles [68]. In this last type of encephalocoele, hypertelorism and facial abnormalities of the midline (labial, palatine cleft) may be detected [61, 69].

Sonography is also used to look for potentially associated abnormalities [57, 58, 62, 64, 65, 68, 70–72]:

- Of the face: microcephaly, cleft
- Of the central nervous system: cerebellar hypoplasia, Dandy-Walker malformation, vermian agenesis, gyration abnormalities, corpus callosum agenesis
- Of the kidneys: cysts, renal agenesis
- Of the abdomen: omphalocoele
- Of the limbs: reduction defects, polydactyly

The encephalocoele could be part of a rubella fetopathy or a syndrome, notably Meckel-Gruber and Walker-Warburg syndromes, frontonasal dysplasia and the amniotic adhesion form of the amniotic con-stricting band syndrome. In this last case, the defect is generally irregular, asymmetrical and in an atypi-cal location [63].

Varied chromosomal abnormalities may also be observed, notably trisomy 18, in up to 44% of cases [58, 64, 65, 70, 71, 73, 74]. As an indication, in a series of 58 encephalocoeles diagnosed at birth, 35 were isolat-ed, two were associated with trisomy 18 and 21 with other malformations. Interestingly, on the 35 isolated cases, seven antenatal US examinations were deemed normal, and another diagnosis had been suggested in four cases [74].

Contribution of Fetal MRI

Given the rarity of this pathology, it is hardly surpris-ing that no series studying the contribution of fetal MRI to the diagnosis of meningocoeles and encepha-locoeles has been published. A few cases have been reported in some series [75–77]. We have personally observed five cases: two encephalocoeles and three meningocoeles.

Fetal MRI is only really useful where an apparent-ly isolated meningocoele or encephalocoele with no karyotypic abnormality is diagnosed in US. In this case, its role is to help precisely determine the con-tents of the malformation. Meningocoeles and ence-phalocoeles are not always easily distinguished in US. In this respect, the higher spatial resolution and con-trast resolution of MRI could be an asset.

Meningocoeles are typically homogeneous in T1 hyposignal and T2 hypersignal. Encephalocoeles have heterogeneous and sometimes gyriform con-tents. With MRI, one can observe the possible conti-nuity between the brain and the encephalocoele or even the presence of a portion of ventricle inside the malformation. Since the cranial vault is hypointense in T1 and in T2, it can prove difficult to ascertain the presence of a small defect, and hence to distinguish an epidermoid cyst from a meningocoele [59] (Fig. 11). The most important matter here is to make sure that there is no intracranial extension. For the same reasons as in US, this diagnosis is also very dif-ficult to establish in MRI in cases of cephalic presen-tation and oligohydramnios, or when the meningo-coele or encephalocoele is too small.

Before 34 weeks of gestation, an analysis of the pe-ricerebral space can be made in order to look for a communication between the brain and the malfor-mation. In this context, however, the pericerebral space is sometimes very thin even before 34 weeks of gestation, thus making it difficult to evaluate gyra-tion.

A small cisterna filled with amniotic fluid adjoin-ing the cranial vault may be mistaken for a meningo-coele or an epidermoid cyst.

MRI can also reveal the splitting of a venous sinus (superior longitudinal sinus, torcular herophili) (Fig. 11), or an associated gyration abnormality or ab-normality of the posterior fossa (notably vermian or cerebellar hypoplasia), rarely detected in US. These last two elements have a determinant influence over the prognosis [57].

Natural History and Prognosis

The natural history of encephalocoeles is very poorly known, as most antenatal diagnoses of such malfor-mations lead to termination of pregnancy.

Some cases studied sequentially during pregnancy with US show that the size of the malformation may change (it may even sometimes temporarily disap-pear [56]). The same applies to the contents, which can go from cystic to solid [56], and vice versa [63].

This explains the difficulties encountered in estab-lishing a prognosis in the antenatal period. Overall, however, the presence of associated malformations or a known broader syndromic context including the malformation, is naturally the sign of a poor progno-sis. In the absence of associated malformations, the main prognostic factors are microcephaly and hydro-cephaly, the pivotal prognostic factor being the pres-ence and amount of brain inside the herniated sac [57, 68, 71]. The quantity of herniated cerebral tissue is linked with the child's intellectual prognosis [57]. When over 50% of the intracranial contents are ex-ternalized, the survival rate is very low [64]. When the cephalocoele diagnosis is established in utero, the survival rate is about 20% (21% for Goldstein et al. [65], 22% for Budorick et al. [64]). The prognosis of meningocoeles, on the other hand, is much better. This explains why every effort should be made to at-tempt to distinguish between these two entities in an-tenatal examinations [66].

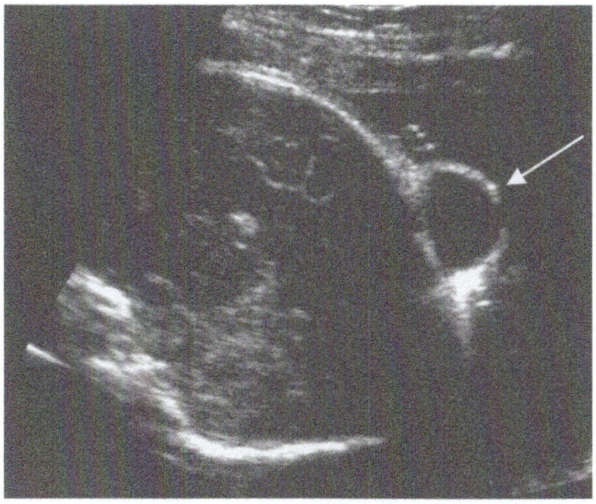

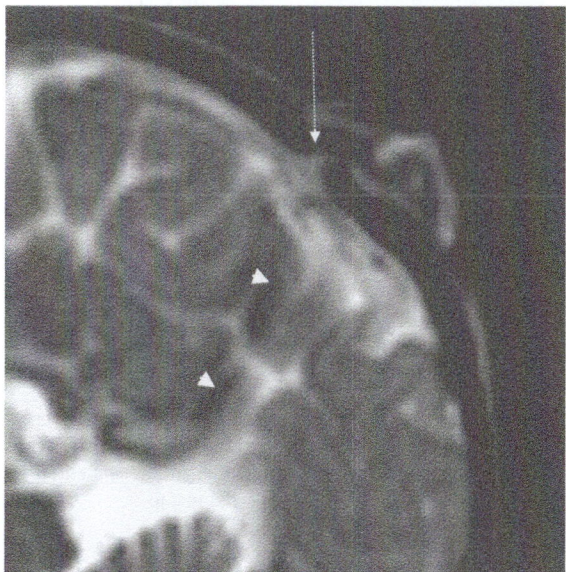

Fig. 11 a–e. Parieto-occipital meningocoele. **a** US at 33 weeks of gestation. Paramedian sagittal slice. Pericranial, extracerebral midline parieto-occipital anechoic formation (*arrow*), with a doubt on the presence of a cranial vault defect. **b, c** Fetal MRI at 33 weeks of gestation. T2-weighted midline sagittal slice (**b**) and axial slice at the level of the vertex (**c**). The fluid-filled lesion is isointense to the cerebrospinal fluid. The calvarial defect is not clearly visible. The superior longitudinal sinus (*arrowhead*) is split in front of the lesion. The diagnosis of meningocoele is suggested. **d, e** Postnatal MRI at 1 month. T1-weighted (**d**) and T2-weighted (**e**) midline sagittal slices. The defect of the cranial vault (*dotted arrow*) is clearly visible in T2. Note the persistence of a falcine sinus (*arrowheads*), not seen in its totality on this slice. The child was operated on at 3 months (Prof. A. Pierre-Kahn, Hôpital Necker-Enfants Malades): excision of the meningocoele, the pedicle is dissected at its point of entry into the skull

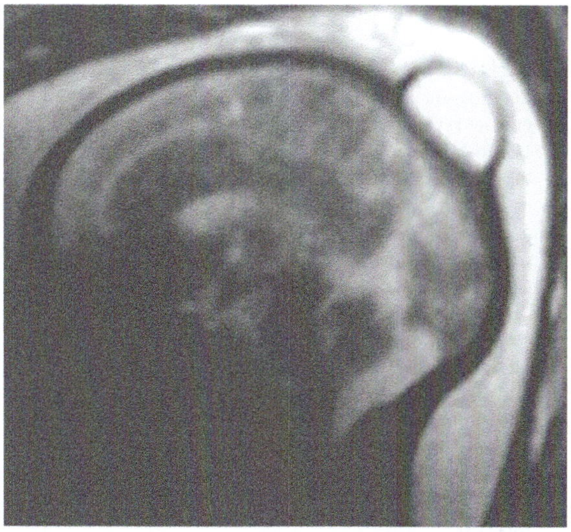

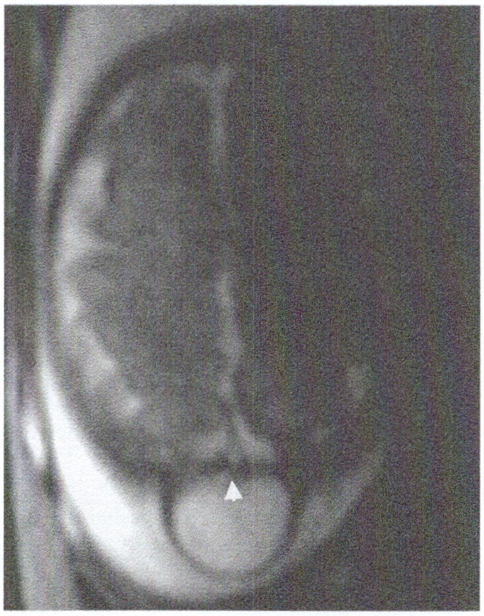

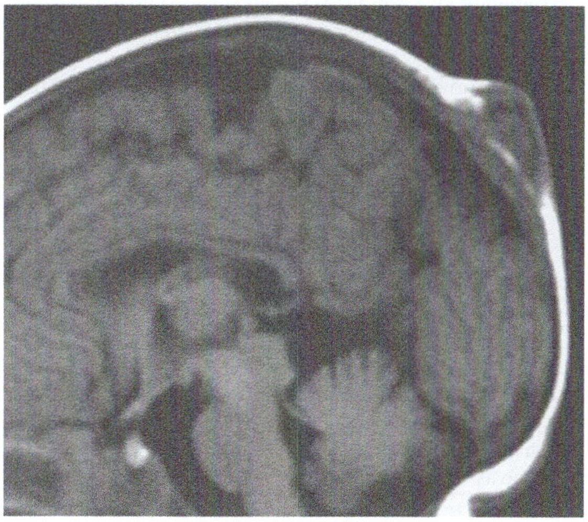

References

1. Heckel S, Favre R, Gasser B, Christmann D (1995) Prenatal diagnosis of a congenital astrocytoma: a case report and literature review. Ultrasound Obstet Gynecol 5:63–66

2. Dören M, Tercanli S, Gullotta F, Holzgreve W (1997) Prenatal diagnosis of a highly undifferentiated brain tumour. A case report and review of the literature. Prenat Diagn 17:967–971

3. Chien YH, Tsao PN, Lee WT, Peng SF, Tsou Yau KI (2000) Congenital intracranial teratoma. Pediatr Neurol 22:72–74

4. Molina CP, Hawkins H, Campbell G, Rowe T, Grafe M (1999) Case of the month: January 1999 – Fetus with echogenic mass in third ventricle. Brain Pathol 9:605–606

5. Suresh S, Indrani S, Vijayalakshmi S, Nirmala J, Meera G (1993) Prenatal diagnosis of cerebral neuroblastoma by fetal brain biopsy. J Ultrasound Med 5:303–306

6. Ferreira J, Eviatar L, Schneider S, Grossman R (1993) Prenatal diagnosis of intracranial teratoma. Pediatr Neurosurg 19:84–88

7. Geraghty AV, Knott PD, Hanna HM (1989) Prenatal diagnosis of fetal glioblastoma multiforme. Prenat Diagn 9:613–616

8. D'Addario V, Pinto V, Meo F, Resta M (1998) The specificity of ultrasound in the detection of fetal intracranial tumors. J Perinat Med 26:480–485

9. Oi S, Tamaki N, Kondo T, Nakamura H, Kudo H, Suzuki H, Sasaki M, Matsumoto S, Ueda Y, Katayama K, Mochizuki M (1990) Massive congenital intracranial teratoma diagnosed in utero. Childs Nerv Syst 6:459–461

10. Peng SS, Shih JC, Liu HM, Li YW, Hsieh FJ (1999) Ultrafast fetal MR images of intracranial teratoma. J Comput Assist Tomogr 23:318–319

11. Weyerts LK, Catanzarite V, Jones MC, Mendoza A (1993) Prenatal diagnosis of a giant intracranial teratoma associated with pulmonary hypoplasia. J Med Genet 30:880–882

12. Sherer DM, Onyeije CI (1998) Prenatal ultrasonographic diagnosis of fetal intracranial tumors: a review. Am J Perinatol 15:319–328

13. Mazouni C, Porcu-Buisson G, Girard N, Sakr R, Figarella-Ballanger D, Guidicelli B, Bonnier P, Gamerre M (2003) Intrauterine brain teratoma: a case report of imaging (US, MRI) with neuropathologic correlations. Prenat Diagn 23:104–107

14. Mitchell D, Rojiani AM, Richards D, Yachnis AT, Powell SZ (1995) Congenital CNS primitive neuroectodermal tumor: case report and review of the literature. Pediatr Pathol Lab Med 15:949–956

15. Yamada T, Takeuchi K, Masuda Y, Moriyama T, Kitazawa S, Maruo T (2003) Prenatal imaging of congenital cerebral primitive neuroectodermal tumor. Fetal Diagn Ther 18:137–139

16. Chung SN, Rosemond RL, Graham D (1998) Prenatal diagnosis of a fetal intracranial tumor. J Ultrasound Med 17:521–523

17. Diguet A, Laquerrière A, Eurin D, Chanavaz-Lacheray I, Ruchoux MM, Rossi A, Marpeau L (2002) Fetal capillary haemangioblastoma: an exceptional tumour. A review of the literature. Prenat Diagn 22:979–983

18. Yuh WTC, Nguyen HD, Fisher DJ, Turgut Tali E, Gao F, Simonson TM, Kao SCS, Weiner CP (1994) MR of fetal central nervous system abnormalities. AJNR 15:459–464

19. Honda M, Toda K, Baba H, Yonekura M (2003) Congenital cavernous angioma of the temporal bone: case report. Surg Neurol 59:120–123

20. Cavalheiro S, de Castro Sparapani FV, Moron AF, Da Silva MC, Stavale JN (2002) Fetal meningeal hemangiopericytoma. J Neurosurg 97:1217–1220

21. Sherer DM, Abramowicz JS, Eggers PC, Metlay LA, Sinkin RA, Woods JR (1993) Prenatal ultrasonographic diagnosis of intracranial teratoma and massive craniomegaly with associated high-output cardiac failure. Am J Obstet Gynecol 168:97–99

22. Romero R, Pilu G, Jeanty P, Ghidini A, Hobbins JC (1988) The central nervous system. In: Romero R, Pilu G, Jeanty P, Ghidini A, Hobbins JC (eds) Prenatal diagnosis of congenital anomalies. Appelton and Lange, Norwalk, CT, pp. 1–80

23. Romero R, Pilu G, Jeanty P, Ghidini A, Hobbins JC (1988) Choroid plexus papilloma in prenatal diagnosis of congenital anomalies. Appelton and Lange, Norwalk, CT

24. Pilu G, Falco P, Perolo A, Sandri F, Cocchi G, Ancora G, Bovicelli L (1997) Differential diagnosis and outcome of fetal intracranial hypoechoic lesions: report of 21 cases. Ultrasound Obstet Gynecol 9:229–236

25. Hassan J, Sepulveda W, Teixeira J, Cox PM (1996) Glioependymal and arachnoid cysts: unusual causes of early ventriculomegaly in utero. Prenat Diagn 16:729–733

26. Rafferty PG, Britton J, Penna L, Ville Y (1998) Prenatal diagnosis of a large fetal arachnoid cyst. Ultrasound Obstet Gynecol 12:358–361

27. Langer B, Haddad J, Favre R, Frigue V, Schlaeder G (1994) Fetal arachnoid cyst: report of two cases. Ultrasound Obstet Gynecol 4:68–72

28. Barkovich AJ (2000) Hydrocephalus. In: Barkovich AJ (ed) Pediatric neuroimaging. Lippincott Williams & Wilkins, Philadelphia, pp 581–620

29. Meizner I, Barki Y, Tadmor R, Katz M (1988) In utero ultrasonic detection of fetal arachnoid cyst. J Clin Ultrasound 16:506–509

30. Diakoumakis EE, Weinberg B, Mollin J (1986) Prenatal sonographic diagnosis of a suprasellar arachnoid cyst. J Ultrasound Med 5:529–530

31. Bannister CM, Russell SA, Rimmer S, Mowle DH (1999) Fetal arachnoid cysts: their site, progress, prognosis and differential diagnosis. Eur J Pediatr Surg 9 [Suppl I]:27–28

32. Lyon G, Evrard P (2000) Hypertensions intracrâniennes non tumorales. In: Lyon G, Evrard P (eds) Neuropédiatrie. Masson, Paris, pp 67–157

33. Pierre-Kahn A, Hanlo P, Sonigo P, Parisot D, McConnell RS (2000) The contribution of prenatal diagnosis to the understanding of malformative intracranial cysts: state of the art. Childs Nerv Syst 16:618–626

34. Hogge WA, Schnatterly P, Ferguson JE (1995) Early prenatal diagnosis of an infratentorial arachnoid cyst: association with an unbalanced translocation. Prenat Diagn 15:186–188

35. Leistikow EA, Costakos DT, Jones NE, Bester SD, Deering WM, Stevens MK (2000) Isolated large third-trimester intracranial cyst on fetal ultrasound: fact or fiction? Pediatrics 106:844–848

36. Sherer DM, Bennett SL, Abramowicz JS (1991) Persistent unilateral intracranial cystic structure in a third-trimester fetus with normal neonatal outcome: another potential sonographic pitfall. J Ultrasound Med 10:246

37. Aletebi FA, Fung KFK (1999) Neurodevelopmental outcome after antenatal diagnosis of posterior fossa abnormalities. J Ultrasound Med 18:683–689

38. Wester K, Hugdahl K (1995) Arachnoid cysts of the left temporal fossa: impaired preoperative cognition and post-operative improvement. J Neurol Neurosurg Psychiatry 59: 293–298

39. Sepulveda W, Platt CC, Fisk NM (1995) Prenatal diagnosis of cerebral arteriovenous malformation using color Doppler ultrasonography: case report and review of the literature. Ultrasound Obstet Gynecol 6:282–286

40. Lasjaunias P (1997) Vein of Galen aneurysmal malformation in vascular diseases in neonates, infants and children. In: Lasjaunias P (ed) Vascular diseases in neonates. Springer-Verlag, Berlin Heidelberg New York, pp 67–202

41. Lee W, Kirk JS, Pryde P, Romero R, Qureshi F (1994) Atypical presentation of fetal arteriovenous malformation. J Ultrasound Med 13:645–647

42. Comstock CH, Kirk JS (1991) Arteriovenous malformations: locations and evolution in the fetal brain. J Ultrasound Med 10:361–365

43. Campi A, Scotti G, Filippi M, Gerevini S, Strigimi F, Lasjaunias P (1996) Antenatal diagnosis of vein of Galen aneurysmal malformation: MR study of fetal brain and postnatal follow-up. Neuroradiology 38:87–90

44. Delezoide AL, Fallet-Bianco C, Narcy F, Frappat S, Esculpavit C (1997) L'anévrysme de la veine de Galien : point de vue du foetopathologiste. Med Fœtale Echogr Gynecol 30:28–32

45. Brunelle F (1997) Arteriovenous malformation of the vein of Galen in children. Pediatr Radiol 27:501–513

46. Reiter AA, Huhta JC, Carpenter RJ, Segall GK, Hawkins EP (1986) Prenatal diagnosis of arteriovenous malformation of the vein of Galen. J Clin Ultrasound 14:623–628

47. Strauss S, Weinraub Z, Goldberg M (1991) Prenatal diagnosis of vein of Galen arteriovenous malformation by duplex sonography. J Perinat Med 19:227–230

48. Dan U, Shalev E, Greif M, Weiner E (1992) Prenatal diagnosis of fetal brain arteriovenous malformation: the use of color Doppler imaging. J Clin Ultrasound 20:149–151

49. Chisholm CA, Kuller JA, Katz VL, McCoy MC (1996) Aneurysm of the vein of Galen: prenatal diagnosis and perinatal management. Am J Perinatol 13:503–506

50. Rodesch G, Hui F, Alvarez H, Tanaka V, Lasjaunias P (1994) Prognosis of antenatally diagnosed vein of Galen aneurysmal malformations. Childs Nerv Syst 10:79–83

51. Martinez-Lage JF, Garcia Santos JM, Poza M, Garcia Sanchez F (1993) Prenatal magnetic resonance imaging detection of a vein of Galen aneurysm. Childs Nerv Syst 9: 377–378

52. Simon EM, Goldstein RB, Coakley FV, Filly RA, Broderick KC, Musci TJ, Barkovich AJ (2000) Fast MR Imaging of fetal CNS anomalies in utero. AJNR Am J Neuroradiol 21:1688–1698

53. Yamashita Y, Abe T, Ohara N, Maruoka T, Toyoda O, Inoue O, Kojima K, Kato H (1992) Successful treatment of neonatal aneurysmal dilatation of the vein of Galen: the role of prenatal diagnosis and transarterial embolization. Neuroradiology 34:457–459

54. Has R, Günay S, Ibrahimoglu L (2003) Prenatal diagnosis of a vein of Galen aneurysm. Fetal Diagn Ther 18:36–40

55. Larsen WJ (1993) The fourth week. In: Larsen WJ (ed) Human Embryology. Churchill Livingstone, New York, pp 65–92

56. Bronshtein M, Zimmer EZ (1991) Transvaginal sonographic follow-up on the formation of fetal cephalocele at 13–19 weeks' gestation. Obstet Gynecol 78:528–530

57. Martinez-Lage JF, Poza M, Sola J, Soler CL, Montalvo CG, Domingo R, Puche A, Ramon FH, Azorin P, Lasso R (1996) The child with a cephalocele: etiology, neuroimaging, and outcome. Childs Nerv Syst 12:540–550

58. Jeanty P, Shah D, Zaleski W, Ulm J, Fleischer A (1991) Prenatal diagnosis of fetal cephalocele: a sonographic spectrum. Am J Perinatol 8:144–149

59. Shahabi S, Busine A (1998) Prenatal diagnosis of an epidermal scalp cyst simulating an encephalocele. Prenat Diagn 18:373–377

60. Ferriman EL, McCormack J (1995) An epidermal scalp cyst simulating an encephalocele. Prenat Diagn 15:981–984

61. Castillo M, Mukherji SK (1996) Developmental anomalies, infratentorial. In: Castillo M, Mukherji SK (eds) Imaging of the pediatric head, neck and spine. Lippincott-Raven, Philadelphia, pp 69–94

62. Drugan A, Weissman A, Evans MI (2001) Screening for neural tube defects. Clin Perinatol 28:279–287

63. Hanley ML, Guzman ER, Vintzileos AM, Leiman S, Doyle A, Shen-Schwarz S (1996) Prenatal ultrasonographic detection of regression of an encephalocele. J Ultrasound Med 15:71–74

64. Budorick NE, Pretorius DH, McGahan JP, Grafe MR, James HE, Slivka J (1995) Cephalocele detection in utero: sonographic and clinical features. Ultrasound Obstet Gynecol 5:77–85

65. Goldstein RB, LaPidus AS, Filly RA (1991) Fetal cephaloceles: diagnosis with US. Radiology 180:803–808

66. Okaro E, Broussin B, Ville Y (1998) Prenatal diagnosis of atypical cystic lesions of the fetal scalp. Ultrasound Obstet Gynecol 12:442–444

67. Bronshtein M (1992) Bar-Hava I, Bulmenfeld Z (1992) Early second-trimester sonographic appearance of occipital haemangioma simulating encephalocele. Prenat Diagn 12:695–698

68. Fleming AD, Vintzileos AM, Scorza WE (1991) Prenatal diagnosis of occipital encephalocele with transvaginal sonography. J Ultrasound Med 10:285–286

69. Chervenak FA, Isaacson G, Rosenberg JC, Kardon NB (1986) Antenatal diagnosis of frontal cephalocele in a fetus with atelosteogenesis. J Ultrasound Med 5:111–113

70. Källen B, Robert E, Harris J (1998) Associated malformations in infants and fetuses with upper or lower neural tube defects. Teratology 57:56–63

71. Wininger SJ, Donnenfeld AE (1994) Syndromes identified in fetuses with prenatally diagnosed cephaloceles. Prenat Diagn 14:839–843

72. Wang P, Chang FM, Chang CH, Yu CH, Jung YC, Huang CC (1999) Prenatal diagnosis of Joubert syndrome complicated with encephalocele using two-dimensional and three-dimensional ultrasound. Ultrasound Obstet Gynecol 14:360–364

73. Coerdt W, Miller K, Holzgreve W, Rauskolb R, Schwinger E, Rehder H (1997) Neural tube defects in chromosomally normal and abnormal human embryos. Ultrasound Obstet Gynecol 10:410–415

74. Boyd PA, Wellesley DG, De Walle HEK, Tenconi R, Garcia-Minaur S, Zandwijken GRJ, Stoll C, Clementi M (2000) Evaluation of the prenatal diagnosis of neural tube defects by fetal ultrasonographic examination in different centres across Europe. J Med Screen 7:169–174

75. Levine D, Barnes PD, Edelman RR (1999) Obstetric MR imaging. Radiology 211:609–617

76. Resta M, Spagnolo P, Dicuonzo F, Palma M, Florio C, Greco P, D'Addario V, Vimercati A, Selvaggi L, Caruso G, Clemente R (1994) La risonanza magnetica del feto. Parte I: Tecnica d'esame ed anatomia normale dell'encefalo. Riv Neuroradiol 7:53–65

77. Levine D, Barnes PD, Madsen JR, Li W, Edelman RR (1997) Fetal central nervous system anomalies: MR imaging augments sonographic diagnosis. Radiology 204:635–642

Ventricular Dilatation

Several terms are used in the literature to describe the increase in size of the cerebral ventricular system. The word "hydrocephalus" refers to the progressive distension of the ventricles caused by the increase in the quantity of cerebrospinal fluid, but carries no indication as to its cause (either production or resorption disorder) [1]. Hydrocephalus causes the cranial perimeter to increase [2]. It is contrasted with the ventricular dilatation linked with a developmental abnormality of the cerebral hemispheres and with the in vacuo dilatation related to lesions of the cerebral parenchyma. The term "ventriculomegaly" is very frequently used in the English-language literature, although it only refers to the widening of one or several ventricles, regardless of the skull dimensions, and the cause of this dilatation.

Ventricular dilatation is a frequent entity, observed, according to various authors, in approximately 0.5%–2% of births [3–9]. It is isolated in 0.39%–0.87% of births [10].

Ventricular dilatation has a very diverse aetiology; it is observed in many fetal cerebral pathologies. It seemed, however, justified to devote a chapter to this subject, as ventricular dilatation very often is the first (and sometimes the only) sign in ultrasonography leading to suspicion of a cerebral abnormality. It is also, in a number of cases, the first indication for fetal MRI (326 cases of ventricular dilatation in the 1,100 fetal cerebral MRIs done in our institution).

Definition of Ventricular Dilatation

Many articles in the fetal US literature deal with the size of the ventricles [1–17]. Usually, the atria are measured on an axial slice at the level of the septum pellucidum cyst, just above the thalami. On these slices, the atria and the frontal horns can be visualized well. The measurement is made on a line perpendicular to the atrium's major axis and does not include ventricular walls. This dimension is generally quite stable throughout pregnancy at around 7.6 ± 0.6 mm for some authors (on 100 fetuses between 14 and 38 weeks of gestation [11]), and 6.5 ± 1.5 mm for others (on 537 fetuses between 13 and 42 weeks of gestation [13]).

Measuring the deepest ventricle is usually quite easy, whereas the inevitable artefacts in the hemisphere closest to the probe make measurements of the most superficial ventricle far less reliable. This is why many articles dealing with ventricular dilatation in ultrasonography only offer measurements of the deepest ventricle, thus leaving ground for numerous classification errors between uni- and bilateral dilatations. Every time the presentation allows it, and it almost always does, this measurement should also be made on a coronal plane. The difference between the distances measured on an axial slice and on a coronal slice does not exceed 2 mm; the mean value is 6.5 mm on the axial plane and 6.6 mm on the coronal plane (in a series of 506 fetuses between 13 and 42 weeks of gestation [13]).

The ventricles are said to be dilated when the atrial diameter is greater than 10 mm. The dilatation is called "mild" under 15 mm, and "severe" above that figure.

Ventricular dilatation can also be evaluated by measuring the distance between the choroid plexus and the ventricular wall. It is said to be mild when this dimension is between 3 and 8 mm [9]. The atrial diameter/diameter of the hemisphere ratio has also been studied and seems to be constant at approximately 0.35 [13]. This ratio could be used to evaluate ventricular dilatation, but the atrial diameter is by far the most commonly used datum.

It appears useful, however, to assess the atriocerebral ratio (atrial diameter/cerebral BPD). In our experience on 225 MR examinations of normal fetuses, this ratio decreases physiologically during pregnancy (13.6% at 22 weeks of gestation, 8% at 38 weeks of gestation), which gives a good idea of the fetal brain's growth while the size of the lateral ventricles remains stable [18].

Moreover, the width of the lateral ventricles is statistically significantly higher in males than in fe-

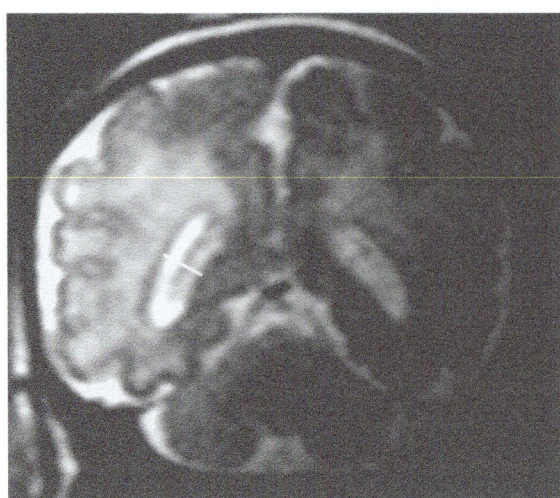

Fig. 1. Atrial diameter measurement in MRI. T2-weighted coronal slice at the level of the atria. The atrium is measured at mid-height on a line perpendicular to its major axis

males, although the difference seems too small (0.1 mm) to be clinically relevant [16]. Several authors [19–21] have noted a large proportion of males among fetuses with ventricular dilatation, some [19] even suggested that, in males, ventricles are only really dilated above 12 mm.

The 10-mm upper limit defining ventricular dilatation is also used in MRI. The main advantages of MRI over ultrasonography are its better reliability and better contrast resolution, the latter of which provides a more precise measurement whatever the position of the fetus's head. We usually take this measurement on a coronal slice at the level of the choroid plexuses, on a plane parallel to the brain stem [18] (Fig. 1).

Ventricular asymmetry without dilatation may be observed in normal fetuses [22]. Asymmetrical dilatation has been defined by some as a size difference between the two atria exceeding 2 mm [3] or 2.4 mm [22, 23].

The third and fourth ventricles' diameters have been evaluated in antenatal US [24, 25] and in fetal MRI [18]. The third ventricle was measured on an axial slice in US [24] and on a coronal slice in MRI [18]. A third ventricle diameter in excess of 3.5 mm in US, or 4 mm in MRI, should be regarded as pathological. The fourth ventricle diameter was measured on an axial slice in US [25] and on a sagittal slice in MRI [18]. The fourth ventricle's anteroposterior diameter normally should not exceed 4.8 mm in US and 7 mm in MRI.

Aetiological Diagnosis of Ventricular Dilatation: Limits of Ultrasonography and Contribution of MRI

The detection of a ventricular dilatation raises a number of questions. Answering these questions should advance towards the aetiology of the dilatation.

Which Ventricles Are Affected by Dilatation? Is This Dilatation Unilateral or Bilateral?

Ultrasonography generally gives a satisfactory answer to these questions, provided however, as we have seen above, that one manages to avoid the artefacts on the most superficial lateral ventricle and obtains coronal slices. When the lateral ventricles are dilated, one must determine whether the frontal horns are dilated. In the normal state, the frontal horns are thin. On an anterior coronal slice, their floor is concave towards the bottom. When they are dilated, the floor is rectilinear, sometimes even convex. One should also determine whether the dilatation is unilateral or bilateral, symmetrical or asymmetrical.

In most cases, MRI only confirms the answers obtained in US. It does not provide any complementary

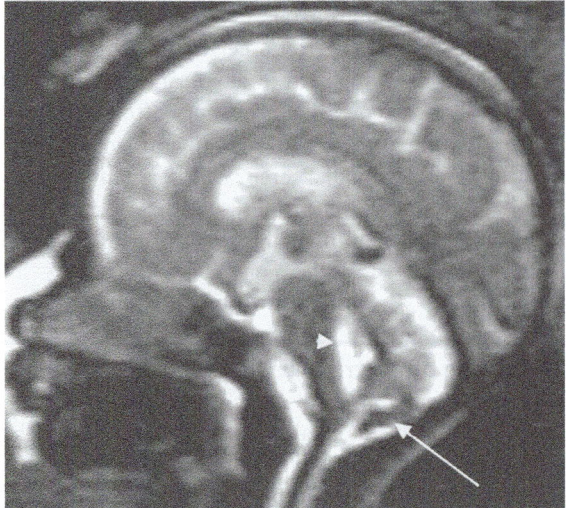

Fig. 2. Trapped fourth ventricle. Fetus at 32 weeks of gestation. T2-weighted midline sagittal slice. Intraventricular haemorrhage resulting in an obstruction of the foramina of Magendie and Luschka and a dilatation of the fourth ventricle (*arrowhead*). The haemorrhage is visible in hyposignal in the cisterna magna (*arrow*)

information, except perhaps regarding the dilatation of the fourth ventricle, which is often better evaluated in MRI (Fig. 2).

What Do the Ventricular Walls Look Like?

One should look for a hyperechoic lining around the ventricles, primarily reminiscent of a haemorrhage, of which it is sometimes the only stigma (Fig. 3).

Also, thick or indented walls can suggest the presence of migration abnormalities (heterotopia) (see Chap. 9, Fig. 5). Here, MRI is often more accurate than US. In our experience of subependymal heterotopia (four cases), ventricular dilatation was always very mild (10–12 mm); the diagnosis was suggested in US in only one case.

Contents of the Ventricles. How Do the Choroid Plexuses Look?

In normal fetuses, the contents of the ventricles are transonic in ultrasonography and homogeneous, T1 hypointense and T2 hyperintense in MRI. One must carefully look for a fluid-fluid level inside the ventricles that would show bleeding (Fig. 4). An abnormally voluminous and heterogeneous choroid plexus can also point to a haemorrhage. MRI, in this case, shows signal abnormalities that clearly indicate bleeding (see Chap. 14, Fig. 1; hence the importance of looking for a hyposignal in an echoplanar T2* sequence).

One should also look for a septation of the ventricles, clearly seen both in US and in MRI, which tends to point to an infectious cause (see Chap. 13, Fig. 3).

Are the Corpus Callosum and Leaves of the Septum Pellucidum Present?

In common practice, it is often ventricular dilatation that leads to a diagnosis of corpus callosum agenesis (CCA). Hence, all the direct and indirect signs of CCA, including parallel atria and increased distance between the frontal horns (see Chap. 8), should be looked for. MRI is often more accurate than US in this analysis.

Depending on the context, the lack of visibility of the septum leaves and fusion of the frontal horns indicate either septal agenesis or clastic destruction of the leaves of the septum (see Chap. 8). It is important to evaluate the morphology of the frontal horns,

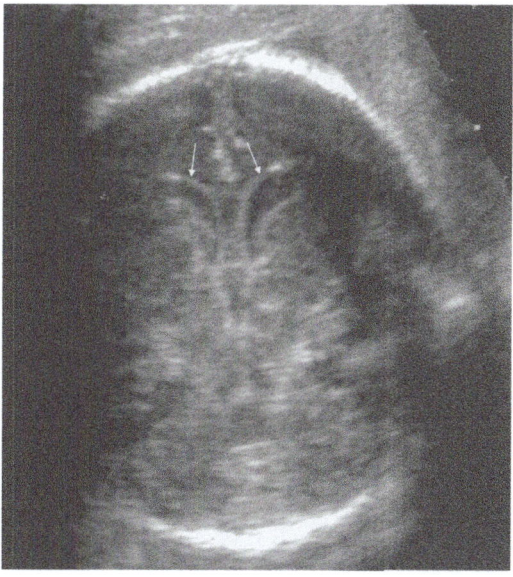

Fig. 3. Fetus at 32 weeks of gestation (same as in Fig. 2). Echoic periventricular lining (*arrows*) linked with an intraventricular haemorrhage

which are usually larger and rounded in cases of clastic destruction of the septum leaves (Fig. 5). MRI often provides little information in addition to that obtained in US. However, it provides a better evaluation of the position of the fornix.

How Does the Cerebral Parenchyma Look? Study of the Germinal Zone, the Signal of the Cerebral Parenchyma and Gyration

Analysis of the germinal zone makes it possible to search for signs of haemorrhage and for subependymal pseudocysts, which would point more to an infectious cause (see Chap. 13) or another type of aetiology such as Zellweger syndrome.

The cerebral parenchyma may manifest lesions reminiscent of ischaemia and/or haemorrhage. MRI contributes much more than US in this context (see Chap. 14).

The cerebral parenchyma may also show signs of signal abnormalities or echogenicity, suggesting a migration abnormality (see Chap. 9, Figs. 4–6). We have diagnosed several cases of lissencephaly in fetuses referred to MRI for ventricular dilatation. It is established that MRI is far more effective than ultrasonography in this field, but it is still important to look for the gyration abnormalities potentially associated with ventricular dilatation in ultrasonography.

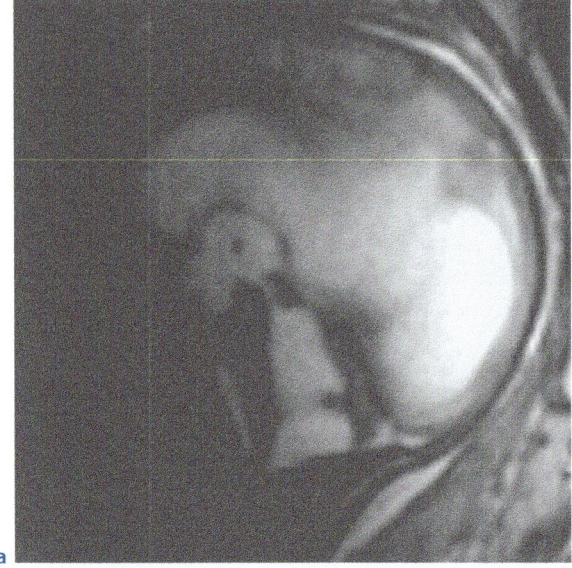

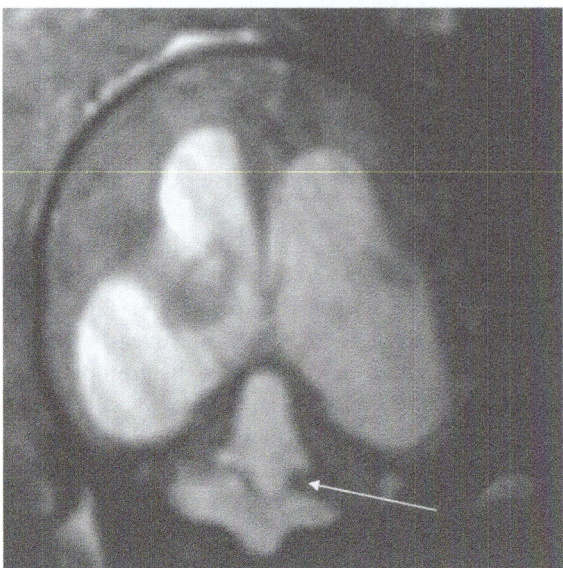

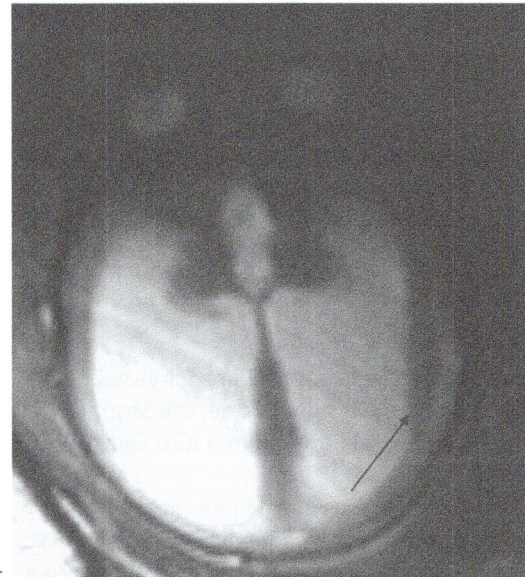

Fig. 4 a–c. Tetraventricular dilatation. Fetus at 34 weeks of gestation referred to MRI following the detection of an apparently isolated triventricular dilatation (the atria measured 36 mm each). T2-weighted sagittal (a), coronal (b) and axial (c) slices. MRI confirms the very severe dilatation of the lateral ventricles (at 33.5 and 36 mm) and of the third ventricle (12 mm). It also detects a dilatation of the fourth ventricle, whose inferior recess is visible on the coronal slice (b; *arrow*). The cause of the dilatation appears on the axial slice (c), which shows a fluid-fluid level in the deepest lateral ventricle (*arrow*), indicating an intraventricular haemorrhage. On the same figure, an artefact causes the marked hypersignal on the most superficial ventricle's occipital horn. No other haemorrhage stigma was visible in either US or MRI

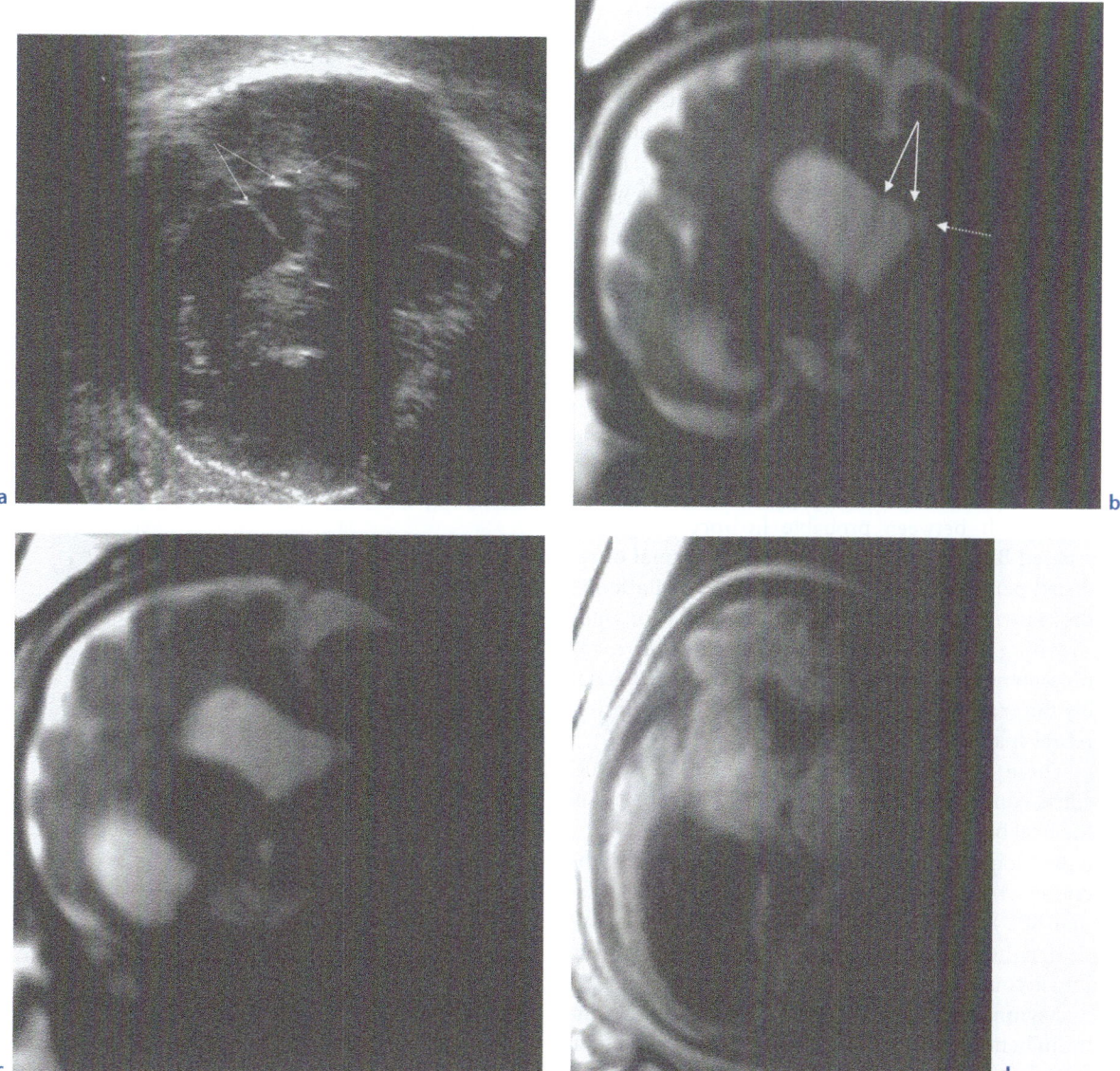

Fig. 5a–d. Unilateral ventricular dilatation. No sonographic abnormality is detected until 33.5 weeks of gestation. **a** US at 33.5 weeks of gestation. Anterior coronal slice showing a dilatation of the right frontal and temporal horns. Both leaves of the septum are visible (*arrows*). The left frontal horn is thin (*dotted arrow*). **b** MRI at 33.5 weeks of gestation. T2-weighted coronal slice at the same level as **a** showing the same abnormalities. **c** On a slightly posterior coronal slice, the right septal leaf is no longer visible, probably ruptured. **d** T1-weighted ax-ial slice showing the significant thinning of the cerebral parenchyma in front of the dilated right occipital horn (atria measured at 38 mm). The left lateral ventricle is thin. The neurofetopathological examination confirms the rupture of the septum leaves and the marked right ventricular dilatation relative to ischaemo-haemorrhagic changes, with calcified leucomalacia in the internal capsule and pallidum and periventricular haemorrhagic lesions

How Is the Posterior Fossa?

Numerous pathologies of the posterior fossa may associate with ventricular dilatation (see Chap. 12). Here too, MRI provides a far more precise analysis than US. Moreover, a herniated cerebellum should lead to suspicion of a myelomeningocoele, which should in any case be looked for in a context of ventricular dilatation.

What Are the Biparietal Diameter, Head Circumference and Width of the Pericerebral Space?

Studying biparietal diameter (BPD), head circumference (HC) and width of the pericerebral space can distinguish between probable hydrocephalus (increased BPD and head circumference, normal or reduced pericerebral space) and in vacuo dilatation of the ventricles (no increase in HC and BPD, possible widening of the pericerebral space). However, many unknowns remain in the antenatal period, and notably the exact significance of a widening of the pericerebral space.

These measurements greatly benefit from MRI since, contrary to US, it can establish a biometry of the fetal brain and not merely one of the skull. The fronto-occipital diameter, the cerebral BPD and the craniocerebral index (cranial BPD-cerebral BIP/cranial BPD) are evaluated this way [18]. The progression in these biometrical parameters should be taken into account.

Asymmetry and excessive development of one brain hemisphere and a widening of the homolateral lateral ventricle probably indicate hemimegalencephaly.

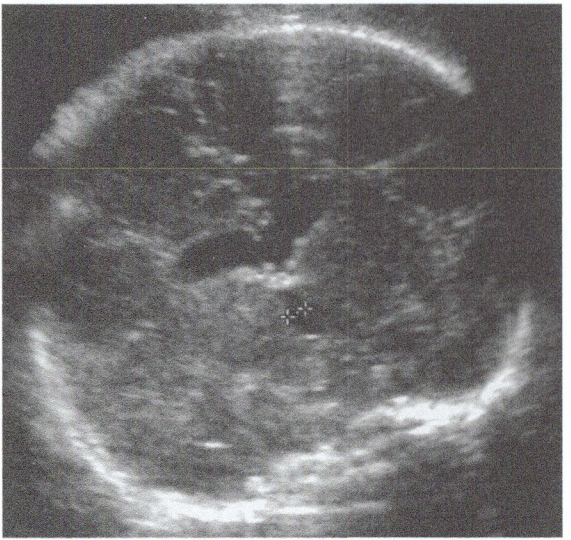

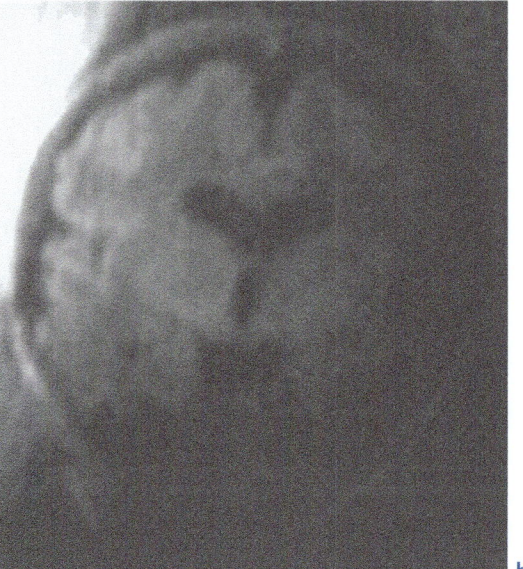

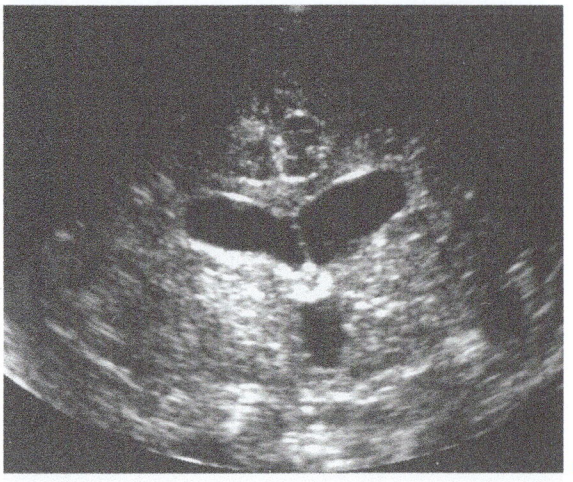

▶

Fig. 6 a–c. Triventricular dilatation in Crouzon disease. **a** Sonography performed at 34 weeks of gestation. Anterior coronal slice showing mild dilatation of the frontal horns (5 mm) and of the third ventricle (4 mm). The atria (not seen on this view) are measured at 14 and 15 mm. Absence of adducted thumbs. **b** Fetal MRI at 34 weeks of gestation. T1-weighted anterior coronal slice showing a biometry and morphology of the ventricles superimposable on those seen in US. **c** Transfontanellar sonography on the 1st day of life. Anterior coronal slice. The frontal horns measure 8 mm each, and the third ventricle is 7.5 mm wide. The atria (not shown) measure 17 and 18 mm. The progression of ventricular dilatation in the postnatal period required the placement of a shunt. At 37 months, the psychomotor development was evaluated at 24–30 months

The shape of the skull should also be studied, as craniostenosis and craniofaciostenosis may be associated with ventricular dilatation (Fig. 6).

A bilateral flattening of the frontal vault (lemon sign in US) should instigate a search for a myelomeningocoele.

Are There any Extracerebral Abnormalities?

The prognosis of ventricular dilatation depends for the most part on the answer to this question, which is primarily dealt with in ultrasonography, as MRI examinations usually focus on the brain in cases of ventricular dilatation. The search for chromosomal aberrations and biological infection stigmas is of course essential, but only fetal imaging shall be dealt with here.

Answering these questions gives the best possible approach to the aetiological diagnosis of ventricular dilatation.

The proportion of chromosomal abnormalities in the literature varies from 1.5 % to 12 % in isolated ventricular dilatations [7, 21, 26, 27], whereas this proportion is higher in dilatations associated with other malformations, varying from 9 % to 36 % [7, 19, 28, 29]. The frequency of associated cerebral or extracerebral abnormalities varies from 41 % to 78 % [7, 19, 29, 30].

The apparent discrepancies between these figures result from different recruiting methods, as the published series are not homogeneous, and some authors only study mild ventricular dilatations, whereas others consider all types of ventricular dilatation.

Among all the cerebral malformations observed, the most frequent are myelomeningocoeles, aqueductal stenosis and corpus callosum dysgenesis.

The proportion of myelomeningocoeles reaches 60 % in some series [8].

Some authors [31, 32] have evaluated the contribution of MRI (at 1.5-T in T2 single-shot fast spin-echo acquisition, 5-mm section thickness) to the precise evaluation of the topography of the myelomeningocoele with a view to antenatal operation. According to the authors of the most recent series [32], antenatal MRI (in 60 fetuses) was roughly equivalent to US in the assignment of the lesion level.

We personally base the diagnosis of myelomeningocoele on the classic sonographic signs:

- Direct signs: visibility of the rachischisis
- Indirect signs: herniated cerebellum, flattening of the frontal vault (lemon sign), lack of mobility of the lower limbs

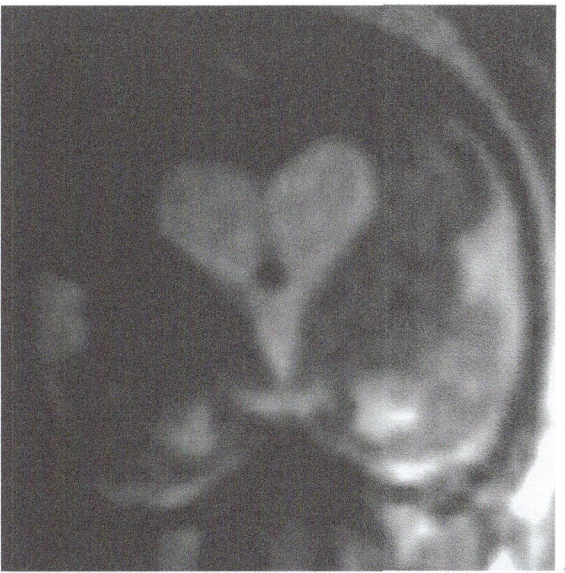

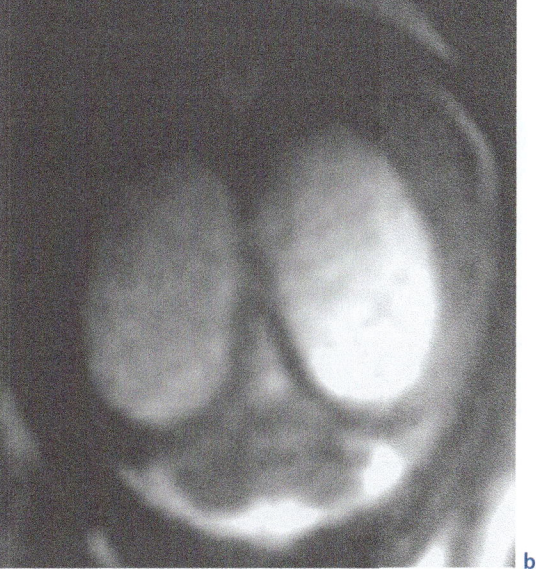

Fig. 7 a, b. Triventricular dilatation, aqueductal stenosis. At 27 weeks of gestation, the US examination detected a dilatation of the frontal horns (7.5 mm), atria (20 and 17 mm) and third ventricle (7 mm) with no visible associated abnormality. MRI at 27.5 weeks of gestation (on T2-weighted anterior (a) and posterior (b) coronal slices) shows an apparently isolated dilatation of the frontal horns (approximately 13 mm), atria (24 and 23 mm) and third ventricle (6 mm). The fronto-occipital diameter is at the 10th percentile, the cranial BPD and cerebral BPD at the 50th percentile, and the craniocerebral index is normal (10%)

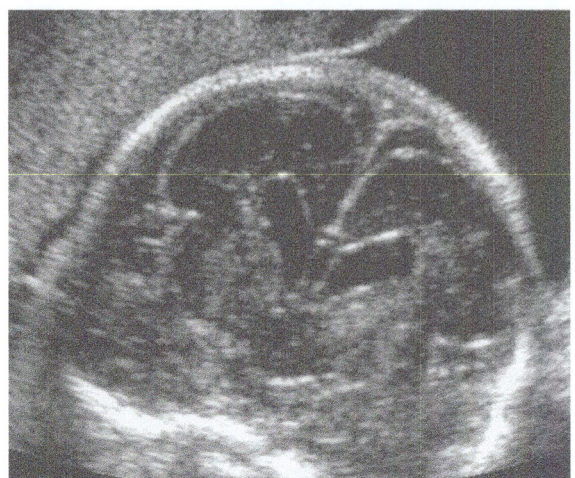

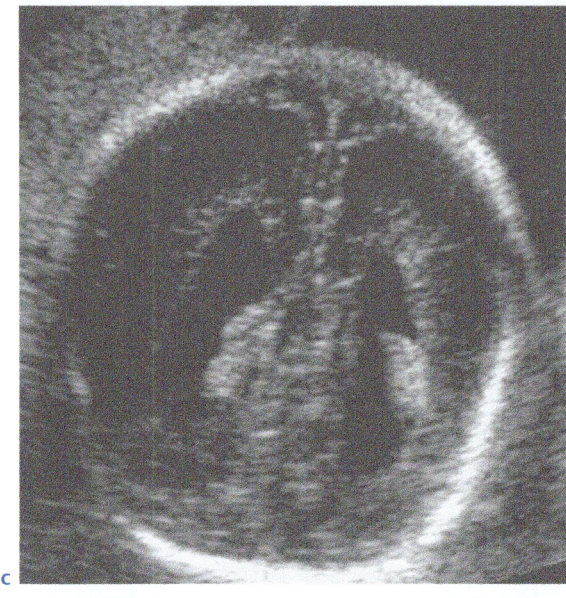

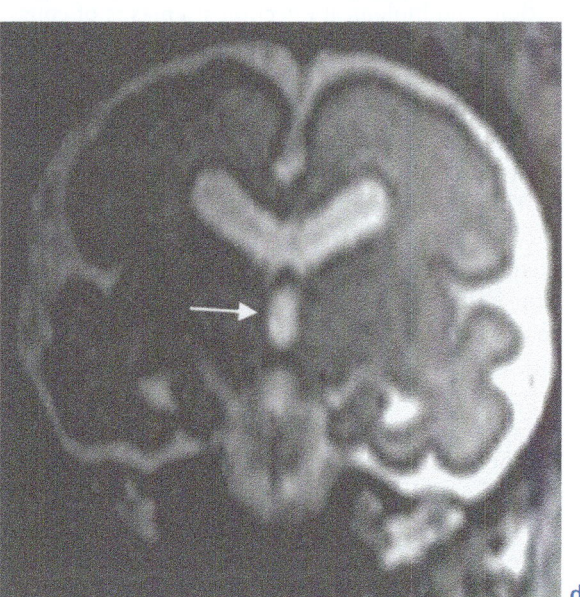

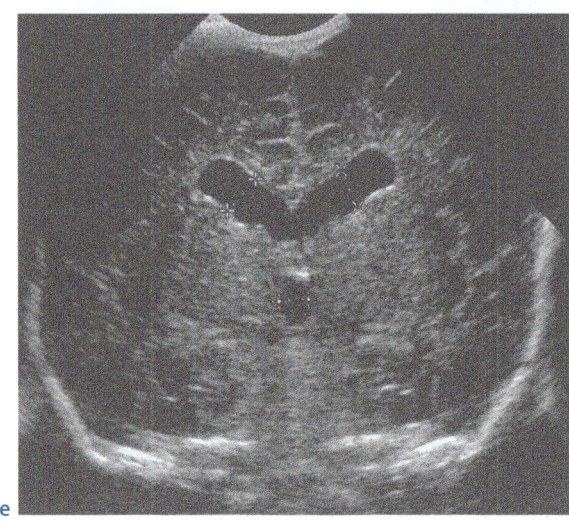

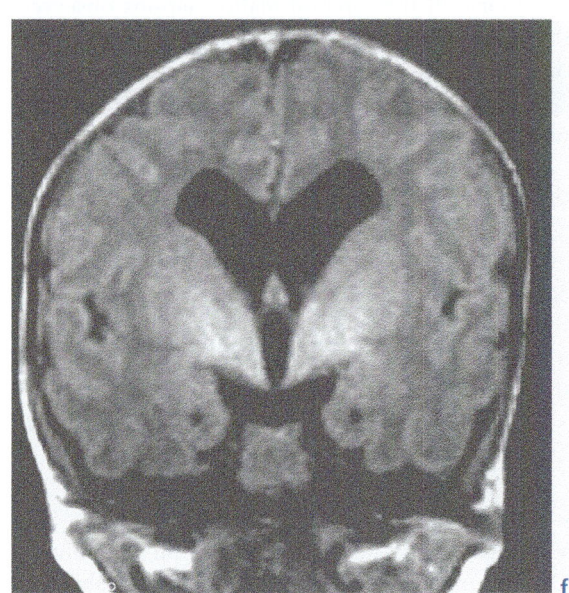

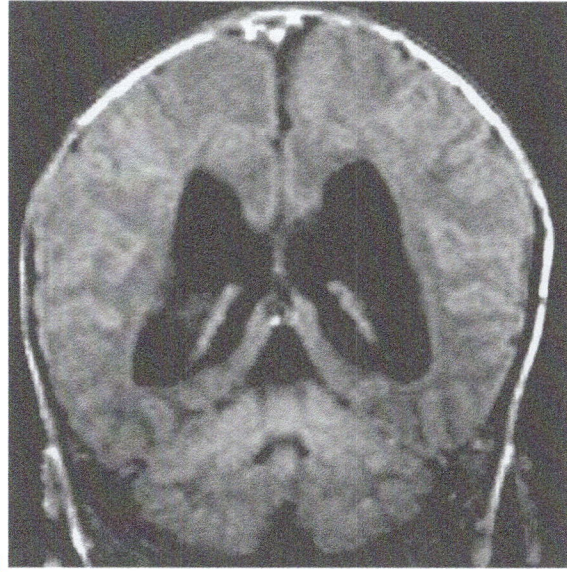

g

Fig. 8a–g. Triventricular dilatation, aqueductal stenosis. **a–c** US performed at 26 weeks of gestation. **a** Axial slice. Only the deepest ventricle is measurable, since the most superficial ventricle cannot be analysed owing to the usual artefacts on the most superficial hemisphere. **b, c** Anterior (**b**) and posterior (**c**) coronal slices in transfontanellar sonography with very good visibility of the ventricles and cerebral parenchyma. **d** The fetal MRI taken at 30 weeks of gestation shows a dilatation of the atria (13.5 and 14.5 mm) and of the frontal horns. On this T2-weighted coronal slice, the third ventricle is a bit too visible (*arrow*). The fronto-occipital diameter is at the 75th percentile, the cerebral BPD is at the 50th percentile, the cranial BPD at the 80th percentile and the craniocerebral index is 14% (the standard value at this stage is 9%). Hence, there is a widening of the pericerebral space. **e** On the 1st day of life, the atria are measured at 16 and 18 mm in transfontanellar sonography, which also shows a mild dilatation of the third ventricle and frontal horns. **f, g** At 3 weeks of life, MRI displays a similar pattern. T1-weighted anterior (**f**) and posterior (**g**) coronal slices. Ventricular dilatation is stable during the following months. In this case, aqueductal stenosis is diagnosed. At 15 months, this child had a normal psychomotor development

We do not proceed to fetal MRI and suggest terminating pregnancy.

As an indication, in our series of 326 cases of ventricular dilatation studied in fetal MRI, excluding myelomeningocoeles (which are not studied in MRI in our institution), one of the following associated cerebral pathologies was found in 41% of cases. These were distributed as follows:

- CCA: 7.6%
- Cerebral ischaemic lesion: 7.6%
- Abnormality of the posterior fossa: 5.5%
- Aqueductal stenosis: 3.7%
- Haemorrhagic lesion: 2.8%
- Septal agenesis: 2.1%;
- Septal destruction: 1.8%
- Arachnoid cyst: 1.9%
- Lissencephaly: 1.2%
- CMV infection: 1.2%
- Subependymal heterotopias: 1.2%
- Holoprosencephaly: 1.2%
- Others (tumours, metabolic disease): 2.7%

In the remaining 193 cases (59%), ventricular dilatation was the only cerebral abnormality detected.

Aqueductal stenosis can be congenital (Figs. 7–9): the recessive X-linked transmission described by Bickers and Adams accounts for approximately 2% of the cases of congenital hydrocephalus. Ventricular dilatation often appears relatively late in pregnancy. The presence of adducted thumbs is not constant [33]. Other forms of aqueductal stenosis with an autosomal recessive transmission have been reported [5, 34, 35]. Aqueductal stenosis can also be acquired or consecutive to an infection, an intraventricular haemorrhage or amniotic band disease. It is always associated with ventricular dilatation, whatever its cause may be. It has been suggested that aqueductal stenosis could result from a hyperpressure exerted on the midbrain by a voluminous communicating hydrocephalus, and therefore that it could be a consequence of ventricular dilatation rather than its cause [1, 34]. A few rare cases of membranes in the aqueduct have been described. In many cases, the cause of aqueductal stenosis remains undetermined.

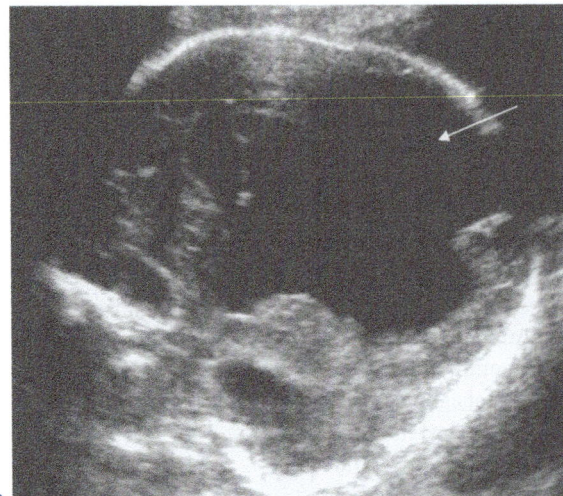

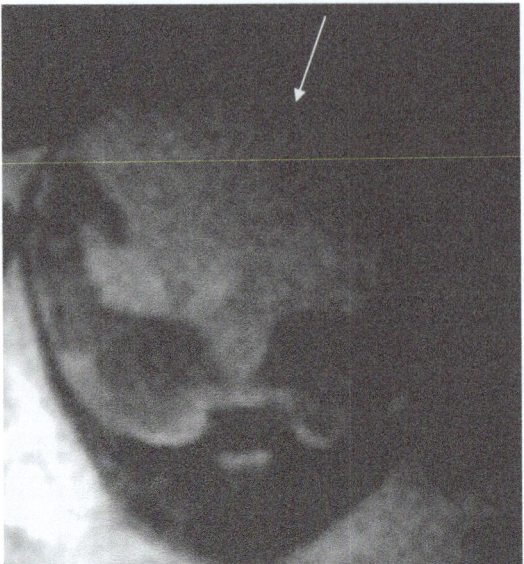

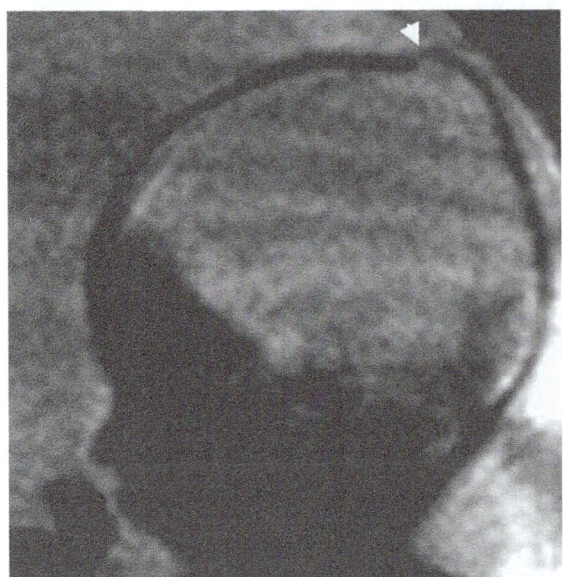

Fig. 9 a–c. Aqueductal atresia. Bichorial and biamniotic twin pregnancy. One of the twins shows a VACTERL-type malformation association with major hydrocephaly. **a** US at 30 weeks of gestation. **b** MRI at 30 weeks of gestation. T2-weighted coronal slice. On these two views, the third ventricle and the lateral ventricles are very dilated. No commissural structure is visible. The frontal horns are far apart, and they communicate with a voluminous interhemispheric cyst (*arrow*). The cerebral biometry is markedly superior to the 90th percentile. **c** T2-weighted midline sagittal slice. Under the pressure of the hydrocephalus, the sutures are disjoint (*arrowhead*). A selective termination of pregnancy is performed. The neurofetopathological examination shows a massive triventricular dilatation linked with aqueductal atresia. The septum and corpus callosum are not visible

Natural History of Ventricular Dilatation, Effect on the Cerebral Parenchyma and Prognosis

The physiology of cerebrospinal fluid (CSF) during pregnancy is inadequately known. CSF is essentially (75%) produced by the choroid plexuses. The capillaries' endothelium also participates in this production. A major part of the CSF is reabsorbed by the cerebral capillaries [33]. The natural history of ventricular dilatation is very incompletely defined in the antenatal context.

Apart from ventricular dilatations of obstructive origin, ventricular dilatation may result from an imbalance in the production and resorption of CSF. Excessive production of CSF (as in choroid plexus papillomas, for instance) is very rare; in most cases, CSF resorption disorders are responsible for ventricular dilatation [29]. The hypothesis of an occlusion of the resorption channels occurring early in fetal life could be envisaged, although it does not seem very plausible, particularly as some cases of hydrocephalus may only develop at a late stage, i.e. towards the end of the second trimester [2, 36]. Another possible explanation is that the CSF resorption channels develop later, or more slowly, than the CSF production. This would explain the resolution of some ventricular dilatations during pregnancy. Up to now, however, no evidence has been presented to support this theory. It seems plausible that the imbalance between production and resorption of CSF has to reach a critical level for the ventricular dilatation and the increased head circumference to become apparent.

Delayed proliferation of the germinal zone neuroblasts has been observed in hydrocephalic rats, but it is not known whether the proliferation is inhibited by an increase in intraventricular pressure or by another factor of genetic origin. This may explain why, in these rats as well as in fetuses with a myelomeningocoele, ventricular dilatation is often associated with a small head circumference [2, 37]. Furthermore, when ventricular dilatation progresses gradually, the pressure increase results first in a compression of the cerebral tissue, then in a constraint of the blood flow and ultimately in cerebral atrophy [29].

In fact, ventricular dilatation often does not seem to result from an intracranial pressure increase, since in many cases the dilatation is only mildly progressive, or even stable or resolvent, and the head circumference is often normal [9]. Does the counterpressure exerted by the amniotic fluid play a role?

Ventricular dilatation may also result from an atrophy of the cerebral parenchyma (in vacuo dilatation) or from a developmental abnormality of the cerebral hemispheres.

The progression of isolated ventricular dilatations in utero, analysed in a review of the literature by Kelly et al. [9] on 295 fetuses studied in published series [2, 7, 19, 21, 23, 26, 28, 38–42], leads to spontaneous resolution in 29 % of cases; the dilatation is stable in 57% of cases, and it keeps increasing in 14 % of cases.

It is very difficult to establish a prognosis for these ventricular dilatations, as the studies published are often based on a small number of fetuses in very heterogeneous cohorts [43]. They often mix unilateral and bilateral, progressive, stable and resolvent, isolated and associated dilatations. One should also keep in mind that, in numerous series, the diagnosis of ventricular dilatation is based on the measurement of just one atrium [27].

In a great majority of articles dealing with ventricular dilatation in antenatal imaging, the diagnosis is based on ultrasonography only. Fetal MRI is rarely even mentioned [19, 40, 44, 45] and only in very small series. The contribution of MRI to the aetiological diagnosis of ventricular dilatation, and hence its influence on the prognosis, has only been studied in one article so far [45], where MRI showed abnormalities that were overlooked in US in seven cases out of 14 (five cases of CCA, one of lissencephaly, one of heterotopia). Yet, several authors [10, 44] have pointed out that associated abnormalities are often detected in postnatal examination (in 25 % [10] or even 36 % [44] of cases) in cases where the US examination led to the belief that the ventricular dilatation was isolated. However, it is regrettable that in most articles the skill of the sonographer (referring or not) is usually not stated, although this is known to have a great influence on the effectiveness of US in detecting some abnormalities.

The various series in postnatal imaging are also often heterogeneous. The imaging technique used is variable (US, computed tomography, MRI), and furthermore it is not always stated.

The neurological follow-up of children is also often made on exceedingly short periods. The normality of a neurological examination at 6 months or 1 year of life is evidently no guarantee of a good prognosis over the long term. Moreover, the methods used to evaluate the potential delay in acquisitions differ greatly from one series to another. Some make do with a mere conversation on the telephone with the treating doctor, or even with the parents, others use neuropsychomotor development tests, others do not even mention the nature of the follow-up [9].

While taking into account all these limitations regarding the literature in this field, we can nonetheless sketch a broad outline of the prognostic factors of ventricular dilatation:

- The presence of associated abnormalities is for many authors a sign of a poor prognosis [2, 3, 29, 30, 38, 39].
- The fetus's gender: many studies report some measure of male predominance in cases of ventricular dilatation [40]. The influence of the fetus's sex on the prognosis, however, remains controversial. To some [19], males have a better prognosis than females, while others [21] maintain that the gender factor bears no significant influence as to the child's progression.
- The type of the dilated ventricle: some authors hold the presence of a dilatation of the third or fourth ventricle to be a negative prognostic factor [42], but the origin of the dilatation is not taken into account.

Aqueductal stenosis, regardless of its cause, heavily burdens the progression of ventricular dilatation [10,

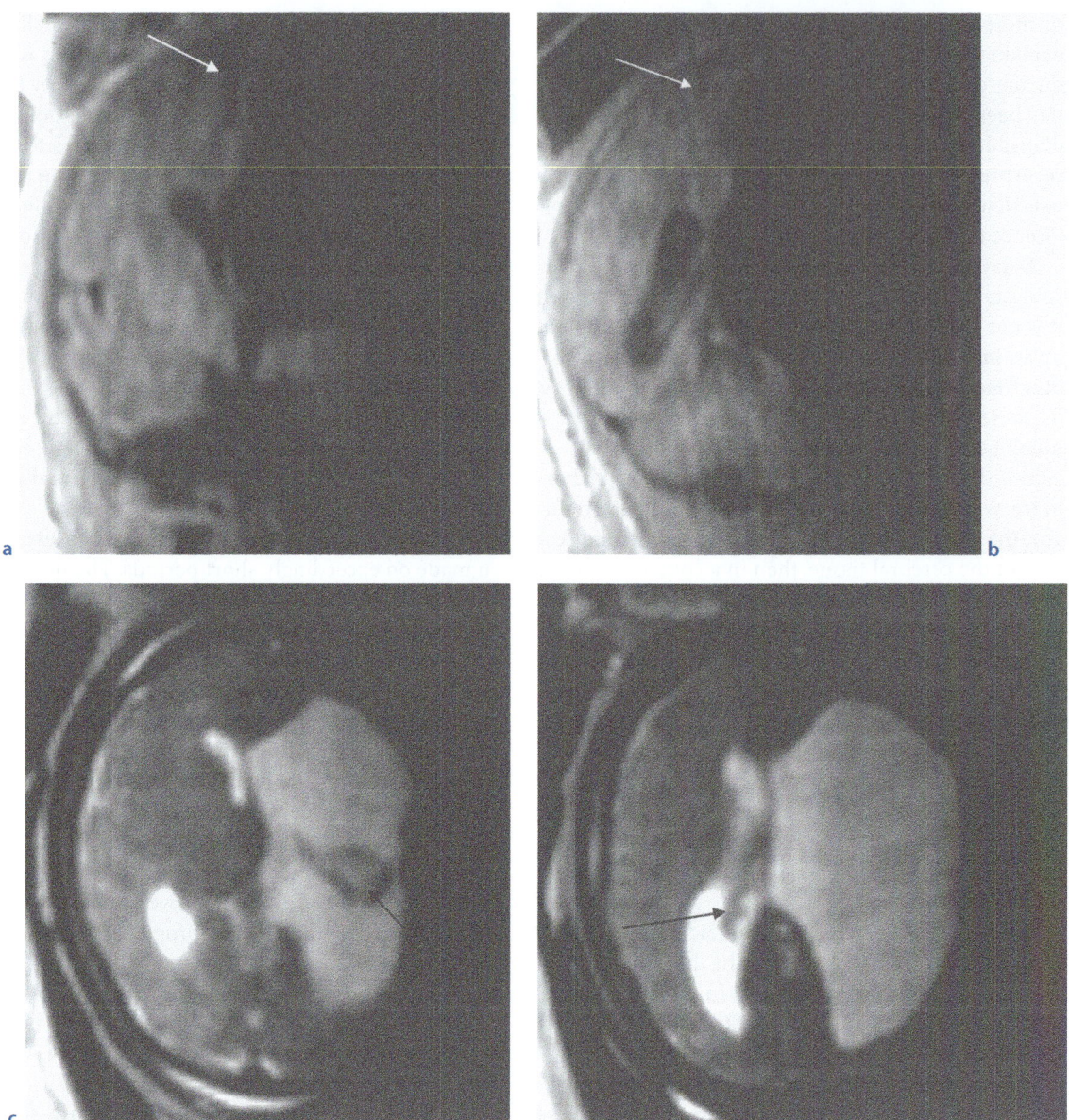

Fig. 10a–g. Unilateral ventricular dilatation. Detection of a unilateral left ventricular dilatation in US at 32 weeks of gestation (no prenatal care). **a, b** MRI performed at 32 weeks of gestation. T1-weighted anterior (**a**) and posterior (**b**) coronal slices. The left lateral ventricle is very dilated (atrium measured at 32 mm) and puffed up, with a thin parenchyma in the periphery. The interhemispheric fissure is deviated to the right (*arrow*). **c, d** T2-weighted axial slices showing a hyposignal of both choroid plexuses (*arrows*), probably resulting from an old haemorrhage. Termination of pregnancy is suggested be- cause of the magnitude of the dilatation and is carried out at 33 weeks of gestation. **e, f** Macroscopic coronal slices at the levels of the thalami (**e**) and of the occipital horns (**f**). The macroscopic examination confirms the asymmetrical ventricular dilatation of the left lateral ventricle, with a rupture of the left leaf of the septum and stigmas of a bilateral intraventricular haemorrhage (*arrows*). The Monro foramina are permeable (*arrowheads*). **g** Histological slice at the level of the aqueduct, showing a gliosis partially obstructing the aqueduct lumen

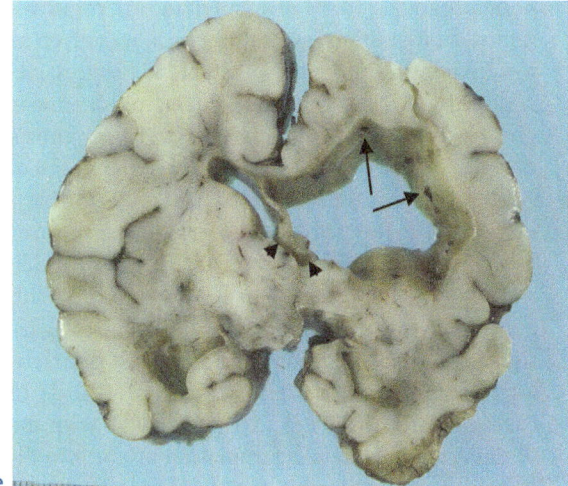

e

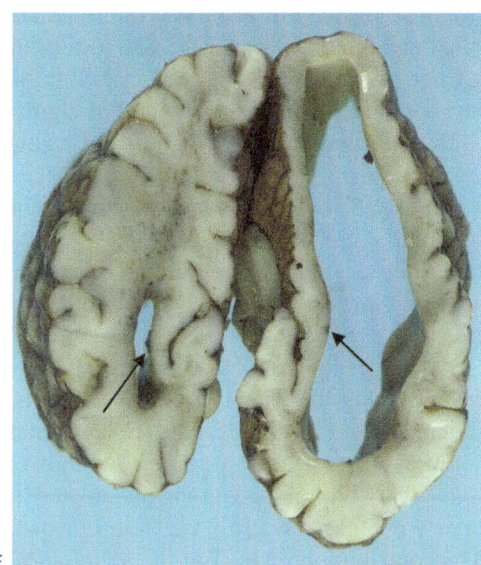

f

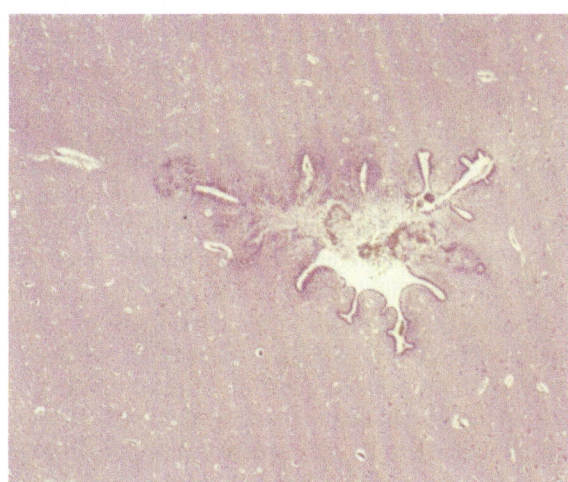

g

46]. The mortality rate here is on the order of 40 %; normal development is only observed in 10 % of cases [46].

- The unilateral or bilateral character of the dilatation: this distinction is made in very few articles that report series, or isolated cases, of mostly mild unilateral ventricular dilatation [3, 23, 40, 47–49] (Figs. 5, 10). The left ventricle is the most often affected [47]. Progression is generally good (in approximately 86 % of cases in the articles cited above), except when there are associated malformations, or when the dilatation progresses rapidly [3]. Two children with one ventricle measured at 14 mm have been reported to progress favourably [3].

- The influence of the asymmetrical or symmetrical character of the dilatation on the prognosis has yet to be studied. The only article dealing with this aspect [3] in fact mostly reports cases of unilateral dilatation.

- The scale of ventricular dilatation: the relation between the size of the ventricles and the prognosis is disputed. Some [50] consider that there is a significant correlation between the ventricles' size and the degree of developmental retardation, while for others [10] this relation depends on the physiopathology of ventricular dilatation. Indeed, a mild in vacuo dilatation resulting from cerebral atrophy carries a much worse prognosis than that of a larger dilatation of obstructive origin with a normal cerebral parenchyma (Fig. 11). Severe dilatations (AD > 15 mm), however, often have a poor prognosis. Regarding the milder dilatations (10 mm < AD < 15 mm), the difficulty lies in determining a threshold under which the prognosis is significantly better. Some [21] evaluate this threshold at 11 mm (92 % good prognoses under 11 mm, only 58 % above), others [19, 39] at 12 mm (80 % good prognoses under 12 mm [39]; still others [42] situate the limit at 13 mm. One may wonder why this threshold should not be established in MRI, since it is a more precise and more reliable method.

- The progression of ventricular dilatation in the course of pregnancy raises the question of the measurements' reliability. The more quickly the dilatation progresses, the worse the prognosis [2, 8, 10, 30, 42]. In such cases, Gupta et al. [10] and Bannister et al. [2] have reported a poor prognosis in 33 % and 66 % of patients, respectively. Some authors [51] have reported persistent dilatations of

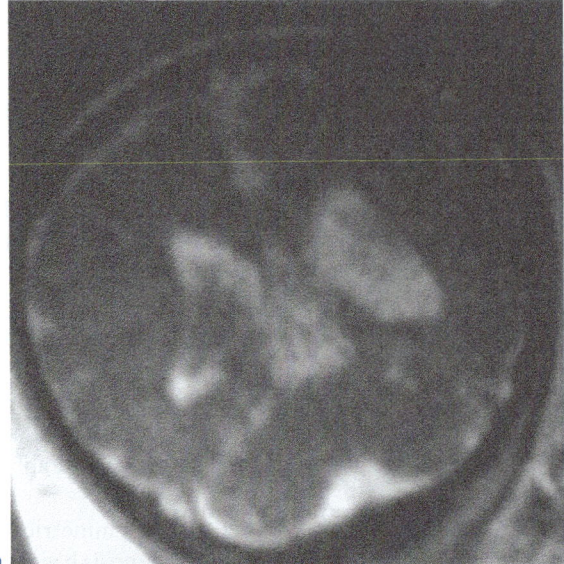

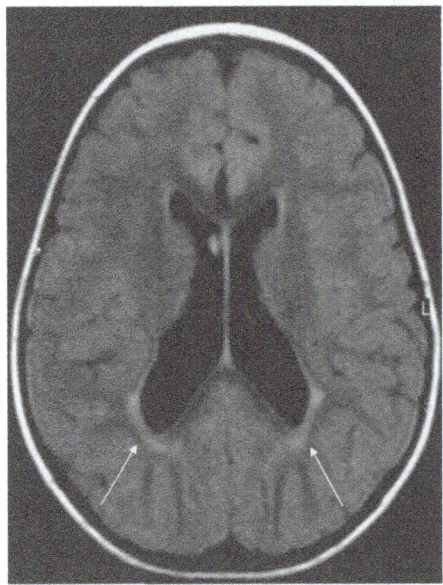

Fig. 11 a, b. Mild bilateral ventricular dilatation. Periventricular leucomalacia. Detection at 38 weeks of gestation of a non-evolutive, moderate, bilateral and asymmetrical ventricular dilatation evaluated at 11 mm on the left and 14 mm on the right. **a** MRI at 38 weeks of gestation. T2-weighted coronal slice. The dilatation seems to be isolated. **b** Postnatal MRI at 2.5 years. Axial slice in FLAIR sequence at the level of the lateral ventricles. The atria measure at 15 mm on the right and 12 mm on the left. The lateral ventricles are square-shaped at the back, and the posterior periventricular white matter is hyperintense (*arrows*). This pattern is compatible with sequelae of periventricular leucomalacia. At 3 years, the child shows pyramidal syndrome, hypertonia of the lower limbs and equinus feet

poor prognosis (67 % of mental and/or cognitive retardation), but no further precision was given as to whether the dilatation was stable or progressive. A resolution of the dilatation during pregnancy is observed in one-third of cases [19]. The prognosis of resolvent dilatations is generally better (70 % of good prognoses for Arora et al. [42], 80 % for Bannister et al. [2]). The resolution of some severe, 16-mm dilatations has been reported [2, 42], but such a resolution is not necessarily synonymous with good prognosis. Cases of developmental retardation have been reported in children with ventricular dilatation [50]; some of them (two-thirds of cases for Bannister et al. [2]) were linked with the discovery at postnatal examination of abnormalities that were not seen in antenatal examination. The prognosis of stable dilatations is intermediate between those of the progressive and resolvent forms. Good progression is observed in 50 %–71 % of cases [2, 42]. Some authors [21] found no significant difference between the prognoses of stable and resolvent forms.

- Some authors [8] hold the early appearance of ventricular dilatation to be a sign of poor prognosis. In another series [20], however, the regressive and very mild forms appear early in the course of pregnancy.

Although ventricular dilatation is the most commonly encountered cerebral abnormality in antenatal findings, it remains, as seen above, largely unknown. Its aetiology is very diverse, and it remains isolated in approximately 60 % of cases [9] (55.7 % in our own series). The contribution of MRI to the aetiological diagnosis of ventricular dilatation, and hence to the evaluation of its prognosis, which essentially depends on the associated abnormalities, has yet to be studied in large series. However, in light of our own experience, it seems certain that, since the analysis of the brain is more precise with MRI than in ultrasonography, MRI can at least help refine the aetiological diagnosis of ventricular dilatation. By gathering the data provided in the different, very inhomogeneous series published on mild isolated dilatation, which can only provide an exclusion diagnosis, developmental retardation affects 0 %–36 % of cases, with an average of 10.4 %. The postnatal follow-up of these children is generally very short, and therefore this last figure will certainly have to be reconsidered as soon as a long-term follow-up of children diagnosed in the antenatal period with ventricular dilatation is available. Late-arising neurodevelopmental disorders (between

3.5 and 7 years of life) have recently been reported in such children [52]. The resolution of a ventricular dilatation in the antenatal period is no guarantee of a good prognosis.

References

1. Lyon G, Evrard P (2002) Hydrocéphalies, collections liquidiennes péricérébrales chroniques. In: Lyon G, Evrard P (eds) Neuropédiatrie, 2nd edn. Masson, Paris
2. Bannister CM, Russel SA, Rimmer S, Arora A (2000) Prenatal ventriculomegaly and hydrocephalus. Neurol Res 22: 37–42
3. Durfee SM, Kim FM, Benson CB (2001) Postnatal outcome of fetuses with the prenatal diagnosis of asymmetric hydrocephalus. J Ultrasound Med 20:263–268
4. Koga Y, Tahara Y, Kida T, Matumoto Y, Negishi H, Fujimoto S. Prenatal diagnosis of congenital unilateral hydrocephalus. Pediatr Radiol 1997 ; 27 : 319–320.
5. Brady TB, Kramer RL, Qureshi F, Feldman B, Kupsky WJ, Johnson MP, Evans MI (1999) Ontogeny of recurrent hydrocephalus: presentation in three fetuses in one consanguineous family. Fetal Diagn Ther 14:198–200
6. Beke A, Csabay L, Rigo J Jr, Harmath A, Papp Z (1999) Follow-up studies of newborn-babies with congenital ventriculomegaly. J Perinat Med 27:495–505
7. Nicolaides KH, Berry S, Snijders JM, Thorpe-Beeston JG, Gosden C (1990) Fetal lateral cerebral ventriculomegaly: associated malformations and chromosomal defects. Fetal Diagn Ther 5:5–14
8. Wilhelm C, Keck C, Hess S, Korinthenberg, Breckwoldt M (1998) Ventriculomegaly diagnosed by prenatal ultrasound and mental development of the children. Fetal Diagn Ther 13:162–166
9. Kelly EN, Allen VM, Seaward G, Windrim R, Ryan G (2001) Mild ventriculomegaly in the fetus, natural history, associated findings and outcome of isolated mild ventriculomegaly: a literature review. Prenat Diagn 21:697–700
10. Gupta JK, Bryce FC, Lilford RJ (1994) Management of apparently isolated fetal ventriculomegaly. Obstet Gynecol Surv 49:716–721
11. Cardoza JD, Goldstein RB, Filly RA (1988) Exclusion of fetal ventriculomegaly with a single measurement: the width of the lateral ventricular atrium. Radiology 169:711–714
12. Filly RA, Goldstein RB (1994) The fetal ventricular atrium: fourth down and 10 mm to go. Radiology 193:315–317
13. Hilpert PL, Hall BE, Kurtz AB (1995) The atria of the fetal lateral ventricles: a sonographic study of normal atrial size and choroid plexus volume. AJR 164:731–734
14. Browning PD, Laorr A, McGahan JP, Krasny RM, Cronan MS (1994) Proximal fetal cerebral ventricle: description of US technique and initial results. Radiology 192:337–341
15. Farrell TA, Hertzberg BS, Kliewer MA, Harris L, Paine SS (1994) Fetal lateral ventricles: reassessment of normal values for atrial diameter at US. Radiology 193:409–411
16. Kramer RL, Yaron Y, Johnson MP, Evans MI, Treadwell MC, Wolfe HM (1997) Differences in measurements of the atria of the lateral ventricle: does gender matter? Fetal Diagn Ther 12:304–305
17. Patel MD, Goldstein RB, Tung S, Filly RA (1995) Fetal cerebral ventricular atrium: difference in size according to sex. Radiology 194:713–715
18. Garel C, Chantrel E, Sebag G, Brisse H, Elmaleh M, Hassan M (2000) Le développement du cerveau fœtal : atlas IRM et biométrie. Sauramps Médical, Montpellier
19. Vergani P, Locatelli A, Strobelt N, Cavallone M, Ceruti P, Paterlini G, Ghidini A (1998) Clinical outcome of mild fetal ventriculomegaly. Am J Obstet Gynecol 178:218–222
20. Mercier A, Eurin D, Mercier PY, Verspyck E, Marpeau L, Marret S (2001) Isolated mild fetal cerebral ventriculomegaly: a retrospective analysis of 26 cases. Prenat Diagn 21: 589–595
21. Patel MD, Filly AL, Hersh DR, Goldstein RB (1994) Isolated mild fetal cerebral ventriculomegaly: clinical course and outcome. Radiology 192:759–764
22. Achiron R, Yagel S, Rotstein Z, Inbar O, Mashiach S, Lipitz S (1997) Cerebral lateral ventricular asymmetry: is this a normal ultrasonographic finding in the fetal brain? Obstet Gynecol 8:233–237
23. Lipitz S, Yagel S, Malinger G, Meizner I, Zalel Y, Achiron R (1998) Outcome of fetuses with isolated borderline unilateral ventriculomegaly diagnosed at mid-gestation. Ultrasound Obstet Gynecol 12:23–26
24. Hertzberg BS, Kliewer MA, Freed KS, McNally PJ, DeLong DM, Bowie JD, Kay HH (1997) Third ventricle: size and appearance in normal fetuses through gestation. Radiology 203:641–644
25. Baumeister LA, Hertzberg BS, Mc Nally PJ, Kliewer MA, Bowie JD (1994) Fetal fourth ventricle: US appearance and frequency of depiction. Radiology 192:333–336
26. Tomlinson MW, Treadwell MC, Bottoms SF (1997) Isolated mild ventriculomegaly: associated karyotypic abnormalities and in utero observations. J Maternal-Fetal Med 6:241–244
27. Pilu G, Falco P, Gabrielli S, Perolo A, Sandri F, Bovicelli L (1999) The clinical significance of fetal isolated cerebral borderline ventriculomegaly: report of 31 cases and review of the literature. Ultrasound Obstet Gynecol 14:320–326
28. Robson S, McCormack K, Rankin J (1998) Prenatally detected mild/moderate cerebral ventriculomegaly: associated anomalies and outcome. Eur J Pediatr Surg 8 [Suppl I]: 70–71
29. Drugan A, Krause B, Canady A, Zador IE, Sacks AJ, Evans MI (1989) The natural history of prenatally diagnosed cerebral ventriculomegaly. JAMA 261:1785–1788
30. Twining P, Jaspan T, Zuccollo J (1994) The outcome of fetal ventriculomegaly. Br J Radiol 67:26–31
31. Mangels KJ, Tulipan N, Tsao LY, Alarcon J, Bruner JP (2000) Fetal MRI in the evaluation of intrauterine myelomeningocele. Pediatr Neurosurg 32:124–131
32. Aaronson OS, Hernanz-Schulman M, Bruner JP, Reed GW, Tulipan NB (2003) Myelomeningocele: prenatal evaluation-comparison between transabdominal US and MR Imaging. Radiology 22:839–843
33. Schrander-Stumpel C, Fryns JP (1998) Congenital hydrocephalus: nosology and guidelines for clinical approach and genetic counselling. Eur J Pediatr 157:355–362
34. Castro-Gago M, Alonso A, Eiris-Punal J (1996) Autosomal recessive hydrocephalus with aqueductal stenosis. Childs Nerv Syst 12:188–191

35. Hamada H, Watanabe H, Sugimoto M, Yasuoka M, Yamada N, Kubo T (1999) Autosomal recessive hydrocephalus due to congenital stenosis of the aqueduct of Sylvius. Prenat Diagn 19:1067–1069

36. Reece EA, Goldstein I (1997) Early prenatal diagnosis of hydrocephalus. Am J Perinatol 14:69–73

37. Weller RO, Mitchell J, Griffin RL, Gardner MJ (1978) The effects of hydrocephalus upon the developing brain. J Neurol Sci 36:383–402

38. Goldstein RB, La Pidus AS, Filly RA, Cardoza J (1990) Mild lateral cerebral ventricular dilatation in utero: clinical significance and prognosis. Radiology 176:237–242

39. Bromley B, Frigoletto FD, Benacerraf BR (1991) Mild fetal lateral cerebral ventriculomegaly: clinical course and outcome. Am J Obstet Gynecol 164:863–867

40. Senat MV, Bernard JP, Schwärzler P, Britten J, Ville Y (1999) Prenatal diagnosis and follow-up of 14 cases of unilateral ventriculomegaly. Ultrasound Obstet Gynecol 14:327–332

41. Hudgins RJ, Edwards MSB, Goldstein R, Callen PW, Harrison MR, Filly RA, Golbus MS (1988) Natural history of fetal ventriculomegaly. Pediatrics 82:692–697

42. Arora A, Bannister CM, Russell S, Rimmer S (1998) Outcome and clinical course of prenatally diagnosed cerebral ventriculomegaly. Eur J Pediatr Surg 8 [Suppl I]:63–64

43. Den Hollander NS, Vinkesteijn A, Schmitz-Van Splunder P, Catsman-Berrevoets CE, Wladimiroff JW (1998) Prenatally diagnosed fetal ventriculomegaly: prognosis and outcome. Prenat Diagn 18:557–566

44. Valat AS, Dehouck MB, Dufour P, Dubos JP, Djebara AE, Dewismes L, Robert Y, Puech F (1998) Ventriculomégalie cérébrale fœtale. Etiologie et devenir, à propos de 141 observations. J Gynecol Obstet Biol Reprod 27:782–789

45. Greco P, Vimercati A, De Cosmo L, Laforgia N, Mautone A, Selvaggi L (2001) Mild ventriculomegaly as a counselling challenge. Fetal Diagn Ther 16:398–401

46. Levitsky DB, Mack LA, Nyberg DA, Shurtleff DB, Shields LA, Nghiem HV, Cyr DR (1995) Fetal aqueductal stenosis diagnosed sonographically: how grave is the prognosis? AJR 164:725–730

47. Kinzler WL, Smulian JC, McLean DA, Guzman ER, Vintzileos AM (2001) Outcome of prenatally diagnosed mild unilateral cerebral ventriculomegaly. J Ultrasound Med 20:257–262

48. Farrell SA (1998) Transient unilateral cerebral ventriculomegaly. Prenat Diagn 18:303–306

49. Tsao PN, Teng RJ, Wu TJ, Tsou Yau KI, Wang PJ (1996) Nonprogressive congenital unilateral ventriculomegaly. Pediatr Neurol 14:66–68

50. Bloom SL, Bloom DD, Dellanebbia C, Martin LB, Lucas MJ, Twickler DM (1997) The developmental outcome of children with antenatal mild isolated ventriculomegaly. Obstet Gynecol 90:93–97

51. Low JA, Galbraith RS, Sauerbrei EE, Muir DW, Killen HL, Pater E, Karchmar EJ (1986) Motor and cognitive development of infants with intraventricular hemorrhage, ventriculomegaly, or periventricular parenchymal lesions. Am J Obstet Gynecol 155:750–756

52. Gilmore JH, Van tol JJ, Streicher HL, Williamson K, Cohen SB, Greenwood RS, Charles HC, Kliewer MA, Whitt JK, Silva SG, Hertzberg BS, Chescheir NC (2001) Outcome in children with fetal mild ventriculomegaly: a cases series. Schizophr Res 30:219–226

Abnormalities of the Posterior Cerebral Fossa

Laurent Guibaud

The abnormalities of the posterior fossa (PF) observed in antenatal examinations include the small posterior fossa associated with a defect of neural tube closure in Chiari II malformation (see Chap. 11), the congenital cystic abnormalities of the PF, and a heterogeneous group of exceptional abnormalities such as rhombencephalosynapsis, tumoral lesions and vascular malformations.

Congenital Cystic Abnormalities of the Posterior Fossa

Congenital cystic abnormalities of the PF are usually diagnosed in US upon discovery of an increase in the size of the cisterna magna (>10 mm). These abnormalities include Dandy-Walker malformation, cerebellar ageneses and hypoplasias, mega cisterna magna and arachnoid cysts of the posterior fossa.

Anatomical and Embryological Data

The knowledge of a few anatomical and above all embryological facts is a prerequisite to the practice of antenatal diagnosis [1, 2]. Such knowledge provides a better understanding of the so-called cystic patterns of the posterior fossa and the stages at which they appear, particularly when facing a proband.

- The cerebellum and the brain stem derive from a single primordium: the rhombencephalon.
- The cerebellum is composed of a midline structure, the vermis, and two hemispheres.
- The surface of the vermis and of the hemispheres displays a characteristic folding. Thus, a deep fissure, the primary fissure, separates the anterior and posterior parts of the vermis. The posterior vermis shows characteristic fissures. These are, in a craniocaudal direction, the prepyramidal fissure, the secondary fissure, and the posteronodular fissure at the back of the nodulus (Fig. 1).

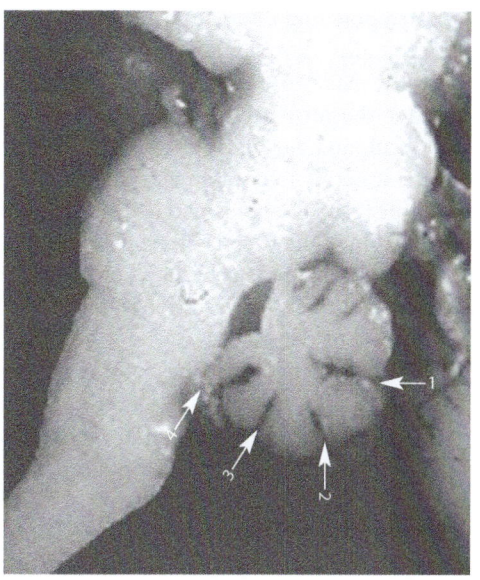

Fig. 1. Midline sagittal slice on an embryo at 20–21 weeks of gestation. Primary fissure (1); prepyramidal fissure (2); secondary fissure (3); posteronodular fissure (4)

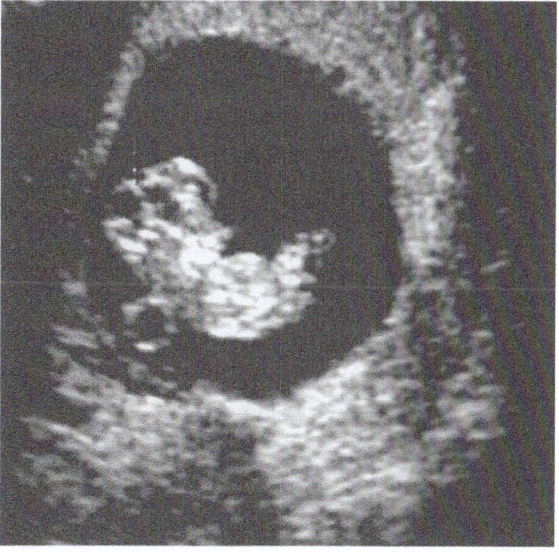

Fig. 2. Ultrasonography. Normal embryo at 8–9 weeks of gestation. Visualization of a physiological cistern inside the future PF (rhomboid fossa)

- The appearance of a transitory fluid-filled structure inside the future posterior fossa at 8–9 weeks of gestation is physiological (Fig. 2). It corresponds to a cisterna or rhomboid fossa located at the back of the pontine flexure that is not found after 10 weeks of gestation. Before 10 weeks of gestation, this 2–3-mm-wide cisterna must not be mistaken for a congenital cystic abnormality of the posterior fossa. The persistence of a fluid-filled structure after 10 weeks of gestation should, however, draw attention to a potential PF cystic abnormality [3].
- The embryological development of the vermis is, schematically, made in a craniocaudal direction. Indeed, after the formation of the archicerebellum, or flocculonodular lobe at 9 weeks of development, the anterior lobe (cranial), and then the posterior lobe (caudal) are formed. A US follow-up of the formation of the vermis has shown that the vermis was still incomplete in 56% and 23% of cases at 14 and 15 weeks of gestation, respectively, and in only 6% of cases at 17 weeks of gestation [4]. Hence, the vermis should be complete after 17 weeks of gestation (15 weeks of development). The sonographic diagnosis of vermian agenesis is therefore possible as early as 18 weeks of gestation [4].
- The embryological developments of the hemispheres and of the vermis are not concomitant, as the hemispheres usually develop a few weeks after the vermis.
- The proliferation of neuroblasts, which eventually leads to the formation and cell differentiation of the cerebellar cortex, reaches its maximum in the 6th month of pregnancy. This explains why the rule in sonography, according to which transverse cerebellar diameter (TCD) = number of weeks of gestation ± 1 mm, applies between 18 and 24 weeks of gestation but is no longer true after 24 weeks of gestation [5, 6]. Indeed, after the 6th month, the cerebellum has asymptotic growth. The TCD is approximately 30 mm at 27 weeks of gestation, and 42 mm at 32 weeks of gestation [5, 6].

Cerebellar hypoplasia is diagnosed based on a diminution of the TCD. It can therefore not be ruled out on the basis of one normal sonography at 20–22 weeks of gestation, contrary to vermian agenesis. This fact stresses the importance of the systematic measurement of the cerebellum in the third trimester, and above all that of the biometrical follow-up of the cerebellum after 25 weeks of gestation in proband cases of cerebellar or pontocerebellar hypoplasia.

Ultrasonographic Analysis of the Posterior Cerebral Fossa

It is essential, particularly in the second trimester, and should not be replaced by MRI too early as, except in some special cases, MRI has no diagnostic indication before 26 weeks of gestation.

In a majority of cases, sonography provides for a good analysis of the posterior fossa, particularly between 18 and 26 weeks of gestation. The examination consists of one axial slice, on which the biometry is evaluated (TCD and cisterna magna), and a strict midline sagittal slice (i.e. showing the nasal bone and corpus callosum), on which the vermis and tentorium cerebelli are analysed (Figs. 3, 4). The vermis is characteristically hyperechoic compared to the hypoechoic cerebellar hemispheres (Fig. 5). This difference in echogenicity also makes it possible to recognize a potential partial volume on the hemispheres in the anatomical study of the vermis. The tentorium cerebelli is not directly visible in US, but the normality of its orientation can be evaluated by assessing the position of the overlying occipital lobe. The vermian fissures, and particularly the primary fissure, are clearly seen from 25 weeks of gestation.

Sonography is also used in looking for associated cerebral and extracerebral abnormalities, particularly for abnormalities of the midline (corpus callosum) at the encephalic level, and for sylvian fissure opercularization abnormalities, ventriculomegaly and alterations of the cephalic biometry in the supratentorial space. The presence of associated extracerebral abnormalities can point to a syndromic pathology.

When there are suspicions of a congenital cystic abnormality of the posterior fossa, MRI is put to good use, as it can determine the precise location of the tentorium cerebelli, to study the anatomy and biometry of the vermis, hemispheres and brain stem, and to look for potential associated cerebral lesions.

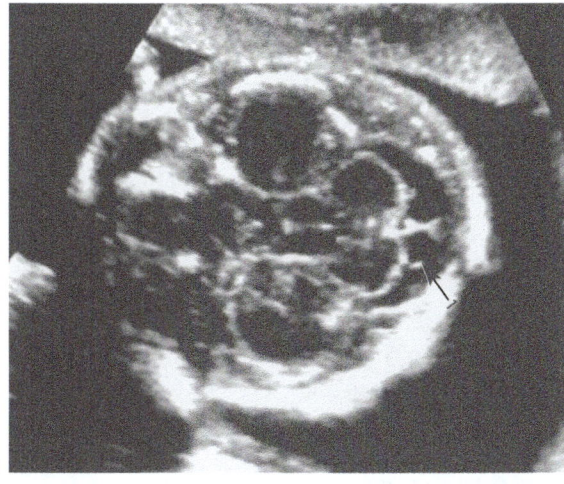

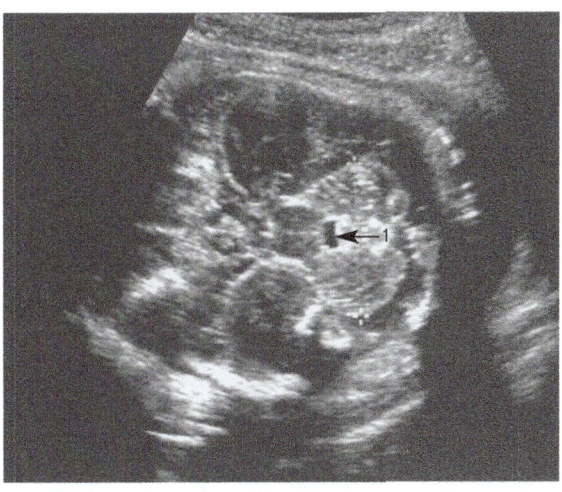

Fig. 3a,b. Ultrasonography. Axial slice on the posterior fossa (PF). a At 20–21 weeks of gestation, visualization of arachnoid veins (1) at the back of the vermis forming a bridge inside the cisterna magna. b 27 weeks of gestation. Visualization of the hemispheric sulci and 4th ventricle (1)

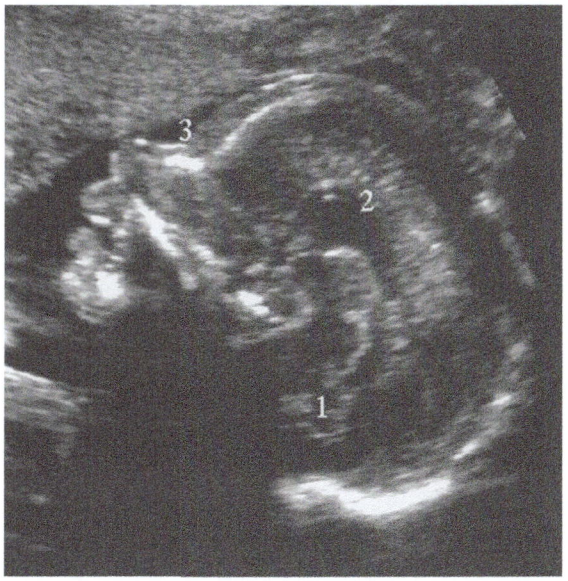

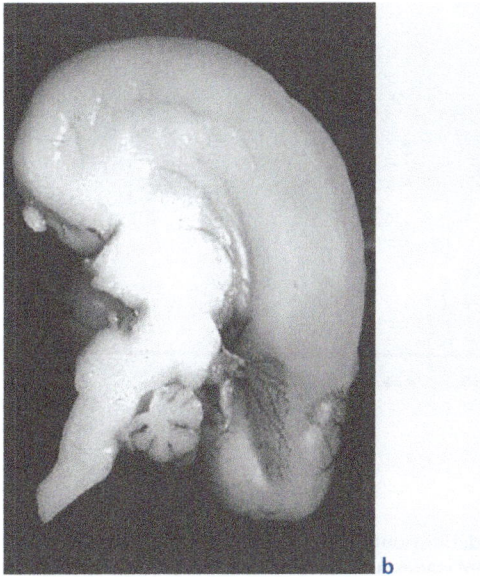

Fig. 4a,b. Median sagittal slice at 20–21 weeks of gestation. a US slice showing the hyperechoic vermis (1). The fissures cannot be individualized at this stage. The presence on this slice of the corpus callosum (2) and nasal bone (3) shows that it is strictly median. b Corresponding anatomical view

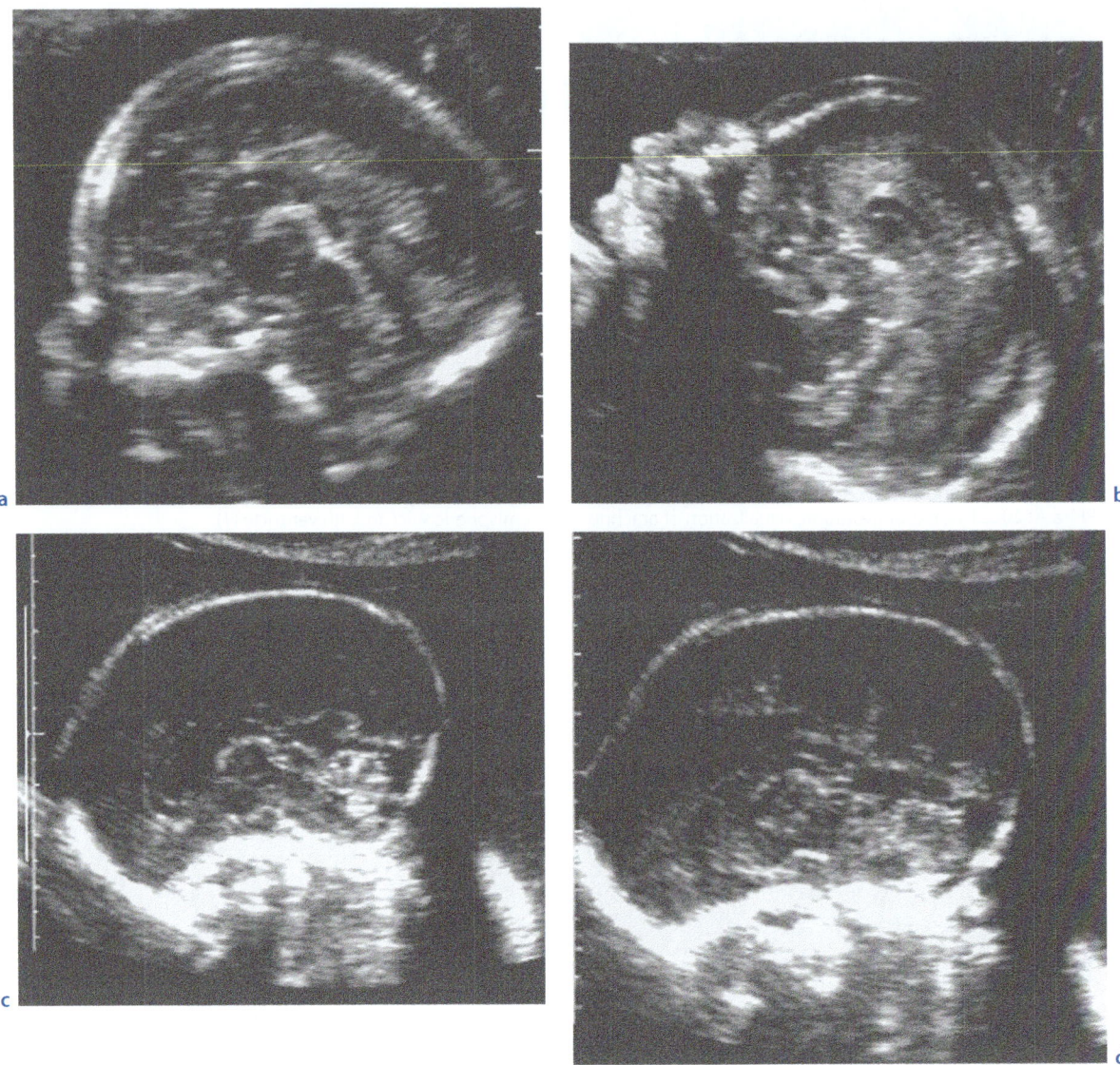

Fig. 5 a–d. Ultrasonography. Sagittal slices of the cerebellum at different stages. **a** At 18 weeks of gestation, the hyperechoic vermis is complete. **b** Same at 20 weeks of gestation. **c, d** At 25 weeks of gestation, beginning of the identification of fissures. The vermis is hyperechoic on a midline sagittal slice (**c**) compared with the adjacent hemisphere, visualized on a parasagittal slice (**d**). At all these terms, the 4th ventricle is identified, and completely covered by the vermis

MRI Analysis of the Posterior Cerebral Fossa

MRI examination of the posterior fossa is performed in the three planes of space on fast (FSE of TSE) or ultrafast (single-shot) T2-weighted sequences with thin slices (3–4 mm), completed by T1- and T2*-weighted sequences to look for possible ischaemo-haemorrhagic lesions (in T1 hypersignal and T2* hyposignal).

MRI can evaluate the global volume of the posterior fossa and the position of the tentorium cerebelli (and particularly that of its insertion at the level of the torcular). It also enables a biometrical and morphological analysis of the cerebellum (vermis and hemispheres), brain stem, cisterna magna and ventricle (Fig. 6). The cerebellum biometry is evaluated according to the standards published [7, 8]. The height of the vermis is over 15 mm from 28 weeks of gestation, and on the order of 20 mm at 30 weeks of gestation. The vermis is studied morphologically, starting with the identification of the anterior lobe and the larger posterior lobe of the primary fissure (from 30 weeks of gestation) and of the prepyramidal and secondary fissures after 32 weeks of gestation [9]. Such identification may, however, remain difficult, particularly in case of partial volume on the adjacent hemispheres.

MRI seems to be the most efficient examination in the analysis of the brain stem. One must look for a loss of the anterior bulge of the pons (absence of pontine flexure) objectively indicating pontocerebellar hypoplasia [9]. This sign is rather important since, in the absence of published standards, the brain stem biometry remains quite subjective.

MRI is also efficient in looking for associated cerebral malformations, and particularly supratentorial malformations (notably migration abnormalities) and abnormalities of the midline.

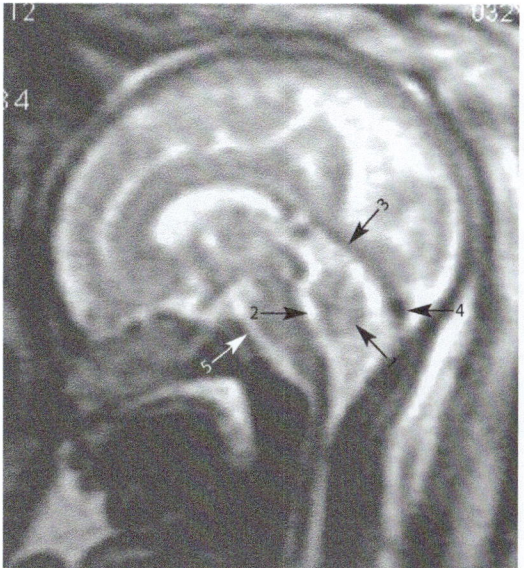

Fig. 6. T2-weighted midline sagittal slice in MRI at 31–32 weeks of gestation. Vermis (*1*), 4th ventricle (*2*), tentorium cerebelli (*3*), torcular herophili (*4*). Anterior bulge of the pons (*5*)

Classification of Congenital Cystic Abnormalities of the Posterior Fossa

Dandy-Walker Malformation

Dandy-Walker (DW) syndrome results from a development abnormality of the rhombencephalon appearing between the 7th and the 10th week of development [2]. It can therefore be diagnosed early in the antenatal period. Its frequency is on the order of 1/25,000 or 30,000 births. It is essentially sporadic, although a few familial cases have been reported [10]. The aetiology of this malformation is not established, but a viral or toxic (alcohol, Coumadin) origin has been suggested [2].

Dandy-Walker malformation is defined by the following triad (Fig. 7):

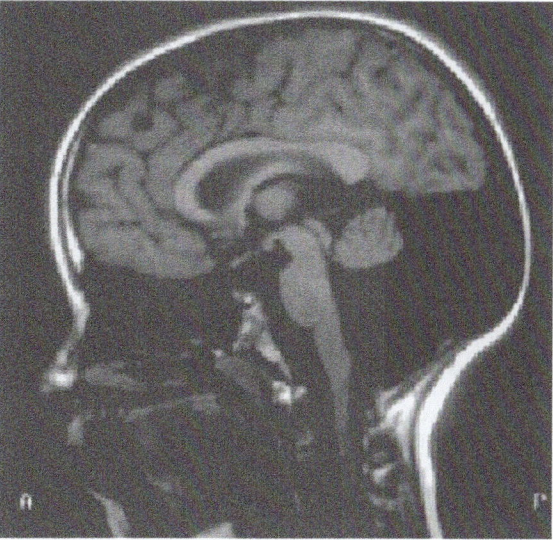

Fig. 7. Dandy-Walker malformation (postnatal MRI). Globally enlarged PF with high tentorium, cystic dilatation of the 4th ventricle and partial vermian agenesis

- Global widening of the posterior fossa, with an ascent of the tentorium cerebelli and its insertion and the ascent of the torcular herophili
- Cystic dilatation of the 4th ventricle (no connection with the subarachnoid space)
- Partial or complete vermian agenesis

The diagnosis of DW rests on the complete triad, with the emphasis laid on the global widening of the PF,

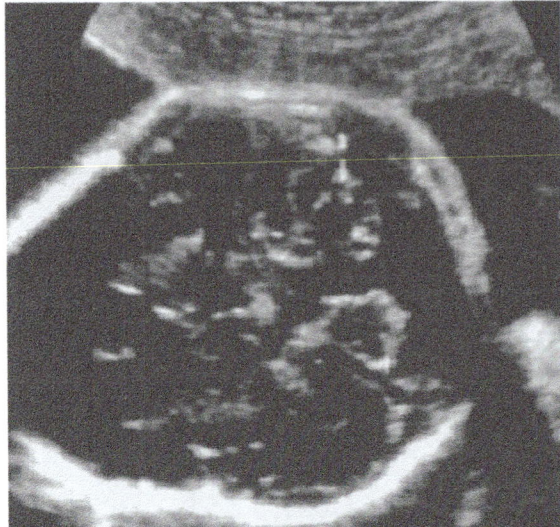

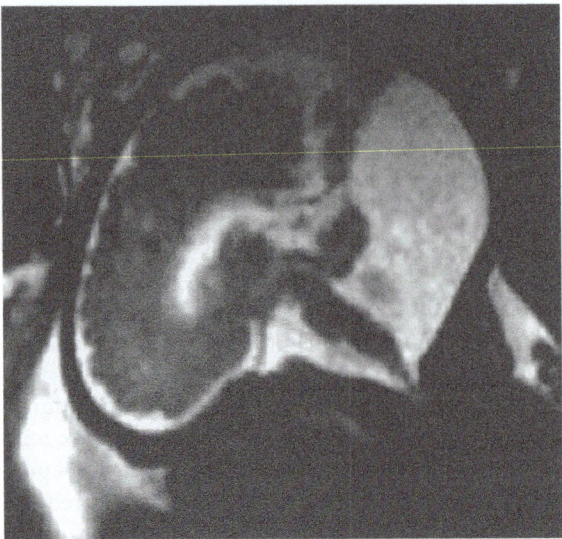

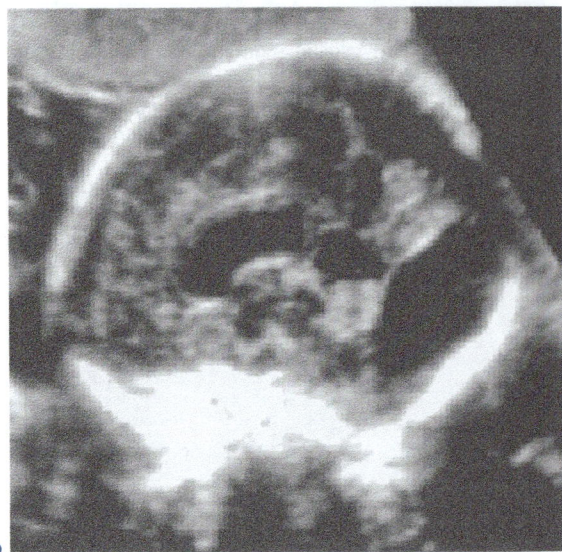

Fig. 9. Fetal MRI at 36 weeks of gestation. Dandy-Walker malformation. Midline sagittal slice. Note the large PF, high tentorium and partial agenesis of the vermis. Good postnatal neurological progression

Fig. 8 a, b. US diagnosis of Dandy-Walker malformation (images courtesy of P. Droullé, Nancy). **a** Abnormal communication between the 4th ventricle and the cisterna magna on an oblique axial slice indicating a vermian agenesis. **b** High tentorium and large PF, clearly seen on a midline sagittal section

pillar of the diagnosis. A tentorium cerebelli in its right place rules out the diagnosis of DW. Widening of the PF is best evaluated on a midline sagittal slice (Figs. 8–10). It may also be suspected on supratentorial axial slices, in the presence of a fluid-filled cisterna secondary to a high tentorium (Fig. 10b). The diagnosis of vermian agenesis is based on the visualization, on an axial slice, of an abnormal midline communication between the 4th ventricle and the cisterna magna, bordered on both sides by the cerebellar hemispheres (Fig. 8a).

Some factors of poor prognosis should be looked for systematically: hydrocephalus (mostly late, sometimes postnatal) and other associated neurological malformations (in particular those of the midline) [1, 11–13] and extraneurological malformations (found in 47%–81% of cases according to Estroff [11]). In a recent series of 50 cases of DW diagnosed in antenatal examinations, Ecker reports associated malformations in 86% of cases, the most frequent being ventriculomegaly (32%) and cardiac abnormalities (38%) [12]. Abnormalities of the limbs (28%), kidneys (28%) and face (26%) have also been observed [12].

DW can be sporadic and isolated, or part of a polymalformation syndrome or a chromosomal aberration (in 46% of cases for Ecker [12]).

A karyotype must therefore be prepared systematically.

Regarding the prognosis, a direct correlation has been reported to exist between the presence of associated extraneurological abnormalities and poor psychomotor development [11, 14, 15]. In a study of 71 cases of DW by Cinalli, 52% of children had an IQ higher than 80. On the other hand, in the same series, poor intellectual development was observed in those children with associated cerebral or maxillofacial malformations. IQ was normal in 54% of the children with isolated DW [3, 16].

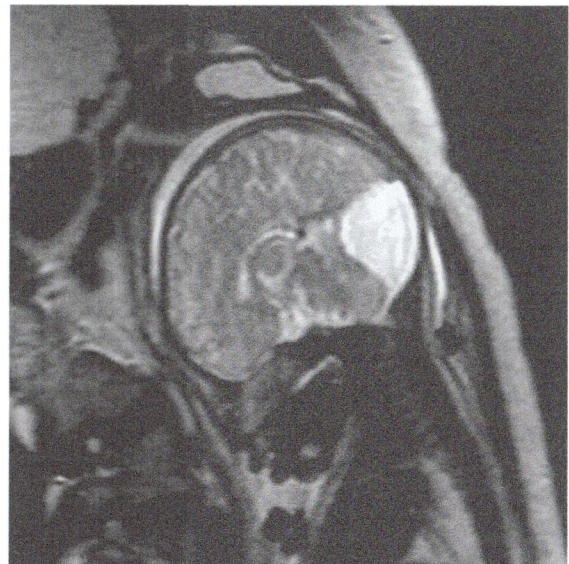

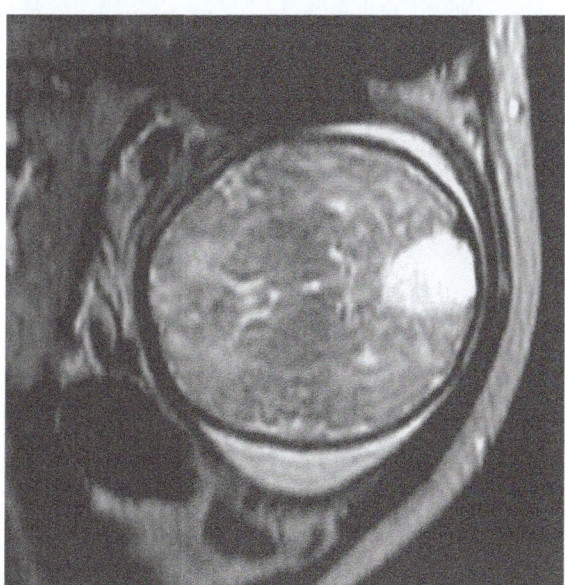

Fig. 10 a, b. Fetal MRI at 36 weeks of gestation. Dandy-Walker malformation. **a** Sagittal slice, global widening of the PF, and high tentorium and torcular herophili. **b** Supratentorial axial slice. Visualization of a cistern indicating a high tentorium. Note the absence of hydrocephalus. Good postnatal neurological progression

Cerebellar Ageneses and Hypoplasias

This group of cerebellar dysplasias must be distinguished from DW. It is heterogeneous, since it includes ageneses, hypoplasia and even early cerebellar atrophies. These are very different entities, sometimes gathered in the literature under the term "Dandy-Walker variant". The malformation can affect the vermis, or the hemispheres (often bilaterally), and, potentially, the brain stem [17]. In all these cases, however, the posterior fossa is not enlarged and the tentorium cerebelli is in its proper place [2]. The increase in size of the cisterna magna is relative and secondary to the decrease, in size or in volume, of the cerebellum.

The difference in the terminology between agenesis and hypoplasia must be stressed, given the implications of this distinction in antenatal management.

Vermian Ageneses

The types of vermian ageneses not associated with large posterior fossa have been gathered by Barkovitch under the name "Dandy-Walker variant" [13], but this designation has often been applied to all kinds of cystic malformations of the normal-volume posterior fossa, which include both agenesis and hypoplasia.

Agenesis is strictly speaking defined as an either complete or partial absence of an anatomical structure. In complete agenesis, the vermis is absent, whereas in partial agenesis a part of the vermis is present; the present part is anatomically of normal volume (Fig. 11). As mentioned in the introduction, partial agenesis is always inferior (caudal). It can be diagnosed in US as early as 18 weeks of gestation. Therefore, in the presence of a proband, a normal US examination at 20–22 weeks of gestation can rule out the possibility of recurrence.

Parental information in cases of vermian agenesis, particularly in the isolated partial forms, is rather delicate. In imaging, one must look for associated abnormalities of poor prognosis, notably on the midline. A karyotype is indispensable. In a homogeneous series of 49 cases of vermian agenesis, Ecker found abnormalities of the heart and limbs in 41 % and 28 % of cases, respectively, and karyotypic abnormalities in 36 % of cases [12].

Agenesis may be part of a syndrome. It is regularly observed in Joubert and Walker-Warburg syndromes, and in the cerebro-oculo-muscular syndrome. In fact, vermian agenesis is found to be associated occasionally with many syndromic entities [2,

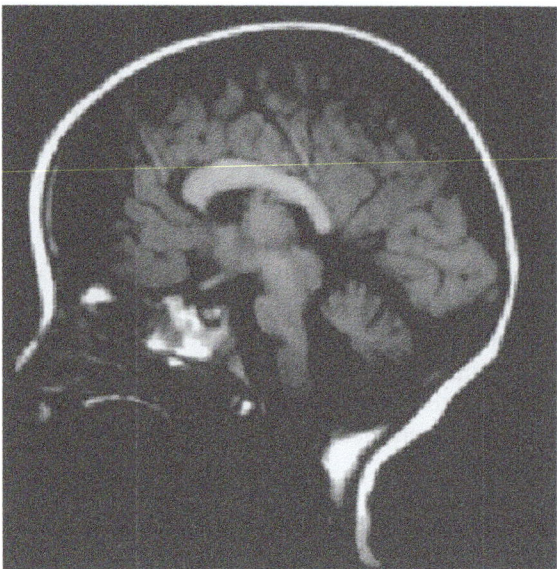

Fig. 11. Partial vermian agenesis (postnatal MRI). The PF is of normal volume. The caudal part of the vermis is present and of normal volume. Note the presence of a thick dysgenic corpus callosum, symptomatic of an associated abnormality of the midline

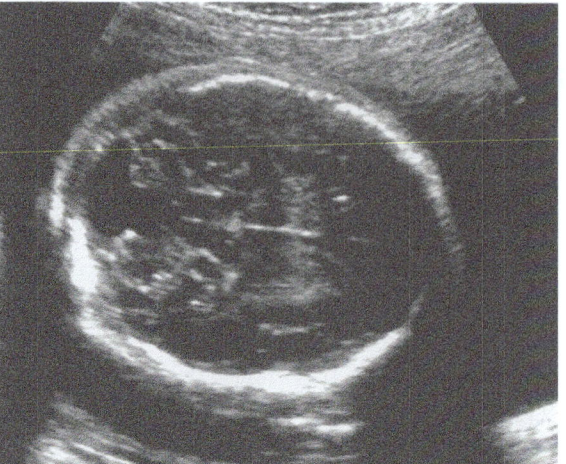

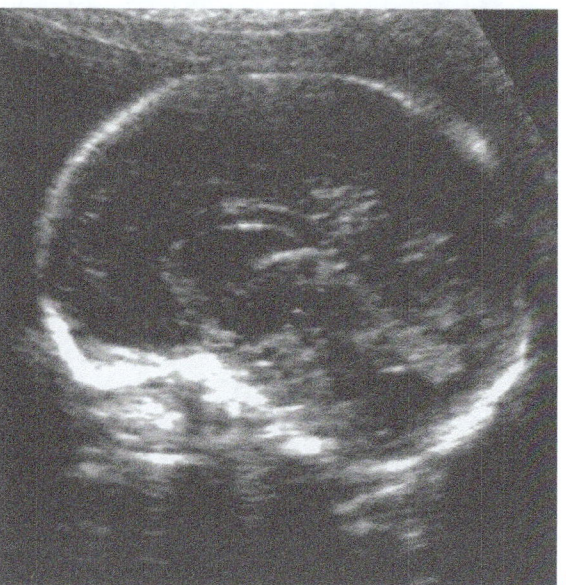

Fig. 12 a, b. US at 21–22 weeks of gestation. Partial vermian agenesis. **a** Abnormal communication between the 4th ventricle and the cisterna magna indicating vermian agenesis (normal TCD). **b** Midline sagittal slice. The partial vermian agenesis and lack of widening of the PF are confirmed. Karyotype: trisomy 21

17]. Finally, vermian agenesis can be isolated, in which case it is most frequently sporadic. However, in the presence of a proband, because a genetic determinism cannot be totally excluded, any further pregnancy must involve a reference ultrasonography at 20–22 weeks of gestation.

The diagnosis of vermian agenesis in US at 20–22 weeks of gestation is made on axial and midline sagittal slices (Figs. 12, 13). The sonographer should look for an increase in size of the cisterna magna, particularly on the midline. On a strict axial slice, the transverse cerebellar diameter is often normal and sometimes slightly reduced. The essential sign is an abnormal communication between the 4th ventricle and the cisterna magna, bordered on both sides by the cerebellar hemispheres, which is visible on coronal and axial slices. Laing [18] has drawn attention to the risk of creating false patterns of partial agenesis on slices that are not strictly axial, but rather axial oblique. When vermian agenesis is suspected, it is essential to take a midline sagittal slice. Indeed, this makes it possible to evaluate the volume of the PF and shows the incompleteness of the vermis (easily identifiable for its hyperechogenicity, contrasting with the hypoechoic hemispheres), as well as the uncovered 4th ventricle (Fig. 12b). The midline sagittal slice may, however, be difficult to obtain, particularly

at a late stage or when the presentation is not favourable.

The search for associated cerebral and extracerebral abnormalities in US must be systematic.

An early MRI may be done before 25 weeks of gestation, although it brings little new information regarding the positive diagnosis of this pathology compared to a well-conducted sonography. Indeed, in our experience, in the 2nd trimester it is sometimes easier to take a perfect midline sagittal slice in US than in

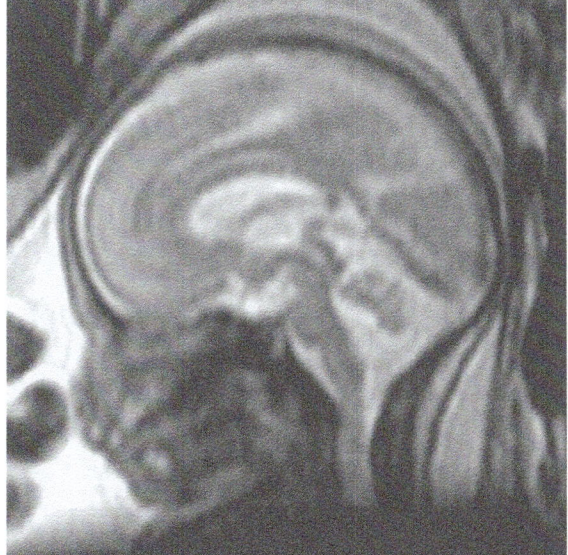

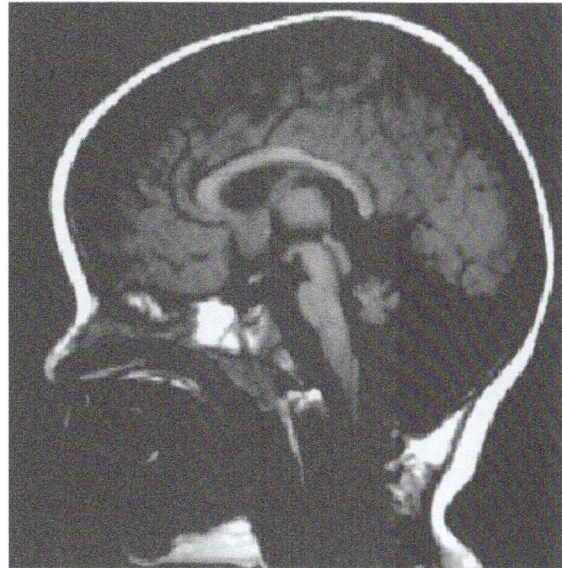

a

Fig. 14. Cerebellar hypoplasia (postnatal MRI). Complete vermis of very reduced size. Normal volume PF. Normal brain stem with anterior bulge of the pons

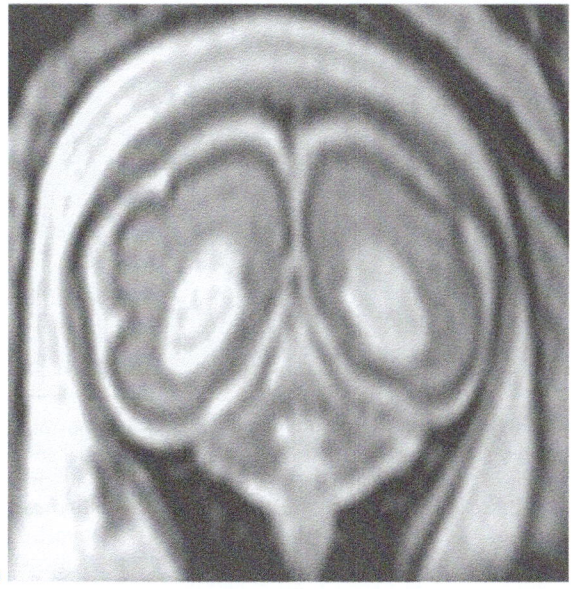

b

Fig. 13 a, b. MRI at 28 weeks of gestation. Partial vermian agenesis. **a** The partial vermian agenesis and the normal volume of the PF with a well-positioned tentorium cerebelli can be seen on the midline sagittal slice. Note the anterior bulge of the annular pons. **b** Abnormal communication between the 4th ventricle and the cisterna magna on a coronal slice. Normal TCD. Associated with a cardiac abnormality (left ventricle hypoplasia). Death at birth

MRI. Moreover, the presence of a partial volume on one hemisphere in MRI may give a false image of partial agenesis [9]. Thin slices reduce this risk because of the better spatial resolution, but at the expense of signal intensity. When suspecting a vermian agenesis in US at a late stage, an MRI ought to be done on prin-ciple, as it can evaluate the extent of the agenesis, particularly in partial forms, and look for associated lesions.

The presence of associated cerebral abnormalities, and particularly migration abnormalities, is best assessed in MRI between 30 and 32 weeks of gestation.

Cerebellar Hypoplasia

Hypoplasia is defined as a complete anatomical structure displaying a congenital volume diminution (as opposed to atrophy, where the diminution of volume is secondary) (Fig. 14). Cerebellar hypoplasia is a heterogeneous group that includes isolated cerebellar hypoplasias and pontocerebellar hypoplasias, which can be primitive or secondary.

Secondary hypoplasias may be part of a polymalformation context, a karyotypic abnormality, or a syndromic or infectious (CMV) complex [17]. It should be noted that hypoplasias secondary to a metabolic pathology have been reported, as in CDG syndrome. It seems, however, that these are early atrophies rather than actual developmental abnormalities of the hypoplasia type.

The group of primitive cerebellar hypoplasias (PCH) associated with an involvement of the pons is classically divided into two groups: the forms with an associated involvement of the anterior horn of the spinal cord, very rapidly lethal (type I PCH in Barth's classification), and the forms with no involvement of

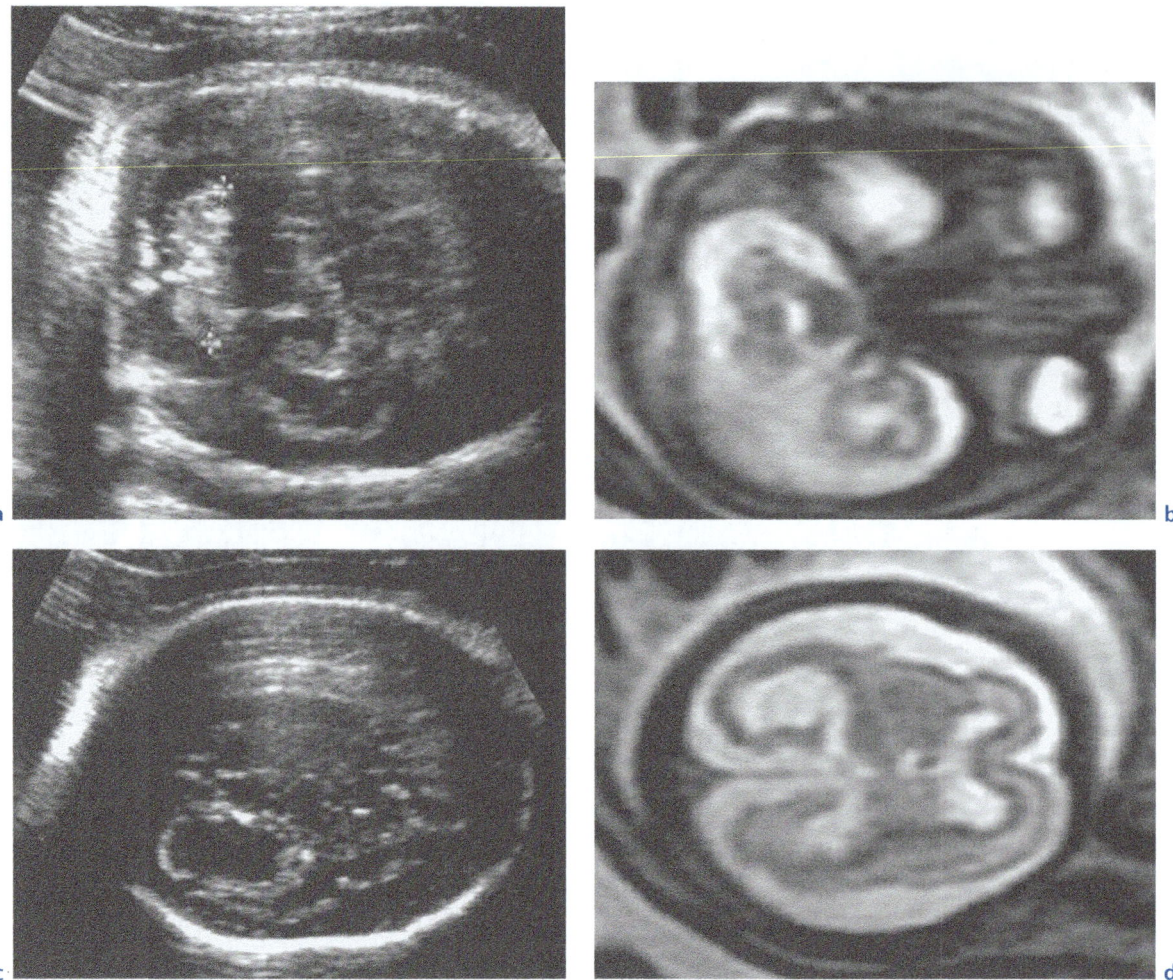

a   b

c   d

Fig. 15 a–d. CMV fetopathy at 25 weeks of gestation. Patient submitted for microcephaly. Subtentorial axial slice in US (**a**) and in MRI (**b**) showing hypoplasia of the cerebellum demonstrated by the diminution of TCD. Supratentorial axial slice in US (**c**) and in MRI (**d**). Major abnormalities of the gyration and organization of the cortex

Fig. 16 a–g. Pontocerebellar hypoplasia (ante- and postnatal ▶ imaging). G3P2 patient. First pregnancy: pontocerebellar hypoplasia (death in neonatal period). Normal second child. **a–c** US follow-up of the third pregnancy (from video captures). **a** At 22 weeks of gestation, normal TCD 22 mm. **b** At 27 weeks of gestation: TCD 27 mm (10th percentile, 50th percentile at 30 mm). **c** At 33 weeks of gestation, TCD 30 mm (3rd percentile, 50th percentile at 42–44 mm). **d–g** Postnatal MRI. Absence of the anterior bulge of the pons (absence of pontine flexure) on the midline sagittal slice (**d**). Severely reduced postnatal TCD on an axial slice (**f**). Pancake-shaped hypoplastic hemispheres on the parasagittal (**e**) and coronal (**f**) slices. The antenatal diagnosis of a recurrence is reached at the end pregnancy and confirmed after birth

the anterior horn, but with an evolutive microcephaly, and death in early childhood (type II PCH) [19, 20]. There probably is a third type, with a variably severe neurological picture, which often associates other supratentorial or midline abnormalities [21].

No early antenatal diagnosis, particularly biological diagnosis, of primitive pontocerebellar hypoplasia is possible without a chromosomal or molecular marker [19]. The absence of biological diagnosis makes the sonographic follow-up particularly necessary in the presence of a proband, given the existence of mostly recessive autosomal familial forms [19, 22].

It is essential to know of the normal progression of cerebellum growth and the intense proliferation at the 6th month of pregnancy (see "Anatomical and Embryological Data" above). Indeed, some cerebellar and pontocerebellar hypoplasias only appear late, after 25 weeks of gestation, in the form of a reduction of

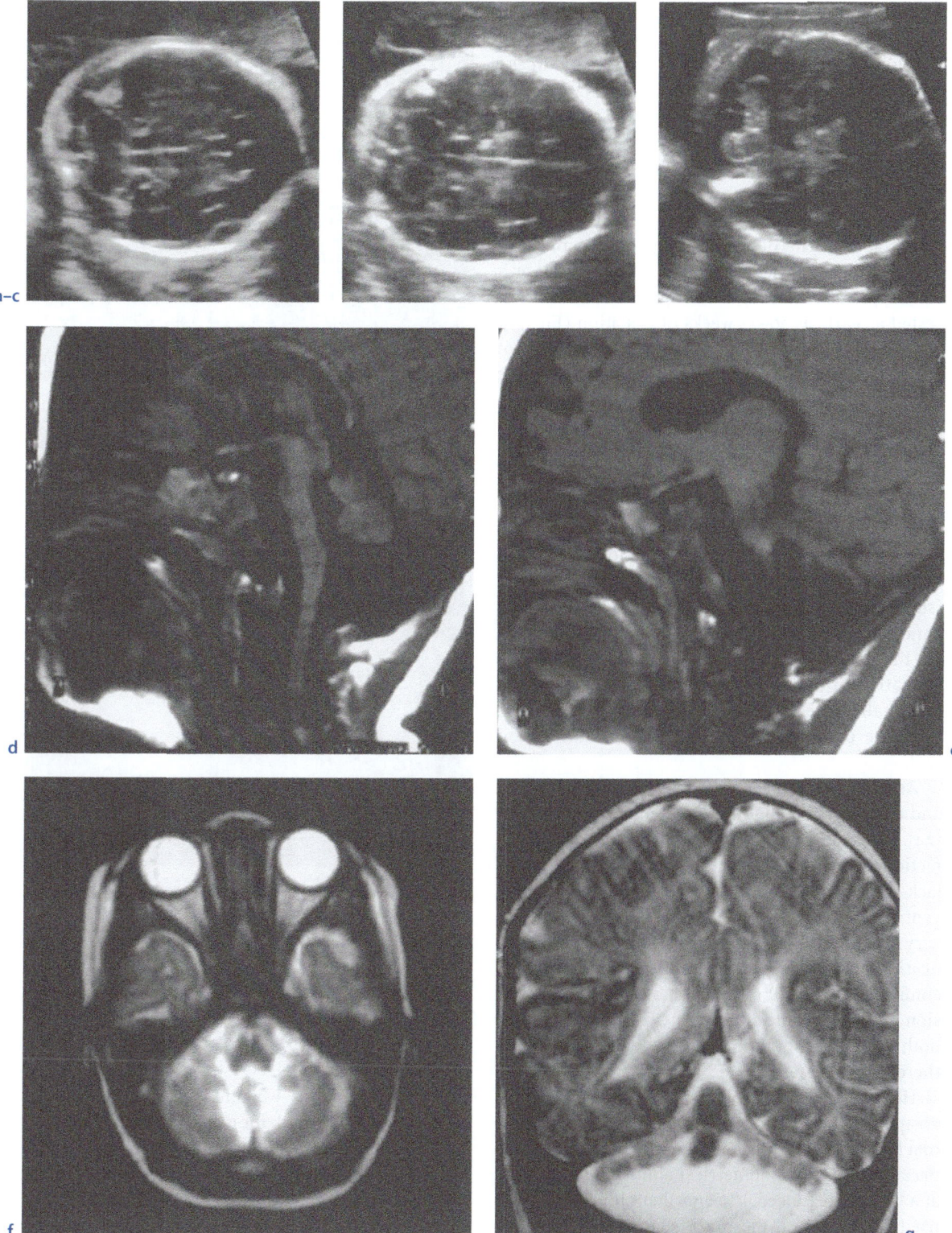

the transverse cerebellar diameter. This fundamental notion justifies the importance of a sonographic follow-up with measurement of the TCD at 20–22 weeks of gestation, 26–27 weeks of gestation and 32 weeks of gestation in the presence of a proband.

The sonographic diagnosis of cerebellar hypoplasia essentially relies on the significant diminution of the TCD, associated in most cases with a relative enlargement of the cisterna magna and a complete vermis. In some forms of cerebellar hypoplasia, particularly in those associated with a CMV fetopathy or a karyotypic abnormality, the diagnosis may be suggested as early as 20–22 weeks of gestation (Fig. 15). However, a normal sonography of the PF cannot guarantee the absence of cerebellar hypoplasia at birth, as illustrated by one personal observation of pontocerebellar hypoplasia (Fig. 16).

Thus, the heterogeneous group of cerebellar hypoplasias probably does not correspond to a uniform physiopathological mechanism [23]. The hypoplasias detected early in antenatal examination, and particularly those associated with an infectious fetopathy, are linked with a pathology of the germinal zones (sub- and supratentorial for CMV). On the other hand, some autosomal recessive genetic hypoplasias are thought to be linked with an abnormality in the formation of the definitive cerebellar cortex arising during the differentiation of the granular layer, and therefore only appear late in the antenatal period [22].

As with vermian ageneses, the search for cerebral and extracerebral abnormalities must be systematic [24]. In the early-arising forms linked with a CMV infection, the supratentorial abnormalities are many: lack of opercularization of the sylvian fissure, mild ventriculomegaly, altered head circumference and very evocative periventricular and perivascular calcifications. In this early form, the infectious fetopathy is confirmed on a PCR of the amniotic fluid. The decision on the outcome of pregnancy is taken, based on both sonographic and biological data. An MRI is therefore not essential.

However, MRI seems indispensable when there is an apparently isolated (negative infectious tests, normal karyotype) significant reduction of the TCD, especially when this biometrical abnormality appears at a late stage. Indeed, it seems that only MRI can be used in evaluating the brain stem and diagnosing possible pontocerebellar hypoplasia. This diagnosis is based on the absence of pontine flexure resulting from a hypoplasia of the pons, and on the pancake-like shape of the hemispheres (sign described in postnatal examinations) [9, 23].

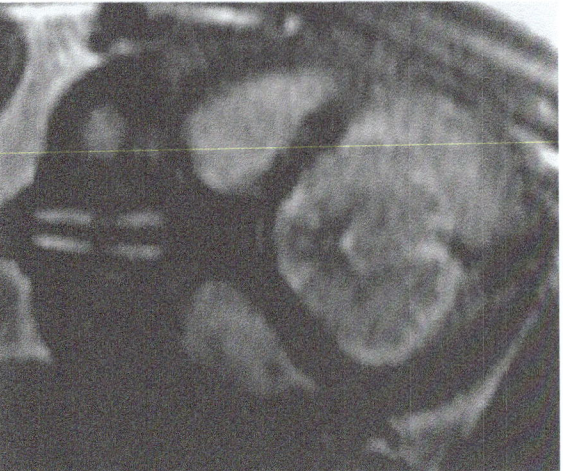

a

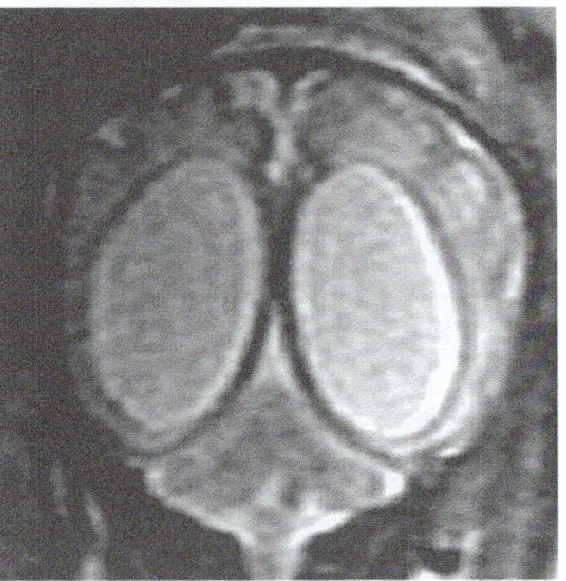

b

Fig. 17 a, b. MRI at 33 weeks of gestation. Pattern of polymicrogyria of the cerebellum. Slight diminution of the TCD (39 mm) and indented pattern of the cerebellar cortex (**a**). Decrease in volume of the left hemisphere on a coronal slice (**b**). Normal cisterna magna. Note the complete corpus callosum agenesis resulting in colpocephaly. Possibility of consanguinity

Using T1- and T2*-weighted slices in MRI should make it possible to look for ischaemo-haemorrhagic-type clastic lesions, which could be responsible for uni- or bilateral asymmetrical hemispheric lesions, or even for a secondary atrophy of the pons. One should also take into account the possibility of (rare) localized dysplasias such as polymicrogyria (Fig. 17), potentially affecting only one hemisphere and associating a diminution of the hemisphere's volume with a passive enlargement of the cisterna magna facing it [25].

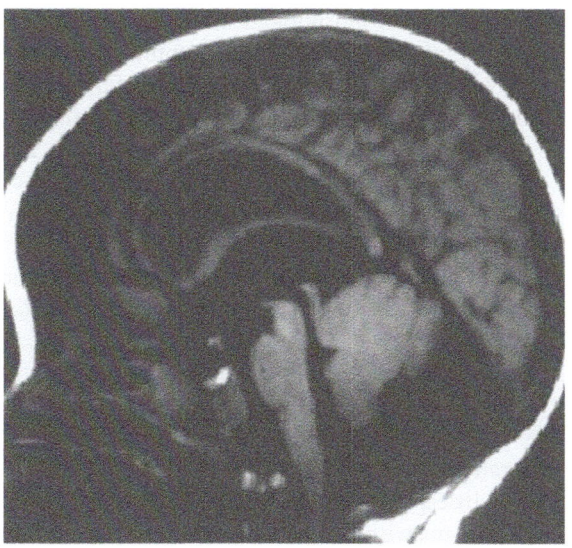

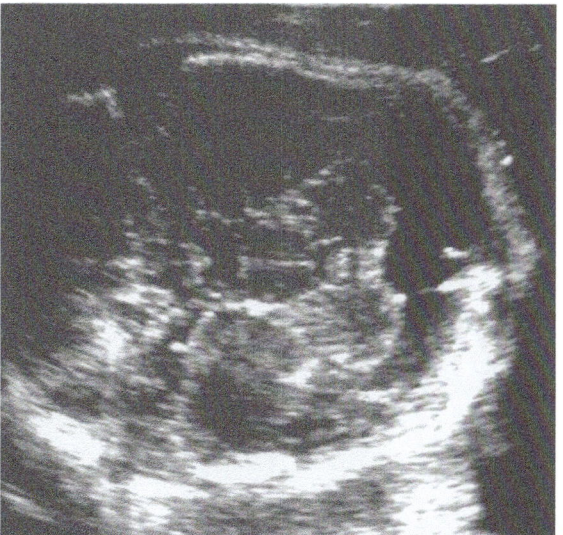

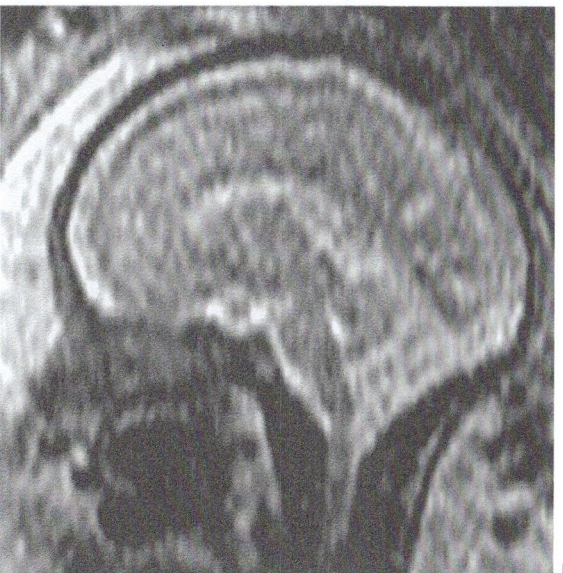

Fig. 18. Mega cisterna magna (postnatal MRI). Isolated enlarged cisterna magna. Normal volume PF and integrity of the cerebellum (complete vermis)

Mega Cisterna Magna, Blake's Pouch Cyst, Retrocerebellar Arachnoid Cysts

Mega cisterna magna, Blake's pouch cyst and retrocerebellar arachnoid cysts are very similar as far as imaging is concerned; they are hence often difficult to distinguish [2, 26, 27].

In all these cases, the volume of the posterior fossa is normal and the tentorium cerebelli and torcular herophili are in a normal position (Fig. 18). The tentorium may potentially be higher than normal because of a compressive cystic formation, but its insertion remains in place [2].

Mega cisterna magna is to be regarded rather as a variant in the normal state corresponding to an expansion of the medullocerebellar cistern, which communicates freely with the perimedullar subarachnoid space. Theoretically, it cannot give rise to a CSF flow disorder or to a mass effect on the adjacent cerebellum. Blake's pouch cysts result from an evagination of the caudal part of the tela choroidea without communication with the perimedullar space. They might give rise to an overlying hydrocephalus [28]. Their posteroinferior location leads to the rotation and horizontalization of the vermis, with an inferior opening of the 4th ventricle that is easily identifiable in imaging [9, 28].

Finally, retrocerebellar cystic formations, often on the midline and sometimes lateralized, are to be regarded as arachnoid cysts. Depending on their size,

Fig. 19a, b. Mega cisterna magna. **a** US at 28 weeks of gestation: large cisterna magna (12 mm). Integrity of the cerebellum. Normal TCD. **b** MRI at 28 weeks of gestation. The enlarged cisterna magna is confirmed. Normal volume PF. Integrity of the vermis. Note the absence of hydrocephalus at the supratentorial level. Normal postnatal progression

they can cause a mass effect on the cerebellar parenchyma and/or hydrocephalus.

In common practice, the diagnosis in fetal imaging is based in all cases on a large cisterna magna (>10 mm) that may be on the midline or lateral, symmetrical or asymmetrical, but always on an anatomically complete cerebellum of normal volume (Fig. 19). Here, one must:

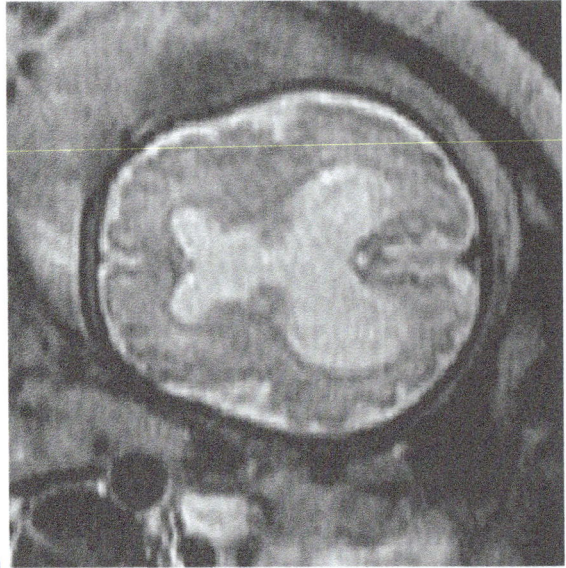

a

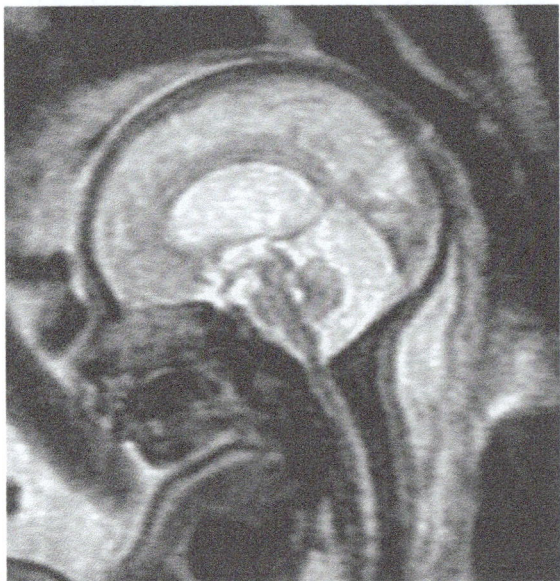

b

Fig. 20 a, b. MRI at 33 weeks of gestation. Compressive retrocerebellar cyst. Patient referred to MRI for ventriculomegaly, confirmed on a supratentorial axial slice (a). Midline sagittal slice (b) showing the presence of a compressive retrocerebellar cyst causing a triventricular dilatation and a slight mass effect on the tentorium cerebelli. The insertion of the tentorium is in its normal position. The vermis is normal. The hydrocephalus is not evolutive after birth. Good clinical progression over 3-year follow-up

- Determine the morphological and biometrical integrity of the cerebellum. Anatomical integrity may be difficult to ascertain, because of the potential compressive action of the cystic formation resulting in a distortion of the cerebellum with, notably, a high or flattened vermis, compressed or wide-apart hemispheres and bulging tentorium cerebelli.
- Look systematically for repercussions on the CSF flow with the formation of a hydrocephalus (Fig. 20).

These cystic formations have a very good prognosis. The possible mass effect on the adjacent cerebellum generally has no clinical repercussion. The presence of a hydrocephalus, however, should require postnatal follow-up, with a possible indication for a derivation.

Diagnostic Difficulties

In common practice, diagnosing certain cystic abnormalities of the posterior fossa may be quite difficult, particularly in the absence of postnatal follow-up and reference images (including a midline sagittal slice in the 2nd trimester).

The diagnosis may be delicate in the following situations:

- Vermian agenesis without cystic pattern.
  In this form, the cerebellar hemispheres are joined, thus hiding the communication between the 4th ventricle and the cisterna magna. This has been reported in some cases of Joubert's syndrome [9, 29]. Two signs can raise suspicion: the abnormal apposition of the hemispheres due to the absence of vermis, or buttocks sign, and the deformation of the 4th ventricle, which looks elongated in anteroposterior in a keyhole pattern. It is, it should be noted, mostly observed in postnatal examinations.
- Voluminous retrocerebellar cyst displacing the vermis or hemispheres with suspicion of a cerebellar abnormality.
  Some voluminous retrocerebellar cysts with distortion of the cerebellar parenchyma and mass effect on the tentorium cerebelli are difficult to diagnose and may lead to suspicion of a Dandy-Walker malformation [30]. The same problem of distortion of the anatomical structures is sometimes still present when postnatal follow-up is done. A de-

crease in volume of one hemisphere is often observed, although in practice the problem is mostly radiological, since this distortion rarely results in cerebellar symptoms, but rather in a hydrocephalus that could necessitate a derivation.

- Abnormal posteroinferior opening of the 4th ventricle with horizontalization, rotation and compression of the vermis.
  This abnormality resembling a Blake's pouch cyst may lead to discussing the possibility of inferior vermian agenesis. Considered as reassuring elements are the anatomical normality of the vermis in US in the 2nd trimester and the anatomical integrity of the cerebellum in the 3rd trimester, which implies normal biometrical (evaluation of the height of the vermis) and morphological (visualization of the secondary fissures after 32 weeks of gestation) analyses.

Conclusion

Congenital cystic abnormalities of the posterior fossa are defined by an increase in the size of the cisterna magna. They correspond to very different entities:

- Dandy-Walker malformation, which can be diagnosed early, is characterized by an enlargement of the posterior fossa with a high tentorium cerebelli.
- When the PF is of normal volume, it is advisable to look for a morphological or biometrical abnormality of the cerebellum.
  Agenesis and hypoplasia, often mistakenly gathered under the misleading term "Dandy-Walker variant", must be distinguished. Cerebellar agenesis can be diagnosed as early as 18 weeks of gestation, whereas hypoplasia may appear as late as in the 6th month of pregnancy (after 25 weeks of gestation). Agenesis and hypoplasia may be isolated, or included in a more complex, sporadic or familial picture.
- Dandy-Walker malformation, cerebellar agenesis and cerebellar hypoplasia demand a search for associated neurological and extraneurological malformations and the preparation of a karyotype.
- Isolated agenesis and hypoplasia can be sporadic or genetic (often autosomal recessive). The follow-up schedule for further pregnancies will depend on whether the proband is a case of agenesis or hypoplasia.

- Mega cisterna magna, Blake's pouch cyst or arachnoid cysts of the posterior fossa are diagnosed on the basis of an enlarged cisterna magna with a normal biometry and morphology of the cerebellum. One must always look for a CSF flow disorder with formation of a hydrocephalus. When the cyst is voluminous, the anatomical distortion may impair the analysis of the adjacent cerebellum, in antenatal as in postnatal examinations.

Rhombencephalosynapsis

Rhombencephalosynapsis is an exceptional malformation. Since its original description by Obersteiner [31], approximately 40, all diagnosed postnatally, have been reported in the literature. Most of these are paediatric observations. This malformation is defined as a fusion of the cerebellar hemispheres with vermian agenesis. Associated with it are a fusion of the cerebellar peduncles and of the dentate nuclei, and occasional supratentorial abnormalities, in particular septal agenesis and hydrocephalus [1, 32]. Some associated extraneurological abnormalities, mainly musculoskeletal, have also been reported [33].

In embryology, rhombencephalosynapsis is thought to result from a disorder of vermian differentiation occurring precociously at the 12th week of development. According to Utsunomiya, it corresponds to a lack of division of the cerebellar hemispheres rather than to an actual fusion (in connection with holoprosencephaly at the supratentorial level) [32]. One mutation or several mutations on the genes that code for the acquisition of a dorsal identity at the level of the midline of the mesencephalon–metencephalon junction region, among which the *Lmx1a* gene, which takes part in the early individualization of the ponto-mesencephalic junction, could be involved in the genesis of this malformation [34].

Imaging data, and particularly MRI data, show a flat and continuous pattern on the base of the hemispheres (as opposed to two distinct cerebellar hemispheres separated by the vermis). The transverse folding is highly characteristic [32, 35, 36]. The transverse cerebellar diameter is classically reduced, but the degree of hypoplasia varies from case to case [1]. A rhomboid deformation of the 4th ventricle is visible on axial slices, with a characteristic fusion or joining of the dentate nuclei and of the cerebellar peduncles. The posterior fossa is often abnormally small, with no identifiable cystic formation.

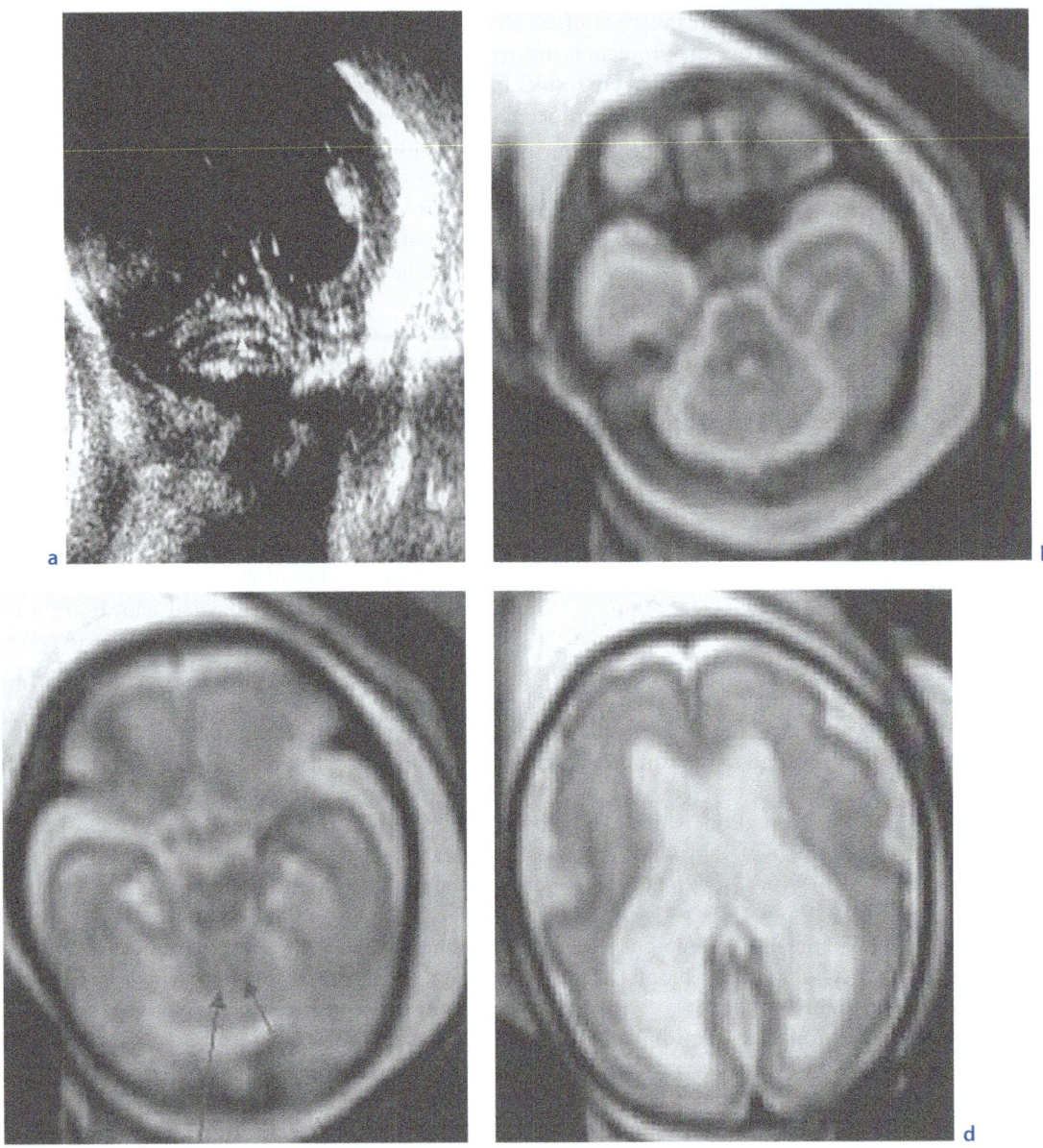

In a case of vermian agenesis associated with a very small transverse cerebellar diameter (13 mm) diagnosed at 18 weeks of gestation in antenatal US, rhombencephalosynapsis was diagnosed a posteriori in fetopathology [37]. Some exceptional cases (not reported in the literature) have been diagnosed antenatally, including one personal observation where rhombencephalosynapsis was strongly suspected in US, and later confirmed in fetal MRI (Fig. 21): in ultrasonography at 28 weeks of gestation, the cerebellum appeared in the form of a single block, since the two hemispheres were not individualized and the vermis was not visible. This block displayed a single

Fig. 21 a–d. Rhombencephalosynapsis. **a** US at 28 weeks of gestation, coronal slice displaying a cerebellum formed of a single block with a characteristic transverse folding. **b, c** MRI, axial slices showing a single cerebellar block with apposition of the dentate nuclei (*arrows*). Reduced TCD. **d** MRI, supratentorial axial slice showing ventriculomegaly associated with septal agenesis

transverse folding (Fig. 21a) associated with a significantly reduced transverse cerebellar diameter. Fetal MRI confirmed the fusion of the hemispheres, and more importantly the apposition of the dentate nuclei (Fig. 21c). Also associated in this case were septal agenesis and ventriculomegaly, clearly identified in US and MRI.

Clinically, rhombencephalosynapsis is accompanied by cerebellar manifestations and motor impairment [38]. The intellectual handicap is variable from one case to another. It appears to be rather accurately correlated with a reduction in volume of the cerebellum [1]. In the vast majority of cases, patients die in early childhood, although in some exceptional occurrences it has been described in adult patients.

Capillary Telangiectasia of the Rhombencephalon

Cerebral vascular malformations are classically categorized in arteriovenous, venous (cavernoma and venous development abnormalities) and capillary malformations [39]. Capillary telangiectasia is a vascular malformation of capillary vessels, initially described by pathologists [40]. Indeed, this lesion is usually not identifiable in angiography or with computed tomography, but it can be identified in MRI [40–43]. It is in most cases located in the rhombencephalon, particularly in the pons. In a series of 12 cases identified in MRI, Barr reports three cases of pontine lesions that are isointense to the adjacent parenchyma on T1 and T2 spin-echo sequences, and hence not visible in the absence of an injected sequence [41]. The lesion is described as hypointense in T1 spin-echo and slightly hyperintense in T2 spin-echo in, respectively, three and eight cases. A lesion showing in hyposignal was found in all seven patients for whom a T2-weighted gradient echo sequence had been performed. In every case, the postgadolinium T1 sequence showed a contrast enhancement inside a lesion with an irregular outline described as a brush-like pattern, associated in eight cases out of 12 with the visualization of a drainage vein.

No mass effect or haemorrhage has been described.

This description of capillary telangiectasia has been confirmed by other authors since then [40, 42, 43]. In particular, the hypointense spot in gradient echo and the contrast enhancement were observed in every case in a series of 18 cases reported by Lee [40].

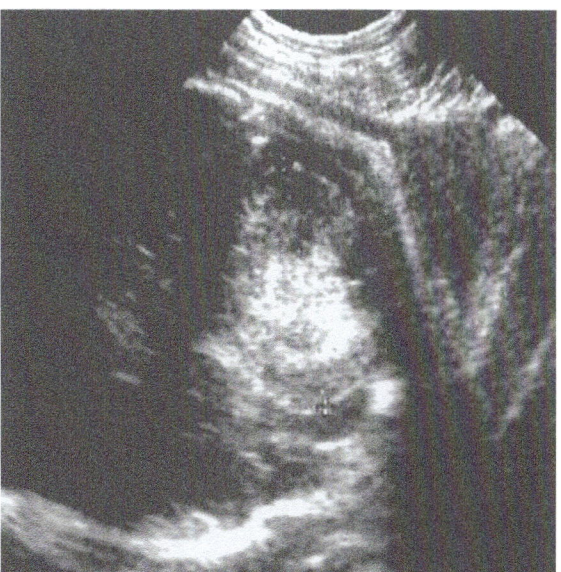

a

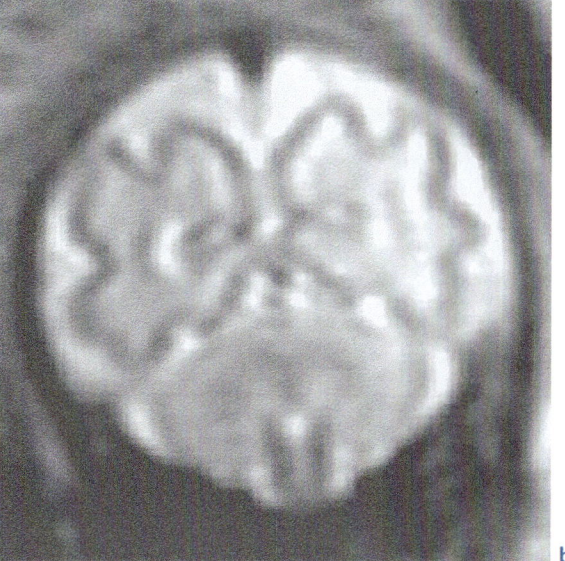

b

Fig. 22 a, b. Capillary telangiectasia of the rhombencephalon (case 1). **a** US at 30 weeks of gestation: presence of a large hyperechoic area centred on the vermis and extending to the adjacent hemispheres. **b** MRI, T2-weighted coronal slice. Complete absence of identifiable lesions (same as in T1 sequence)

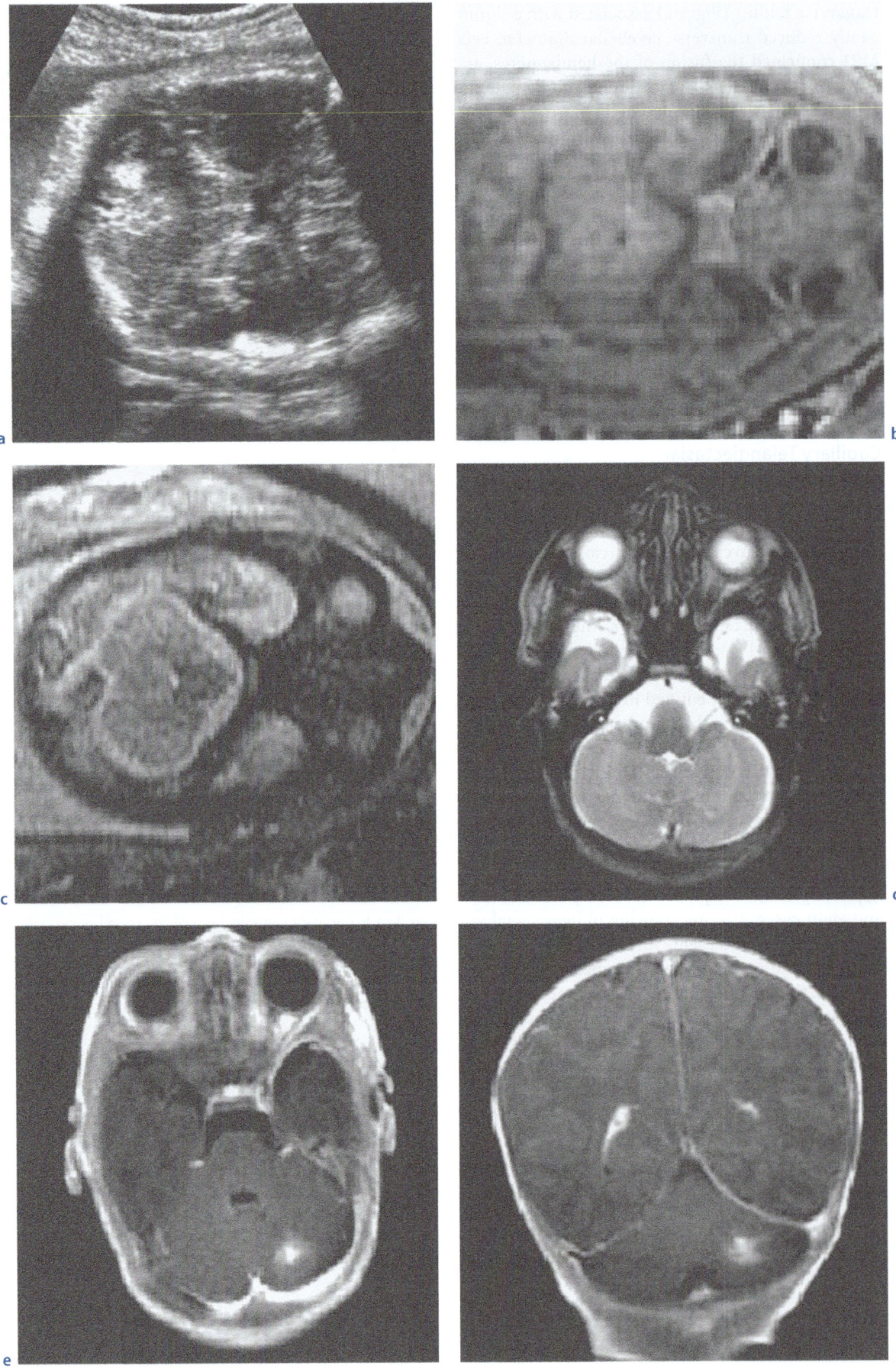

◄ **Fig. 23 a–f.** Capillary telangiectasia of the rhombencephalon (case 2). **a** US at 34 weeks of gestation. Hyperechoic area on the internal aspect of the left cerebellar hemisphere. **b, c** MRI at 34 weeks of gestation, complete absence of identifiable lesions on T1- (**b**) and T2-weighted (**c**) axial slices. **d–f** Postnatal MRI, complete absence of identifiable lesions on T1- and T2-weighted axial slices (**d**). In postgadolinium T1-weighted slice, contrast enhancement in brush-like pattern on the internal aspect of the left cerebellar hemisphere on axial (**e**) and coronal (**f**) slices

The congenital character of this lesion has been the subject of much discussion; one personal observation on an 18-month-old child with a pontine lesion supports this hypothesis [44]. However, no other case has yet been reported in the antenatal period.

In light of two personal observations, we will attempt to describe the patterns in ultrasonography and MRI that lead to a diagnosis of capillary telangiectasia of the rhombencephalon [45].

In both cases, the initial ultrasonography displayed a hyperechoic cerebellar lesion possibly reminiscent of a focal ischaemo-haemorrhagic lesion. There was no deformation of the anatomical structures, and the Doppler showed no vascularization. In the first case, the lesion, identified at 24 weeks of gestation, was located on the vermis and protruded on the hemispheres (Fig. 22). In the second case, the lesion, identified at 32 weeks of gestation, was located strictly on one cerebellar hemisphere (Fig. 23). In both cases, the lesion did not progress during the sonographic follow-up. Fetal MRI, done with T1 and T2 spin-echo sequences, showed no identifiable cerebellar lesion, thus ruling out the possibility of ischaemo-haemorrhagic lesion. In the first case, termination of pregnancy was decided. The fetopathological study provided the diagnosis of capillary telangiectasia. In the second case, the similarities with the first observation led to suggesting the diagnosis in the antenatal period. The diagnosis was confirmed in postnatal MRI. The lesion was not clearly visualized on T1- and T2-weighted spin-echo sequences. It was identified on the T1 postgadolinium sequence, which showed the typical pattern at the level of the pons, with an increased contrast in a brush-like pattern, and visualization of a drainage vessel.

The diagnosis of capillary telangiectasia of the rhombencephalon may therefore be suggested in antenatal examination by a hyperechoic image, not seen in T1- and T2-weighted fetal and postnatal MRI, that does not deform the anatomical structures and remains stable throughout the sonographic follow-up.

These last two elements make it possible to rule out a potential ischaemo-haemorrhagic lesion that must be envisaged first when faced with a hyperechoic image on the parenchyma.

The diagnosis of this lesion is based on the characteristic contrast enhancement in MRI, and also possibly on the hyposignal on T2-gradient echo sequences (the only sequence capable of displaying the lesion in antenatal MRI) (see Chap. 1, Fig. 2).

Concerning the prognosis, capillary telangiectasia is an occult lesion, discovered fortuitously in most cases [41, 43]. Some lesional associations have been envisaged, particularly capillary telangiectasia with occult cavernous angioma; this association could theoretically entail a risk of haemorrhage of the cavernous angioma [40–43]. Some observations of symptomatic capillary telangiectasia with no associated haemorrhagic phenomena have been reported. Establishing a direct relation between the symptomatology and the lesion observed remains difficult [42, 46].

References

1. Altman NR, Naidich TP, Braffman BH (1992) Posterior fossa malformations. A J Neuroradiol 13:691–724
2. Kollias SS, Ball WS Jr, Prenger EC (1993) Cystic malformations of the posterior fossa: differential diagnosis clarified through embryologic analysis. Radiographics 13:211–1231
3. Bernard JP, Moscoso G, Renier D, Ville Y (2001) Cystic malformations of the posterior fossa. Prenat Diagn 21:1064–1069
4. Bromley B, Nadel AS, Pauker S, Estroff JA, Benacerraf BR (1994) Closure of the cerebellar vermis: evaluation with second trimester US. Radiology 193:61–763
5. Goldstein I, Reece EA, Pilu G, Bovicelli L, Hobbins JC (1987) Cerebellar measurements with ultrasonography in the evaluation of fetal growth and development. Am J Obstet Gynecol 156:1065–1069
6. Hill LM, Guzick D, Fries J, Hixson J, Rivello D (1990) The transverse cerebellar diameter in estimating gestational age in the large for gestational age fetus. Obstet Gynecol 75:981–985
7. Garel C, Chantrel E, Sebag G, Brisse H, Elmaleh M, Hassan M (2000) Le développement du cerveau fœtal. Atlas IRM et biométrie. Sauramps Médical, Montpellier
8. Adamsbaum C, André C, Baron JM, Gelot A (2000) Atlas du cerveau fœtal. Guide d'interprétation des aspects normaux. Masson, Paris
9. Adamsbaum C, Merzoug V, André C, Fallet-Bianco C, Lewin F, Kalifa G, Rolland Y, Moutard M (2002) Prenatal diagnosis of isolated posterior fossa anomalies: attempt at a simplified approach. J Radiol 83:321–328
10. Murray JC, Johnson JA, Bird TD (1985) Dandy-Walker malformation: etiologic heterogeneity and empiric recurrence risks. Clin Genet 28:272–283

11. Estroff JA, Scott MR, Benacerraf BR (1992) Dandy-Walker variant: prenatal sonographic features and clinical outcome. Radiology 185:55–58

12. Ecker JL, Shipp TD, Bromley B, Benacerraf B (2000) The sonographic diagnosis of Dandy-Walker and Dandy-Walker variant: associated findings and outcomes. Prenat Diagn 20:328–332

13. Barkovich AJ, Kjos BO, Norman D, Edwards MS (1989) Revised classification of posterior fossa cysts and cystlike malformations based on the results of multiplanar MR imaging. Am J Roentgenol 153:1289–1300

14. Nyberg DA, Mahony BS, Hegge FN, Hickok D, Luthy DA, Kapur R (1991) Enlarged cisterna magna and the Dandy-Walker malformation: factors associated with chromosome abnormalities. Obstet Gynecol 77:436–442

15. Kolble N, Wisser J, Kurmanavicius J, Bolthauser E, Stallmach T, Huch A, Huch R (2000) Dandy-Walker malformation: prenatal diagnosis and outcome. Prenat Diagn 20:318–327

16. Cinalli G (1995) Pronostic du syndrome de Dandy-Walker. Premières journées de Neurochirurgie Pédiatrique, Pathologie Anténatale, Paris, 2–3 December 1995

17. Ramaekers VT, Heimann G, Reul J, Thron A, Jaeken J (1997) Genetic disorders and cerebellar structural abnormalities in childhood. Brain 120:1739–1751

18. Laing FC, Frates MC, Brown DL, Benson CB, Di Salvo DN, Doubilet PM (1994) Sonography of the fetal posterior fossa: false appearance of mega-cisterna magna and Dandy-Walker variant. Radiology 192:247–251

19. Barth PG (1993) Pontocerebellar hypoplasias. An overview of a group of inherited neurodegenerative disorders with fetal onset. Brain Dev 15:411–422

20. Barth PG (2000) Pontocerebellar hypoplasia–how many types? Europ J Paediatr Neurol 4:161–162

21. Verrier-Beygin A (1999) Syndrome d'hypoplasie pontocérébelleuse congénitale primitive. Hétérogénéité du syndrome. A propos de 16 observations. Dissertation in medicine. Université Claude-Bernard Lyon 1, France

22. Mathews KD, Afifi AK, Hanson JW (1989) Autosomal recessive cerebellar hypoplasia. J Child Neurol 4:189–194

23. Goasdoue P, Rodriguez D, Moutard ML, Robain O, Lalande G, Adamsbaum C (2001) Pontoneocerebellar hypoplasia: definition of MR features. Pediatr Radiol 31:613–618

24. Graber D, Antignac C, Deschenes G, Coulin A, Hermouet Y, Pedespan JM, Fontan D, Ponsot G (2001) Cerebellar vermis hypoplasia with extracerebral involvement (retina, kidney, liver): difficult to classify syndromes. Arch Pediatr 8:186–190

25. Boltshauser E, Steinlin M, Martin E, Deonna T (1996) Unilateral cerebellar aplasia. Neuropediatrics 27:50–53

26. Harwood-Nash DC, Fitz CR (1976) Neuroradiology in infants and children. Vol 3, Mosby, St Louis, pp 1014–1019

27. Raybaud C (1982) Cystic malformations of the posterior fossa. Abnormalities associated with the development of the roof of the fourth ventricle and adjacent meningeal structures. J Neuroradiol 9:103–133

28. Tortori-Donati P, Fondelli MP, Rossi A, Carini S (1996) Cystic malformations of the posterior cranial fossa originating from a defect of the posterior membranous area. Mega cisterna magna and persisting Blake's pouch: two separate entities. Childs Nerv Syst 12:303–308

29. Kendall B, Kingsley D, Lambert SR, Taylor D, Finn P (1990) Joubert syndrome: a clinico-radiological study. Neuroradiology 31:502–506

30. Estroff JA, Parad RB, Barnes PD, Madsen JP, Benacerraf BR (1995) Posterior fossa arachnoid cyst: an in utero mimicker of Dandy-Walker malformation. J Ultrasound Med 14:787–790

31. Obersteiner H (1914) Ein Kleinhirn ohne Wurm. Arb Neurol Inst (Wien) 21:124–136

32. Utsunomiya H, Takano K, Ogasawara T, Hashimoto T, Fukushima T, Okazaki M (1998) Rhombencephalosynapsis: cerebellar embryogenesis. AJNR Am J Neuroradiol 19:547–549

33. Aydingoz U, Cila A, Aktan G (1997) Rhombencephalosynapsis associated with hand anomalies. Br J Radiol 70:764–766

34. Yachnis AT (2002) Rhombencephalosynapsis with massive hydrocephalus: case report and pathogenetic considerations. Acta Neuropathol 103:301–304

35. Simmons G, Damiano TR, Truwit CL (1993) MRI and clinical findings in rhombencephalosynapsis. J Comput Assist Tomogr 17:211–214

36. Truwit CL, Barkovich AJ, Shanahan R, Maroldo TV (1991) MR imaging of rhombencephalosynapsis: report of three cases and review of the literature. AJNR Am J Neuroradiol 12:957–966

37. Litherland J, Ludlam A, Thomas N (1993) Antenatal ultrasound diagnosis of cerebellar vermian agenesis in a case of rhombencephalosynapsis. J Clin Ultrasound 21:636–638

38. Isaac M, Best P (1987) Two cases of agenesis of the vermis of cerebellum, with fusion of the dentate nuclei and cerebellar hemispheres. Acta Neuropathol (Berl) 74:278–280

39. Awad IA, Robinson JR Jr, Mohanty S, Estes ML (1993) Mixed vascular malformations of the brain: clinical and pathogenetic considerations. Neurosurgery 33:179–188

40. Lee RR, Becher MW, Benson ML, Rigamonti D (1997) Brain capillary telangiectasia: MR imaging appearance and clinicohistopathologic findings. Radiology 205:797–805

41. Barr RM, Dillon WP, Wilson CB (1996) Slow-flow vascular malformations of the pons: capillary telangiectasias? AJNR Am J Neuroradiol 17:71–78

42. Auffray-Calvier E, Desal HA, Freund P, Laplaud D, Mathon G, De Kersaint-Gilly A (1999) Capillary telangiectasis, angiographically occult vascular malformations. MRI symptomatology apropos of 7 cases. J Neuroradiol 26:257–261

43. Kuker W, Nacimiento W, Block F, Thron A (2000) Presumed capillary telangiectasia of the pons: MRI and follow-up. Eur Radiol 10:945–950

44. Guibaud L, Pelizzari M, Guibal AL, Pracros JP, Rousselle C (1996) Slow-flow vascular malformation of the pons: congenital or acquired capillary telangiectasia. AJNR Am J Neuroradiol 17:1798–1799; discussion 1799–1800

45. Guibaud L, Garel C, Annie B, Pascal G, Francois V, Vavasseur C, Oury JF, Pracros JP (2003) Prenatal diagnosis of capillary telangiectasia of the cerebellum – Ultrasound and MRI features. Prenat Diagn 23(10):791–796

46. Scaglione C, Salvi F, Riguzzi P, Vergelli M, Tassinari CA, Mascalchi M (2001) Symptomatic unruptured capillary telangiectasia of the brain stem: report of three cases and review of the literature. J Neurol Neurosurg Psychiatry 71:390–393

Antenatal Cerebral Pathologies of Infectious Origin

Cytomegalovirus Infection

Cytomegalovirus (CMV) infection is the most frequent congenital infection; it affects 0.5%–2.5% of live births [1]. Most symptomatic forms arise after a maternal primary infection; the infections arising after reactivation or reinfection are almost always asymptomatic [2]. Among the affected children, the mortality rate can reach 30% [1]. In the surviving children, the most serious sequelae are neurological. Therefore, these neurological complications should be carefully sought in antenatal imaging. Disorders such as neurosensorial hearing loss and chorioretinitis cannot be screened out in antenatal examinations. For this reason, one primarily has to look for direct signs of cerebral involvement, whether or not these are associated with other abnormalities reminiscent of fetal infection: ascites, cardiomegaly, pleural effusion, subcutaneous oedema, intrauterine growth restriction, oligo- or hydramnios, and thick placenta.

Except for the lesions mentioned above such as chorioretinitis, neurosensorial disorders and developmental retardation, the earlier the examination (before 23 weeks of gestation), the lower the diagnostic sensitivity of antenatal US. Many fetal abnormalities may only appear at a late stage; some are even undetectable in antenatal US [3, 4].

Currently, the goal of antenatal imaging is to detect the different forms of disorders as early as possible, based on the descriptions provided by neuropathology: microcephaly, lissencephaly, cortical dysplasia, cerebellar hypoplasia, focal white matter lesions, ventricular dilatation and/or asymmetry, periventricular and/or cortical calcifications, and subependymal cysts.

The type of lesion observed differs depending on the date at which the CMV infection occurs [5].

Early infections (before 16–18 weeks of gestation) occurring during the first phases of neuronal migration lead to lissencephaly (Fig. 1) [6, 7]. The diagnosis

of lissencephaly may be suggested following the observation in US of microcephaly associated with ventricular dilatation [8] and a lack of opercularization of the sylvian fissures.

MRI is much more effective than ultrasonography in this context (see Chap. 9), mainly because the sulci are not always easily analysed in US. The diagnosis of lissencephaly requires extensive knowledge of the chronology of appearance in MRI of the sulci in the fetus [9], even though it is easier when the associated signs mentioned above are present.

Cerebellar hypoplasias are frequently observed in antenatal cases of CMV infection [6]; these seem to be more pronounced the earlier the infection occurs [10]. The cerebellar diameter can be measured in US. MRI provides accurate estimations of the anteroposterior diameter of the vermis and its height and surface, with greater success than US [11]. Given the small size of the structures and the limited spatial resolution of MRI, one cannot distinguish between vermian hypoplasia and partial vermian agenesis (see Chap. 12).

After 26–28 weeks of gestation, focal white matter lesions are observed, which are not linked to an underlying neuronal migration disorder [6]. A normal cortex is a sign of a late infection occurring in the third trimester.

White matter lesions such as periventricular T2 hypersignals have been described in postnatal studies [10]. It is probable that these lesions are not visible in US; nor do they seem to have been reported in fetal MRI. Apart from these myelination abnormalities, lesions due to periventricular leucomalacia and porencephaly have been observed [12]. The areas with calcified necrosis are T1 hyperintense (Fig. 2).

Ventricular dilatation may be the only visible sign of CMV infection in antenatal imaging [13]. Additionally, CMV infection may manifest itself solely in a ventricular asymmetry without dilatation (difference between the ventricles exceeding 2.4 mm, one case out of 21 in Achiron's study [14]). The presence of septae inside the dilated ventricles (Fig. 3) is a good sign

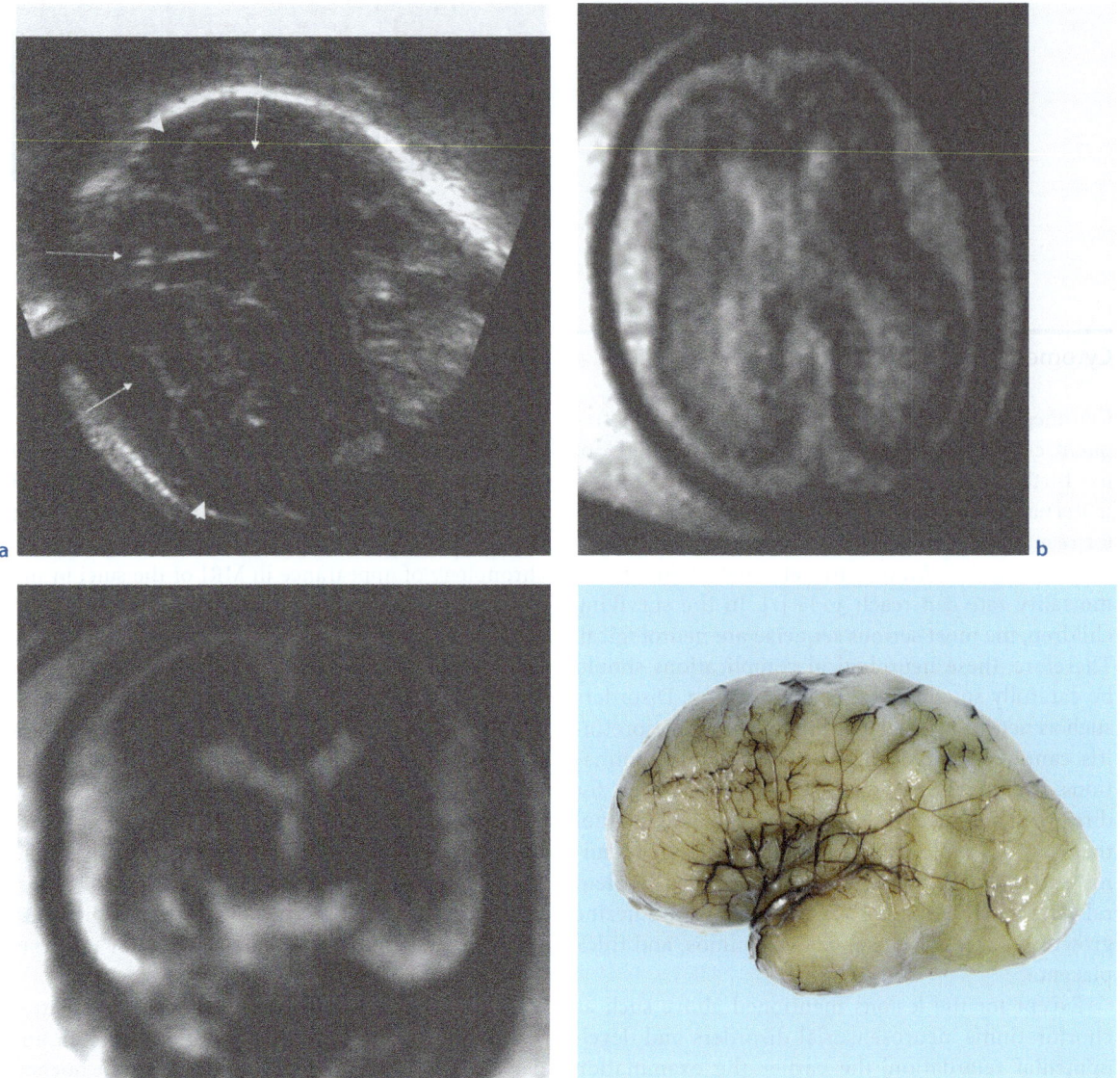

Fig. 1 a–d. CMV fetopathy. Gyration abnormalities. **a** US done at 26.5 weeks of gestation. Coronal slice at the level of the temporal horns. The pericerebral space is widened (*arrowheads*). The sylvian fissures also seem very wide (*arrow*). Additionally, note the linear hyperechogenicity located radially above the frontal horns (*dotted arrows*). **b, c** MRI done at 27 weeks of gestation. T2-weighted axial (**b**) and coronal (**c**) slices. The cerebral biometry reveals subtentorial values far below the 10th percentile, comparable to the standards at 22 weeks of gestation. Gyration is delayed for the stage; the opercularization of the sylvian fissures, notably, has hardly begun. The primary sulci that are normally present at this stage (posterior part of the temporal superior, central and cingular) are not visible. Termination of pregnancy at 28 weeks of gestation. **d** Fetus at 28 weeks of gestation (different from the fetus in **a–c**) Macroscopic view of one hemisphere. Note the pachygyria pattern on the frontal and parietal lobes, and on the incompletely opercularized sylvian fissure

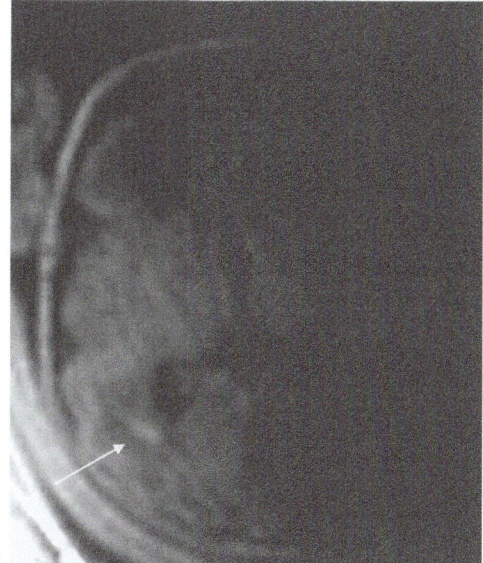

a

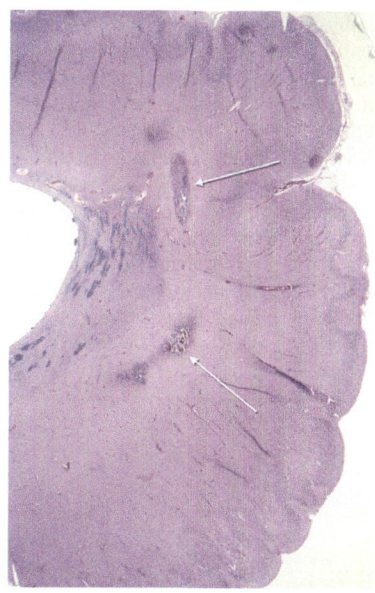

b

Fig. 2 a, b. CMV fetopathy. Cerebral ischaemic lesions. Fetus at 34 weeks of gestation. Ultrasonography consistently displays a mild ventricular dilatation, with atria measured at 12 mm each. **a** MRI done at 34 weeks of gestation. T1-weighted axial slice showing a dilatation of the left atrium. An area in hypersignal is located next to the right ventricle (*arrow*). Pregnancy was terminated at 34 weeks and 4 days of gestation. The histological examination (not shown) confirms the presence of periventricular necrotic lesions; the white matter contains an area of dense gliosis and calcified necrosis, which most probably corresponds to the T1 hypersignal observed in MRI. **b** Fetus at 35.5 weeks of gestation (not the same as in **a**). Frontal histological slice. Enlargement on the higher portion of the frontal horn. Multifocal and calcified white matter necrosis (*arrows*)

of ventriculitis, but these may also be observed following a haemorrhage. There is an entire varied range of ventricular dilatations, from mild dilatation [15] to severe hydrocephalus [16]. The hydrocephalus is either obstructive or communicating. An obstruction of the 4th ventricle by calcifications and arachnoiditis or aqueductal stenosis, both linked to ependymitis, have been blamed in the pathogenesis of these cases of hydrocephalus [12, 17].

The contributions of ultrasonography and MRI to the aetiological diagnosis of ventricular dilatation are detailed in Chap. 11. Let us only mention here that MRI provides a better analysis of the adjacent cerebral parenchyma and of the cortex (gyration abnormalities), this being particularly important in a context of CMV infection. The intraventricular septae are as clearly visible in US as MRI, on condition that the entire ventricle is clearly visible (hence only in the absence of artefacts on the superficial hemisphere).

CMV has an affinity for germinal matrix neuroblasts, which explains the very characteristic periventricular distribution of the lesions it occasions [17, 18]. Subependymal lesions are thought to result either from a direct effect of CMV (direct involvement by CMV of the local vascularization) or from vascular phenomena in relation with a placental involvement linked to CMV. The subependymal region is particularly prone to ischaemia: necrosis and secondary calcification are observed [18, 19].

These periventricular calcifications have been observed both in early- and in late-stage infections. They are visible in antenatal US as hyperechoic areas, usually with no acoustical shadowing [18, 20]. A periventricular hypoechoic ring has also been reported; it could correspond to an early stage of necrosis preceding calcification [18]. MRI, as a rule, is not very effective in the detection of calcifications. In antenatal MRI, areas of calcified necrosis are T1 hyperintense [20, 21]. Calcifications have also been described inside the cortex [12, 22], at the convexity of cerebral gyri. Such calcified necroses of the cortex may be observed in areas of polymicrogyria [12].

The association of microcephaly and periventricular calcifications is therefore very reminiscent of CMV infection, yet the calcifications may not be located in this region, and these signs are by no means specific. A similar symptomatology has been described in relation with the virus of benign lymphocytic choriomeningitis. Moreover, this same association has also been reported in a sibship of consanguineous parents as part of a probably autosomal recessive syndrome; no viral aetiology was found [23].

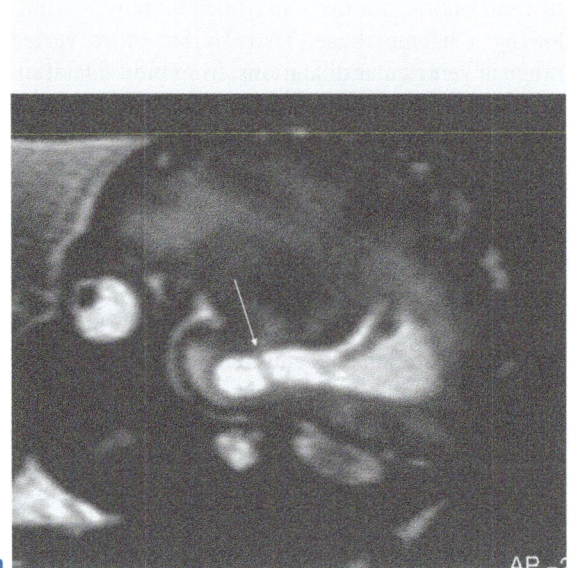

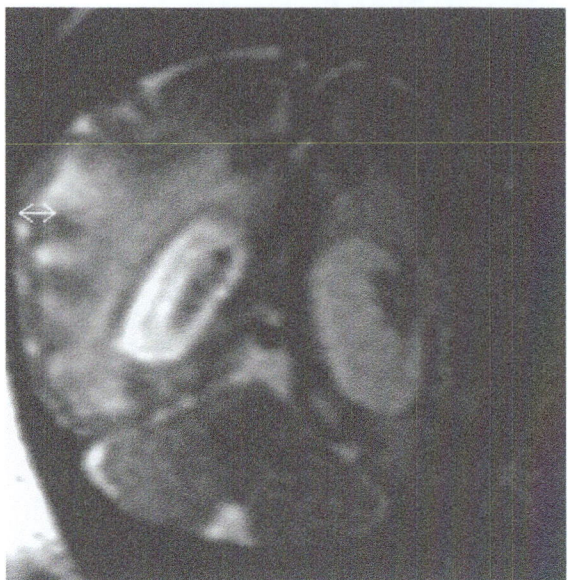

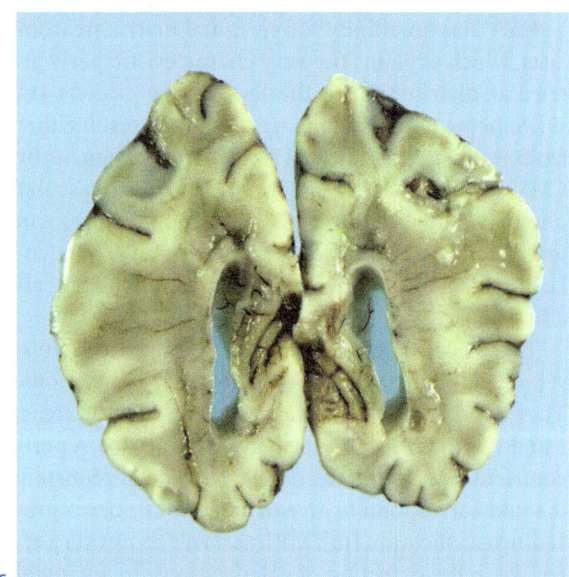

Fig. 3a–c. CMV fetopathy. Fetus at 35.5 weeks of gestation. Same fetus as in Chap. 14, Fig. 6. This fetus displays ventricular dilatation and bilateral subependymal pseudocysts. **a** Note the presence of a septum (*arrow*) within the temporal horns, clearly visible here on this T2-weighted parasagittal slice. This septum was not clearly visible in US. This image can also be interpreted as an anterior temporal lobe cyst [6]. **b** T2-weighted coronal slice. The atria are dilated (left, 16 mm; right, 12 mm). The hyperintensity of the white matter is very pronounced and extends far into the periphery. Termination of pregnancy at 36 weeks of gestation. **c** Coronal macroscopic slice at the level of the atria. The atria are dilated. Greyish areas of softened white matter are visible

In a postnatal study [24], the abnormalities observed with computed tomography (CT) that carry the most severe prognosis seem to be intracerebral calcifications.

Subependymal necrosis may also manifest itself in the presence of subependymal cysts with no associated calcifications. The term "subependymal germinolysis" has been used to describe such cysts [25] (see Chap. 14, Fig. 6).

Ultrasonography does not distinguish between a cystic lesion linked with germinolysis and the progression of a subependymal haemorrhage [15]. Haemorrhages, however, tend to be less often encoun-

tered in antenatal than in postnatal examinations [26].

Other infectious (rubella) or ischaemic pathologies also give rise to similar cystic lesions [26]. These cysts are in fact pseudocysts, as they are not lined with epithelium. They are preferentially located at the level of the caudothalamic groove, but they may also lie around the frontal horns of the lateral ventricles. This last location raises the issue of a differential diagnosis with periventricular leucomalacia, in which the cystic lesions are more external (see Chap. 14). On account of the normal neurological outcome observed in preterm neonates with isolated pseudocysts (19 cases) [26], some authors have expressed doubts on the pathological character of pseudocysts, considering them as a kind of physiological involution of the germinal matrix [26]. Fetal US offers good visibility of pseudocysts; yet it seems MRI is not superfluous when a pseudocyst is detected in US, as one ought to look for potential ischaemo-haemorrhagic lesions pointing to leucomalacia. In the absence of such lesions, and even when the sampling results are persistently negative, the prognosis remains very difficult to evaluate when pseudocysts are detected in antenatal examinations (see Chap. 14).

Other nonspecific abnormalities have been reported in US in cases of antenatal CMV infection; these are mainly linear hyperechoic areas in the thalami resulting from a thickening of the walls of lenticulostriate vessels (candlestick sign). These hyperechoic stripes are related to the deposit of a small quantity of mineralized, amorphous basophilic material. They are not visible in either MRI or CT [17,22]. This pattern has been observed as early as 31 weeks of gestation in a case of CMV infection [22]. It may also be observed in other infectious aetiologies, or in patients with chromosomal aberrations.

Other exceptional abnormalities are reportedly linked with an antenatal CMV infection:

- Hemimegalencephaly [27].
- Hydranencephaly in a child who had probably been infected during the first trimester of pregnancy. Its cause was identified as atheromatous lesions of the aortic arch between the right brachiocephalic artery and the left carotid artery resulting directly from CMV infection [28].
- Schizencephaly [29,30].

The antenatal cerebral imaging of CMV infections is therefore polymorphous; for most lesions, it varies according to the developmental stage at which the infection occurs.

Ultrasonography is efficient in the detection of microcephaly, periventricular calcifications, ventricular dilatation and cerebellar hypoplasia, the latter being the most frequently encountered lesion association, and therefore the most suggestive. Germinolysis and the presence of linear hyperechoic areas in the thalami are not specific to CMV infection.

Ultrasonography therefore plays an essential role in the diagnosis, as it identifies most of the lesions. Some authors have discussed the necessity of a systematic indication for fetal MRI in the event of CMV seroconversion if the US examination is normal [31].

In our experience, in fetuses with CMV seroconversion, when the US examination was normal (21 cases), MRI was always normal. Fetal MRI can refine the diagnosis, notably because of better visibility of gyration abnormalities and the ischaemic impairment of the parenchyma. Consequently, the prognosis is better evaluated, although one must keep in mind that a normal examination cannot guarantee the absence of cerebral involvement, since some abnormalities (cortical dysplasia or polymicrogyria) may easily be overlooked.

Other Infectious Agents

Varicella

The fetopathology of varicella is very rare, as 93% of women in their child-bearing years are already immune against varicella and the risk of fetal involvement is very low after 20 weeks of gestation [32–36]. The fetal varicella syndrome may result either from a haematogenous dissemination of the virus, which accounts for the frequent multiplicity of lesions, or from the development of a herpes zoster, which accounts for the segmental, metameric pattern of some lesions [37,38]. The disorder is characterized by foci of scar or necrotic tissue with calcium deposits in almost every parenchyma, and hence also in the brain [33]. Neurological lesions are observed in 77% of cases [32,33]. These are microcephaly (12%) [32], hydrocephalus [33,39], cerebellar atrophy [33], ischaemic lesions [40], polymicrogyria or intracranial calcifications like those in the other parenchymas (Fig. 4). These abnormalities can be detected in US. In most cases, MRI does not show the calcifications, but it provides a better analysis of cerebellar abnormalities. In our own experience (16 MRI examinations done for varicella contamination early in pregnancy, with disseminate abnormalities in US in only one case), MRI did not provide any more information than what had been obtained in US.

Numerous neurological abnormalities (involvement of the cranial pairs, nystagmus, Horner's syndrome, psychomotor retardation) are undetectable in antenatal US as well as MRI [32,33,35,37], and hence a normal cerebral US or MRI examination does not suffice to rule out all cerebral involvement.

Of course, during the cerebral examination, one must also look for ocular abnormalities. These are frequent (68%) [32], but only microphthalmia can be screened in antenatal MRI. Cataract, chorioretinitis

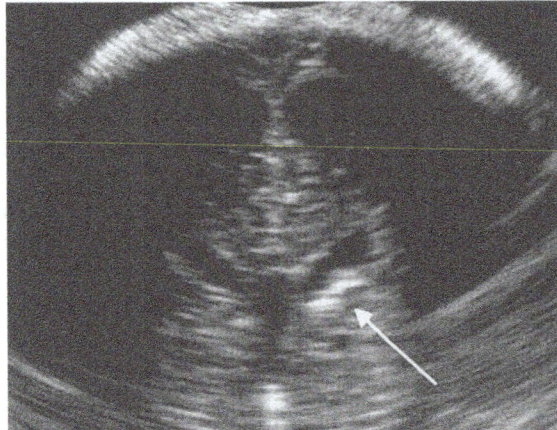

a

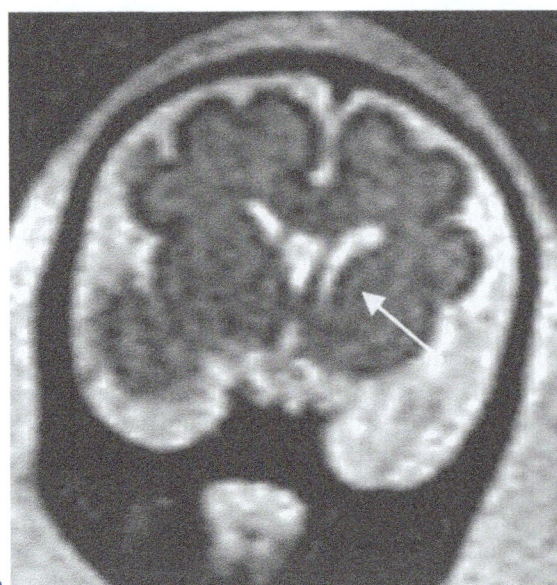

b

Fig. 4 a, b. Varicella. Varicella infection at 15 weeks of gestation. At 21 weeks of gestation, detection of a varus equinus left foot. At 27 weeks of gestation, excess of amniotic fluid and diminution of the fetus's movements. Presence of numerous punctiform hyperechoic formations inside the liver. **a** US cerebral anterior coronal slice at 27 weeks of gestation. Hyperechoic area under the frontal horn of the left lateral ventricle (*arrow*). **b** MRI at 29 weeks of gestation. T2-weighted anterior coronal slice. The presence of a hyposignal under the left frontal horn (*arrow*) is arguable. It supposedly corresponds to the calcification observed in US. No obvious signal abnormality is visible on the T1-weighted slices. Termination of pregnancy is decided at 30.5 weeks of gestation on the basis of a positive test for PCR varicella zoster in the amniotic fluid and the multiplicity of lesions observed in imaging. The fetopathological examination at 30.5 weeks of gestation found numerous foci of calcified necrosis in the lungs, the liver, the adrenal glands and the left germinal zone. There were also small foci of gliosis associated with the microcalcifications

and corneal opacities are all diagnosed postnatally (the diagnosis of cataract is accessible in antenatal US, but has never been reported in fetal MRI; in one personal observation, the cataract was visible in US, but not in fetal MRI).

Toxoplasmosis

Congenital toxoplasmosis (1/3,500–1/1,000 live births [41]) is more severe the earlier transplacental passage of the parasite occurs. The infection may be general or affect essentially the central nervous system. The most commonly observed malformations are neurological disorders consisting in a multifocal necrosis and calcifications. These are generally more marked in the periventricular regions, although they may also be cortical, subcortical, or in the basal ganglia [42–44]. Polymicrogyria and cavitations have also been described [44] (Fig. 5).

When the infection occurs before 20 weeks of gestation, the neurological involvement is severe, generally with microcephaly and ventricular dilatation [41]. Hydranencephaly is also possible. Ventricular dilatation affects the third ventricle and the lateral ventricles; it is linked to an inflammatory reaction around the aqueduct. The aqueduct may be stenosed or obstructed [42, 43]. These abnormalities may also be observed in some patients infected between 20 and 30 weeks of gestation, with variable progression. After 30 weeks of gestation, the calcifications are generally less extensive. Ventricular dilatation may be observed [41].

Ventricular dilatation and calcifications are easily identifiable in ultrasonography. MRI, however, may have a role to play in the detection of some cavitary or polymicrogyric lesions that escape diagnosis in US, although these may also be difficult to visualize in MRI. Chorioretinitis is observed in 85% of the children with congenital toxoplasmosis, but it is not visible in antenatal imaging.

Rubella

Congenital rubella has become very rare in Western countries. Neurological involvement is more frequent when the infection occurs during the first 2 months of pregnancy. These are mainly neurosensorial disorders, which cannot be diagnosed in antenatal imaging.

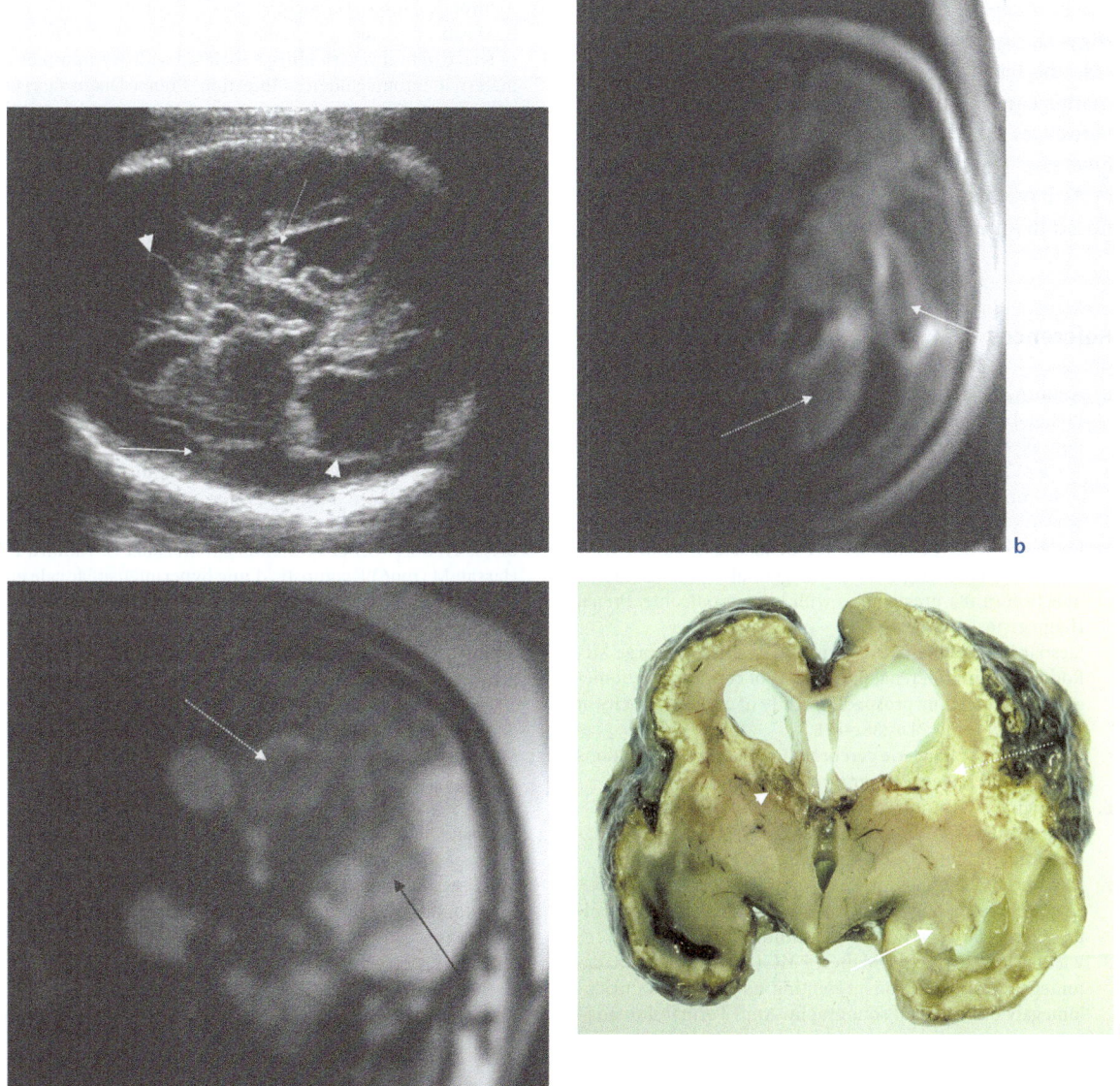

Fig. 5 a–d. Congenital toxoplasmosis. Toxoplasmosis seroconversion at the beginning of pregnancy. Fetus at 31 weeks of gestation. **a** Ultrasonography, axial slice at the level of the thalami. The lateral ventricles are dilated, and surrounded by a hyperechoic lining (*arrowheads*). The left choroid plexus is heterogeneous (*dotted arrow*). The right sylvian fissure is clearly visible (*arrow*), whereas the left one is not easily identifiable, probably because of a temporal atrophy. **b** Fetal MRI, T1-weighted axial slice, at the same level as slice **a**. The left choroid plexus (*dotted arrow*) is abnormally large and hyperintense because of a haemorrhage. The left sylvian infarct is confirmed; it is associated with a temporal atrophy and with a hyperintense parenchyma resulting from a haemorrhagic and/or ischaemic phenomenon (*arrow*). **c** T2-weighted coronal slice, at the level of the third ventricle and of the lateral ventricles' temporal horns. A hypointense blood clot is visible in the left lateral ventricle (*dotted arrow*). The left frontoparietal parenchyma is hyperintense (*black arrow*) and the temporal atrophy is clearly visible. **d** Fetus at 33 weeks of gestation (not the same fetus as in (**a–c**). Macroscopic coronal slice. Note the bilateral cortical necrosis with an involvement of the white matter predominating in the left temporal region (*arrow*), associated with an involvement of the right germinal zone (*arrowhead*) and the head of the left caudate nucleus (*dotted arrow*)

Microcephaly, but also microphthalmia, polymicrogyria, cerebellar heterotopias and calcifications inside the basal ganglia and the periventricular white matter can be observed in neonates in the most severe cases [41, 44]. A gliosis around the aqueduct may give rise to a hydrocephalus. Also, subependymal cysts have been described, which can also be diagnosed in antenatal examinations [44, 45].

References

1. Azam AZ, Vial Y, Fawer CL, Zufferey J, Hohlfeld P (2001) Prenatal diagnosis of congenital cytomegalovirus infection. Obstet Gynecol 97:443–448
2. Tessier V, Mandelbrot L (1998) Epidémiologie de l'infection congénitale à CMV en France. Med Fœtale Echogr Gynecol 35:5–6
3. Enders G, Bäder U, Lindemann L, Schalasta G, Daiminger A (2001) Prenatal diagnosis of congenital cytomegalovirus infection in 189 pregnancies with known outcome. Prenat Diagn 21:362–377
4. Liesnard C, Donner C, Brancart F, Gosselin F, Delforge ML, Rodesch F (2000) Prenatal diagnosis of congenital cytomegalovirus infection: prospective study of 237 pregnancies at risk. Obstet Gynecol 95:881–888
5. Garel C (1998) Imagerie cérébrale anténatale des infections à CMV. Med Fœtale Echogr Gynecol 35:23–26
6. Barkovich AJ, Lindan CE (1994) Congenital cytomegalovirus infection of the brain: imaging analysis and embryologic considerations. AJNR Am J Neuroradiol 15:703–715
7. Hayward JC, Titelbaum DS, Clancy RR, Zimmerman RA (1991) Lissencephaly-pachygyria associated with congenital cytomegalovirus infection. J Child Neurol 6:109–114
8. Twickler DM, Perlman J, Maberry MC (1993) Congenital cytomegalovirus infection presenting as cerebral ventriculomegaly on antenatal sonography. Am J Perinatol 10:404–406
9. Garel C, Chantrel E, Brisse H, Elmaleh M, Luton D, Oury JF, Sebag G, Hassan M (2001) Fetal cerebral cortex: normal gestational landmarks identified using prenatal MR Imaging. AJNR Am J Neuroradiol 22:184–189
10. Steinlin MI, Nadal D, Eich GF, Martin E, Boltshauser EJ (1996) Late intrauterine cytomegalovirus infection: clinical and neuroimaging findings. Pediatr Neurol 15:249–253
11. Garel C, Chantrel E, Sebag G, Brisse H, Elmaleh M, Hassan M (2000) Le développement du cerveau fœtal : atlas IRM et biométrie. Sauramps Médical, Montpellier
12. Perlman JM, Argyle C (1992) Lethal cytomegalovirus infection in preterm infants: clinical, radiological, and neuropathological findings. Ann Neurol 31:64–68
13. Dommergues M, Mahieu-Caputo D, Fallet-Bianco C, Mirlesse V, Aubry MC, Delezoide AL, Dumez Y, Lebon P (1996) Fetal serum interferon-alpha suggests viral infection as the aetiology of unexplained lateral cerebral ventriculomegaly. Prenat Diagn 16:883–892
14. Achiron R, Yagel S, Rotstein Z, Inbar O, Mashiach S, Lipitz S (1997) Cerebral lateral ventricular asymmetry: is this a normal ultrasonographic finding in the fetal brain? Obstet Gynecol 89:233–237
15. Achiron R, Pinhas-Hamiel O, Lipitz S, Heiman Z, Reichman B, Mashiach S (1994) Prenatal ultrasonographic diagnosis of fetal cerebral ventriculitis associated with asymptomatic maternal cytomegalovirus infection. Prenat Diagn 14:523–526
16. Sekhsaria S, Rahbar F, Fomufod A, Mason R, Kosoko O, Trouth J (1992) An unusual case of congenital cytomegalovirus infection with glaucoma and communicating hydrocephalus. Clin Pediatr 31:505–507
17. Kapilivsky A, Garfinkle WB, Rosenberg HK, Peters BD, Kirby CL, Stassi J, Horrow MM (1995) US case of the day. Radiographics 15:239–242
18. Tassin GB, Maklad NF, Stewart RR, Bell ME (1991) Cytomegalic inclusion disease: intrauterine sonographic diagnosis using findings involving the brain. AJNR Am J Neuroradiol 12:117–122
19. Griffith BP, Booss J (1994) Neurologic infections of the fetus and newborn. Neurol Clin 12:541–564
20. Koga Y, Mizumoto M, Matsumoto Y, Hattori T, Tanaka S, Tanaka T, Fujimoto S (1990) Prenatal diagnosis of fetal intracranial calcifications. Am J Obstet Gynecol 163:1543–1545
21. Brisse H, Garel C, Sebag G, Elmaleh M, Fallet C, Vuillard E, Hassan M (1996) Diagnostic d'une hyperintensité focale en pondération T1 en IRM cérébrale fœtale (abstract). J Radiol 77:846
22. Estroff JA, Parad RB, Teele RL, Benaceraff BR (1992) Echogenic vessels in the fetal thalami and basal ganglia associated with cytomegalovirus infection. J Ultrasound Med 11:686–688
23. Monastiri K, Salem N, Korbi S, Snoussi N (1997) Microcephaly and intracranial calcification: two new cases. Clin Genet 51:142–143
24. Boppana SB, Fowler KB, Vaid Y, Hedlund G, Stagno S, Britt WJ, Pass RF (1997) Neuroradiographic findings in the newborn period and long-term outcome in children with symptomatic congenital cytomegalovirus infection. Pediatrics 99:409–414
25. Shaw CM, Alvord EC (1974) Subependymal germinolysis. Arch Neurol 31:374–381
26. Ramenghi LA, Domizio S, Quartulli L, Sabatino G (1997) Prenatal pseudocysts of the germinal matrix in preterm infants. J Clin Ultrasound 25:169–173
27. Jay V, Otsubo H, Hwang P, Hoffman HJ, Blaser S, Zielenska M (1997) Coexistence of hemimegalencephaly and chronic encephalitis. Childs Nerv Syst 13:35–41
28. Kubo S, Kishino T, Satake N, Okano M, Mikawa M, Ishikawa N (1994) A neonatal case of hydranencephaly caused by atheromatous plaque obstruction of aortic arch: possible association with a congenital cytomegalovirus infection? J Perinatol 14:483–486
29. Iannetti P, Nigro G, Spalice A, Faiella A, Boncinelli E (1998) Cytomegalovirus infection and schizencephaly: case reports. Ann Neurol 43:123–127
30. Nuri Sener R (1998) Schizencephaly and congenital cytomegalovirus infection. J Neuroradiol 25:151–152
31. Castanedo B, de Laveaucoupet J, Audibert F, Resten A, Maître S, Aikem N, Musset D (2001) Découverte systématique d'une séroconversion à CMV en cours de grossesse : faut-il faire une IRM cérébrale fœtale lorsque l'échographie cérébrale anténatale est normale ? (abstract) J Radiol 82:1363
32. Dufour P, de Bièvre P, Vinatier D, Tordjeman N, Da Lage B, Vanhove J, Monnier JC (1996) Varicella and pregnancy. Eur J Obstet Gynecol Reprod Biol 66:119–123

33. Pons JC, Vial P, Rozenberg F, Daffos F, Lebon P, Imbert MC, Strub N, Frydman R (1995) Diagnostic prénatal de la foetopathie varicelleuse au deuxième trimestre de la grossesse. J Gynecol Obstet Biol Reprod 24:829–838

34. Higa K, Dan K, Manabe H (1987) Varicella-zoster virus infections during pregnancy: hypothesis concerning the mechanisms of congenital malformations. Obstet Gynecol 69:214–221

35. Kustermann A, Zoppini C, Tassis B, Della Morte M, Colucci G, Nicolini U (1996) Prenatal diagnosis of congenital varicella infection. Prenat Diagn 16:71–74

36. Pons JC, Rozenberg F, Imbert MC, Lebon P, Olivennes F, Lelaidier C, Strub N, Vial M, Frydman R (1992) Prenatal diagnosis of second-trimester congenital varicella syndrome. Prenat Diagn 12:975–976

37. Berrebi A, Assouline C, Ayoubi JM, Parant O, Icart J (1998) Varicelle et grossesse. Arch Pédiatr 5:79–83

38. Petignat P, Vial Y, Laurini R, Hohlfeld P (2001) Fetal varicella-herpes zoster syndrome in early pregnancy: ultrasonographic and morphological correlation. Prenat Diagn 21:121–124

39. Hartung J, Enders G, Chaoui R, Arents A, Tennstedt C, Bollmann R (1999) Prenatal diagnosis of congenital varicella syndrome and detection of varicella-zoster virus in the fetus: a case report. Prenat Diagn 19:163–166

40. Sauerbrei A, Pawlak J, Luger C, Wutzler P (2003) Hints of intracerebral varicella-zoster virus reactivation in congenital varicella syndrome. Eur J Pediatr 162:354–355

41. Barkovich AJ (2000) Infections of the nervous system. In: Barkovich AJ (ed) Pediatric Neuroimaging. Lippincott Williams & Wilkins, Phildadelphia, pp 715–770

42. Friedman S, Ford-Jones LE, Toi A, Ryan G, Blaser S, Chitayat D (1999) Congenital toxoplasmosis: prenatal diagnosis, treatment and postnatal outcome. Prenat Diagn 19:330–333

43. Cotty F, Carpentier MA, Descamps P, Perrotin F, Richard-Lenoble D (1997) Toxoplasmose congénitale avec hydrocéphalie diagnostiquée in utero : évolution sous traitement. Arch Pédiatr 4:247–250

44. Larroche JC, Encha-Razavi F, de Vries L (1997) Central nervous system. In: Gilbert-Barness E. (ed) Potter's pathology of the fetus and infant. Mosby, Saint Louis, pp 1028–1150

45. Makhoul IR, Zmora O, Tamir A, Shahar E, Sujov P (2001) Congenital subependymal pseudocysts: own data and meta-analysis of the literature. Isr Med Assoc J 3:178–183

Abnormalities of the Fetal Cerebral Parenchyma: Ischaemic and Haemorrhagic Lesions

General Information

A number of situations can lead to an impairment of fetal brain perfusion. Schematically, these causes can be of placental, maternal (hypovolaemic shock, hypoxia, abdominal trauma, hypo- or hypertension, drug use) or fetal (infection, anasarca) origin [1, 2]. Aside from these risk situations, one must also consider the monochorial multiple pregnancies, either when one of the fetuses dies in utero, or in the context of a twin-twin transfusion syndrome (TTTS) [3].

Some of these risk situations may result in fetal ischaemic lesions arising via a multifactorial mechanism. This is the case, notably, in monochorial multiple pregnancies following the death of one fetus. Placental vascular anastomoses are observed in 98 % of cases in this type of pregnancy [3]. The severe hypotension resulting from the blood transfusion from the living fetus to the dead one has been blamed, but the placental flow stasis and the release of thromboplastin emboli from the dead twin have also been implicated, as they are responsible for a disseminate intravascular coagulation [1, 3].

In any case, the diminution of fetal brain perfusion can result in ischaemic and/or haemorrhagic lesions, which ought to be sought with even greater attention when one of the above-mentioned situations arises.

In the fetus, the oxygenated blood supplied by the umbilical vein is directed in preference to the liver, the heart and the brain. Consequently, hypoxia results in vasoconstriction in the muscles, skin, lungs, kidneys and intestines, while a maximal flow is preserved in direction of the liver, heart and brain. Fetal hypoxia is accompanied by variations of cerebral vasomotricity consisting in a vasodilatation followed, when the hypoxia persists, by a vasoconstriction [2, 4]. Severe or prolonged hypoxia can provoke fetal death, or definitive cerebral lesions. The existence of such lesions, and their seriousness and distribution, depend on numerous factors, including the nature and duration of the causal mechanism and the fetus'

gestational age. In addition, some developing areas of the brain are particularly sensitive to hypoxia; the areas concerned and their susceptibility vary depending on the stage of pregnancy [5].

Before 34–36 weeks of gestation, white matter, and particularly periventricular white matter, is the most vulnerable zone [1, 5]. The explanation classically offered for this phenomenon is that, until this stage, the periventricular region is essentially perfused by penetrating arteries from the surface of the brain, and hence the boundary zone is located in the ventricles' peripheries. Moreover, the vessels in the periventricular white matter have a limited capacity for vasodilatation at this stage. This increases the vulnerability of this region, which at the same time hosts an intense metabolic activity linked with the considerable proliferation of oligodendrocytes that precedes the myelination process. Around 34–36 weeks of gestation, cerebral vascularization evolves: vessels from the lateral ventricles ensure the perfusion of the deepest regions of the brain. The boundary zone moves closer to the surface; from this moment, the vulnerable zones are the subcortical white matter and the cortex [1]. This watershed regions theory is now being put in doubt, as the vulnerability of periventricular white matter has also been ascribed to vessel muscularization, which progresses from periphery to depth [6]. Furthermore, it seems that other factors can be involved, with infectious, inflammatory, metabolic and even toxic or medicinal sources [6].

The germinal zone located along the lateral ventricles, in which neuroblasts multiply, and from which the nervous cells leave for the cortex in successive migration waves, is also particularly vulnerable. This region is most active between 13 and 26 weeks of gestation; its volume decreases by a half between 26 and 28 weeks of gestation. After 28 weeks of gestation, this diminution is more gradual [7]. Only a few immature cells remain then, at the level of the caudothalamic incisure, under the frontal horns of the lateral ventricles and near the roofs of the temporal horns [8].

Such intense metabolic activity requires a considerable vascular supply, and hence the abundant vascularization (by vessels with very thin muscular walls) in the germinal zone makes it particularly sensitive to variations in blood pressure and to hypoxia and anoxia [1, 2, 9, 10].

Another feature of the fetal brain is its limited capacity for astrocytic reaction to insults. Before 20–21 weeks of gestation, this results in a parenchymal necrosis without gliosis, hence the apparition of a porencephalic cavity, whereas after 26 weeks of gestation, the parenchyma reacts differently. The insults occurring after this stage lead to an intense astrocytic proliferation, which results in a septate cavity with irregular walls. This capacity to trigger such an astrocytic proliferation increases gradually throughout pregnancy, with the result that the later the insult occurs, the more often a pure gliosis with no cystic component is observed [1, 11].

In order to analyse a fetal MRI in a risk situation potentially accompanied by ischaemic and/or haemorrhagic lesions, one must be aware of these facts. Indeed, the patterns and locations of the consequences of a causal mechanism vary during pregnancy. This task also requires good knowledge of the normal appearance of the cerebral parenchyma, which varies depending on the stage of pregnancy, with the successive migration waves and the myelination phenomenon [8, 12, 13]. Following the example of what is recommended for premature neonates [14], a quantitative assessment of the brain, obtained by developing a scoring system in MRI based on myelination, glial cell migration and germinal matrix, could be applied in antenatal examinations.

Actually, the distinction between ischaemic and haemorrhagic lesions is somewhat artificial, as the two phenomena are often mixed. Indeed, during the reperfusion of an ischaemic lesion, especially when the venous pressure increases, capillaries can be ruptured, triggering a haemorrhage [1, 15]. These two types of lesions, however, may also be clearly individualized; pure intraparenchymal ischaemia is actually more frequent in fetuses than in the perinatal period [2]. Furthermore, the symptomatologies of these two types of lesions in MRI are, in our opinion, distinct enough to deserve separate presentations.

Haemorrhagic Lesions

Aside from the risk situations mentioned above, various particular contexts are often associated with fetal cerebral haemorrhagic lesions. This is of course the case with traumas, notably with traffic accidents [16, 17]. Traditional massage techniques intended to perform a version of fetuses in breech presentations have also been blamed [18]. Fetal thrombocytopoenia (linked notably with a coagulation disorder or with fetomaternal platelet alloimmunization) [19, 20] and pre-existing vascular malformations may also cause cerebral haemorrhages.

The location of the haemorrhage is variable. It can be intracerebral and generally supratentorial, but cerebellar haemorrhages have also been reported [21]. Insults on the germinal zone are frequent before 28 weeks of gestation, for the reasons stated above.

The haemorrhage may either be limited to the germinal zone or expand into the lateral ventricles, in which case it may result, at a later stage, in ventricular dilatation caused by an obstructive hydrocephalus linked with the presence of intraventricular clots. At the very last stage, the haemorrhage can spread to the cerebral parenchyma through venous infarcts [1]. An intraventricular haemorrhage may also be secondary to bleeding inside a choroid plexus caused by a rupture of the blood vessels in the plexus [1, 2]. This is relatively frequent.

The haemorrhage may also be purely parenchymal or pericerebral.

The occurrence rate of these antenatal cerebral haemorrhagic lesions has yet to be assessed, but with the recent developments in the MRI field, more and more of these lesions are being identified [11]. It is highly probable that many of the haemorrhages noted in neonates that are usually ascribed to obstetrical manoeuvres have in fact occurred in fetal life.

Signs in Ultrasonography

Many articles report cases of fetal cerebral haemorrhages that were detected in US. These haemorrhages are located mainly at the supratentorial level [9, 10, 15–17, 22–24], but cerebellar [19], pericerebral, subarachnoid and subdural [18, 25, 26] haemorrhages have also been observed. Subdural haemorrhages may be infratentorial [27]. The haemorrhage is in most cases hyperechoic and variably homogeneous. Such hyperechogenicity is also encountered in is-

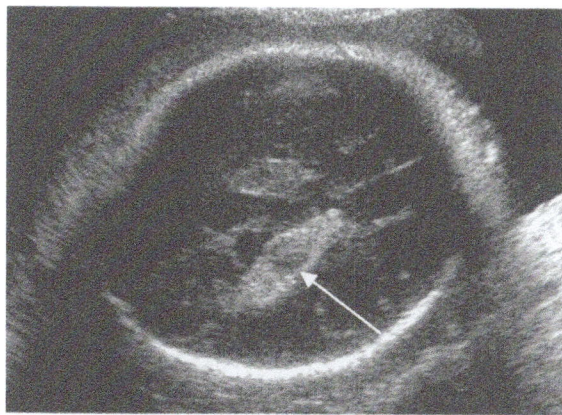

a

◀ **Fig. 1 a–c.** Haemorrhage in a choroid plexus. The patient was being followed closely because of an antecedent of posterior fossa abnormality in the sibship. Normal US at 28 weeks of gestation. At 31 weeks of gestation + 4 days, a haemorrhage was detected in the right choroid plexus. **a** Ultrasonography, axial slice. The right choroid plexus is hyperechoic and heterogeneous (*arrow*). The right lateral ventricle is not dilated. The parenchyma displays a normal pattern. **b** MRI, T1-weighted axial slice. The right choroid plexus appears in hypersignal (*arrow*). **c** MRI, T2-weighted axial slice. The right choroid plexus appears in hyposignal (*arrow*). These signal abnormalities correspond to a semi-recent haemorrhage. The parenchyma's signal is normal. At 1 year, the child's psychomotor development is normal

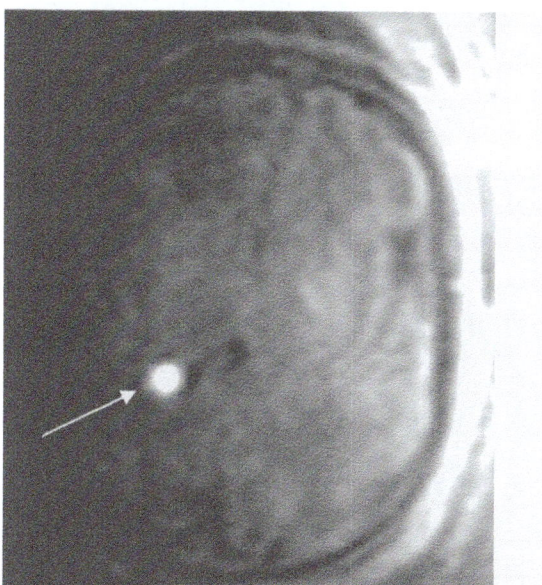

b

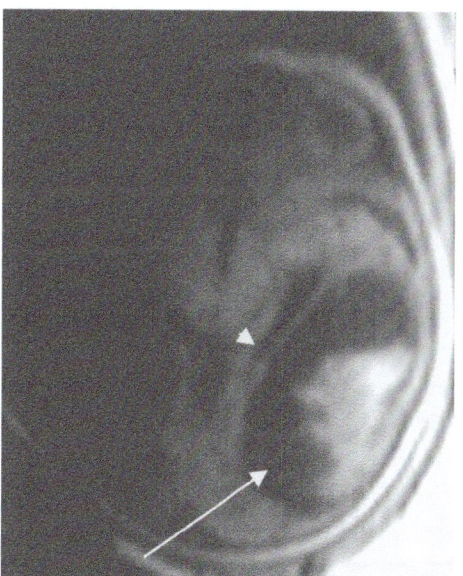

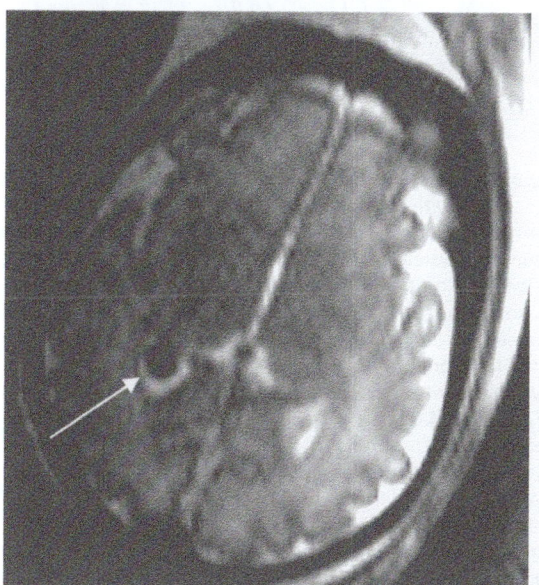

c

Fig. 2. Intraparenchymal haemorrhage. A US examination was done at 36 weeks of gestation following a diminution in fetal movements. On the left, we noted a ventricular dilatation and an ill-defined, probably parenchymal lesion, hardly distinguishable from the lateral ventricle (superficial hemisphere). MRI at 36 weeks of gestation, T1-weighted axial slice. A voluminous, oval-shaped, left temporoparieto-occipital formation (*arrow*) is observed in T1 in mixed signal (hypo- and hyperintense). It is clearly distinct from the lateral ventricle (*arrowhead*). The T1-hypointense component is T2 hyperintense, and the very T1-hyperintense component appears in heterogeneous hyposignal in T2. Additionally, the homolateral choroid plexus is very hyperintense in T1 (not shown) and T2 hypointense. The case is therefore one of voluminous intraparenchymal, and to a lesser extent intraventricular, haemorrhage. This fetus presented thrombocytopoenia, measured 4,000/mm^3, linked with fetomaternal platelet alloimmunization

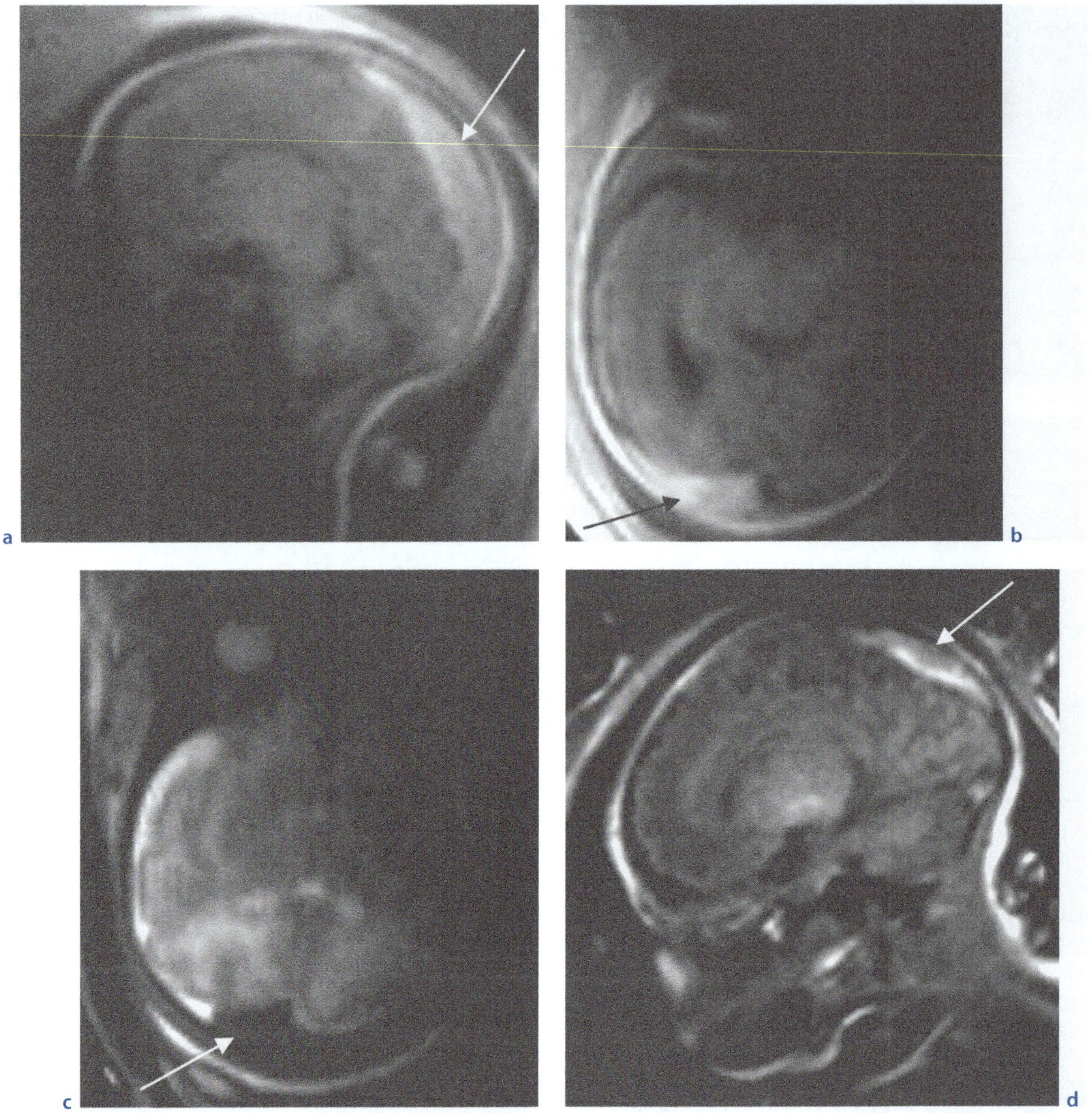

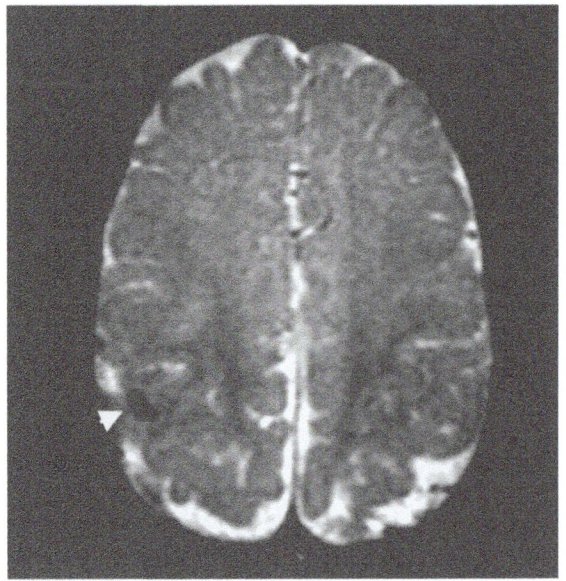

Fig. 3 a–e. Fetal subdural haematoma of traumatic origin. Traffic accident with deceleration at 28 weeks of gestation. No abnormality is detected in US but, because of the violence of the trauma, a systematic MRI examination was scheduled for 32 weeks of gestation. **a, b** T1-weighted sagittal and axial slices. An extended, right parasagittal, T1-hyperintense subdural haematoma (*arrow*) is detected. This haematoma (*arrow*) is located right under the mother's abdominal wall, which possibly explains why the US examination was normal (blind zone). **c** T2-weighted axial slice. The haematoma is hypointense and homogeneous (*arrow*). **d** T1-weighted sagittal slice at 34 weeks of gestation. Cerebral growth is good, the haematoma has decreased in size (*arrow*) and its signal has changed (mixed hypo- and hyperintense in T1, intermediate in T2). The cerebral parenchyma seems to be normal. At birth, the CT scan performed is normal. **e** MRI performed at 8 months of life. T2-weighted gradient echo axial slice. An intraparenchymal T2-hyposignal is visible (*arrowhead*). It may result from an old minor intraparenchymal lesion not seen in antenatal MRI. Normal clinical examination at 1 year of life

chaemic lesions, which demonstrates the limited specificity of US in this field. The US diagnosis of haemorrhage is often rather simple when the lesion is located in the germinal zone, or inside a choroid plexus (Fig. 1) or when the haemorrhage has spread into a lateral ventricle. However, small intraventricular haemorrhages are sometimes completely overlooked because of their size [9] or because the ventricular dilatation is very mild. The ventricular dilatations potentially associated with haemorrhages are generally easily recognizable in US. On the other hand, the poor contrast resolution of US explains why small intraparenchymal haemorrhages, whether in contact with or at a distance from a ventricle, are sometimes missed [9, 10]. Furthermore, the poor visibility of the superficial hemisphere (particularly towards the end of pregnancy, when the fetus is less mobile) can explain the difficulty in diagnosing even the larger intraparenchymal haemorrhages (Fig. 2) and pericerebral haemorrhages (Fig. 3). In the latter case, when the haemorrhage is large enough, the displacement of midline structures may be a useful indirect sign.

Another sign in US is the diminution of the fetus's active movements.

Contribution of MRI

Several articles refer to fetal cerebral [9, 10, 15, 16, 22, 24] or pericerebral [18, 24] haemorrhage. The MRI pattern of haemorrhagic (intra- and pericerebral) lesions is well known in adults. It depends on both intrinsic (macroscopic structure of the clot, hydration state of the clot, location of the haematoma, protein concentration, haemoglobin oxygenation state, presence of an oedema) and extrinsic (magnetic field intensity, type of sequence used) factors [24, 28]. To make it short, the signal differs between recent (< 3 days, T1 hyposignal, T2 hypersignal, then T2 hyposignal), semi-recent (3–14 days, T1 hypersignal, T2 hyposignal, then T2 hypersignal) and old (> 14 days, T1 and T2 hypersignal, then hyposignal) haemorrhages.

At the present time, no such work has been carried out on fetuses, since only a few isolated cases and small series have been published so far and because, in most cases, only one MRI examination is performed per fetus. With time, the haematoma pattern in MRI may become somewhat different, insofar as fetal haemoglobin has a higher affinity with oxygen. Moreover, the degradation process of fetal haemoglobin may well be quicker (scarring, for example, is

quicker in fetuses) [15], but this is only speculative. In any case, MRI offers many advantages over US in this type of indication.

In our own experience (27 cases), MRI facilitates the diagnosis of intraventricular bleeding [9], but above all its better contrast resolution makes it possible to detect intraparenchymal haemorrhages, even those of small size [17] and those that are in contact with a ventricle (Fig. 4). Additionally, MRI offers a good visibility of the whole cerebral parenchyma and pericerebral space, and this whatever the stage (the pericerebral space is distinctly narrower towards the end of pregnancy [12]). Hence, it can detect intraventricular, parenchymal and pericerebral haemorrhages (Figs. 2, 3). By using T1-, T2- and T2*-weighted gradient echo and echoplanar sequences, and with the analysis of signal modifications, haemorrhagic lesions are diagnosed more easily, and their location is more accurately determined in MRI (notably, the detection of an occult bleeding showing in T2* hyposignal inside a vascular malformation; (see Chap. 1, Fig. 2 and the section entitled "Capillary Telangiectasia of the Rhombencephalon" in Chap. 12).

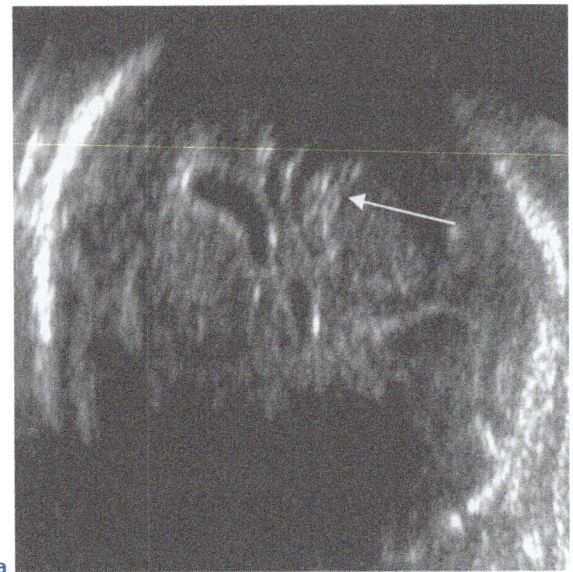

Fig. 4a–e. Intraventricular and intraparenchymal haemorrhage (same fetus as in Chap. 11, Figs. 2, 3). Fetus at 32 weeks of gestation. **a** US. Coronal slice at the level of the frontal horns. Left subependymal haemorrhage (*arrow*). The left frontal parenchyma is not clearly seen (superficial hemisphere). **b, d** MRI, T1-weighted coronal slices, third ventricle (**b**) and atria (**d**). The T1-hyperintense intraventricular haemorrhage is clearly visible in the left lateral ventricle and atrium (*arrow*). There is also a distinct hypersignal at these levels outside the ventricle, which indicates an associated intraparenchymal haemorrhage (*arrowhead*). **c, e** Corresponding macroscopic slices

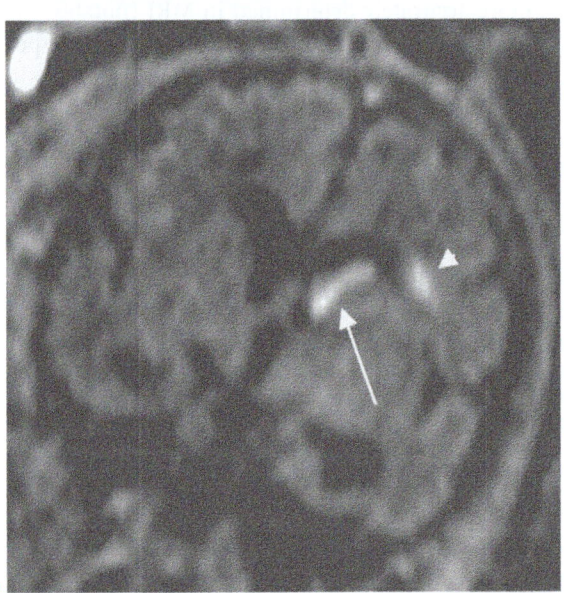

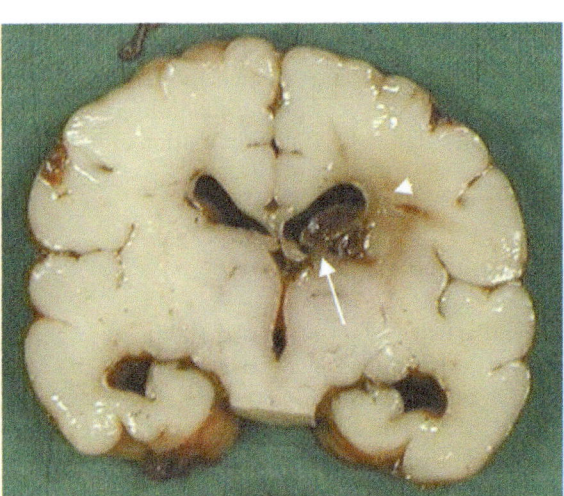

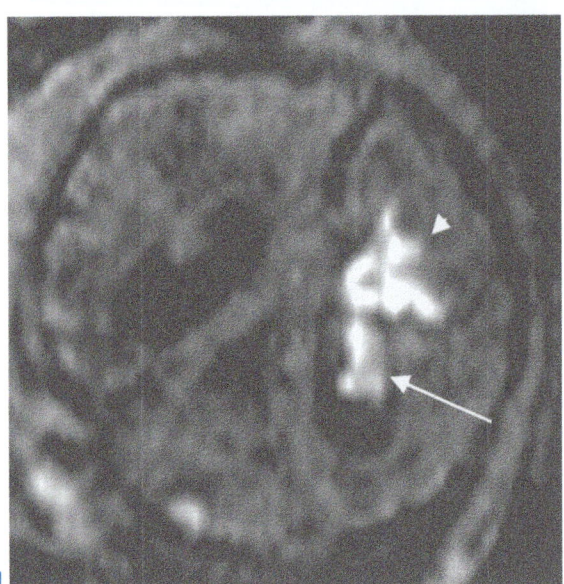

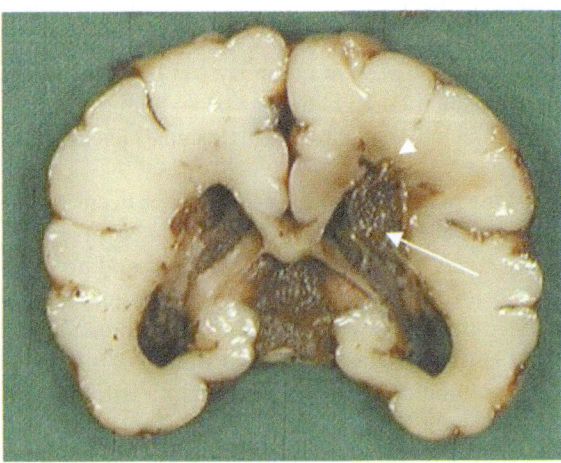

Ischaemic Lesions

Whatever the risk situation one may consider, the repercussions on the fetal brain are different depending on the stage at which the ischaemic lesions have appeared. In the beginning of the second trimester, ischaemic lesions can result in hydranencephaly. When it arises early in pregnancy, before the neuronal migration is complete (i.e. around 20–25 weeks of gestation), ischaemia can give rise to lamination and gyration abnormalities, including polymicrogyria [29]. When the ischaemia occurs in the beginning or in the middle of the second trimester, open-lip schizencephaly may be observed. Closed-lip schizencephaly may result from insults occurring in the middle of the second trimester [30]. After 25–26 weeks of gestation, the periventricular white matter is the most vulnerable (periventricular leucomalacia), and later the subcortical white matter and cortex become sensitive areas. Parenchymal ischaemic lesions may be accompanied by cavitation phenomena, which develop 2–6 weeks (3 weeks on average) after the initial insult [1]. A dilatation in vacuo generally appears rapidly (in 2–4 weeks) on contact with the area affected by leucomalacia. Multicystic encephalomalacia corresponds to an insult occurring late in pregnancy, or even right after birth. Some ischaemic phenomena that occur immediately in prepartum only manifest themselves clinically in peripartum or in immediate postpartum [31].

This section only considers the ischaemic abnormalities of the cerebral parenchyma. The particular issues of schizencephaly and polymicrogyria are further developed in Chap. 9. The subject of hydranencephaly is also not dealt with here. This porencephaly of almost the whole brain only spares the thalami and brain stem (the falx cerebri is present). Even though its origin is very probably ischaemic in some cases, its diagnosis is most often easily reached in ultrasonography, and in any case will not require an MRI.

Signs in Ultrasonography

In its initial phase, a parenchymal ischaemic lesion manifests itself in the form of a variably extensive, and variably homogeneous, hyperechogenicity (isoechoic to the choroid plexus). It can only be detected when it is sufficiently significant and located in an area that is clearly visible in US. This hyperechogenicity is, however, absolutely nonspecific, since oedemas and haemorrhages could lead to similar patterns [1, 5]. Usually, the diagnosis is suggested a few weeks later, when the cavitations and ventricular dilatation possibly accompanied by low growth of the fetal brain appear (Fig. 5). A diminution of fetal active movements and a hydramnios (linked to a swallowing disorder of central origin) can constitute signs in US.

Germinolysis is a somewhat distinct entity. The terms "subependymal cyst" and "pseudocyst" are also used to describe it. It consists in mostly bilateral cystic areas located under the frontal horns, at the level of the caudothalamic groove or at the external angle of the lateral ventricles. In this last location, the cystic areas are often multiple, in a string-of-beads pattern. These cysts are observed in antenatal US [32, 33] or in the immediate postnatal period, sometimes as part of a suggestive context (viral infection, mainly with CMV (Fig. 6) and rubella (see Chap. 13), Zellweger syndrome, antecedent of subependymal haemorrhage), but more often in the absence of a particular context. Pseudocysts may be a marker of chromosomal deletions [33]. Maternal consumption of cocaine has been described as a risk factor [33]. The adjacent parenchyma has a normal echogenicity, no ventricular dilatation is observed (even during progression), and the prognosis is good. Isolated pseudocysts regress spontaneously within 1–12 months after birth in up to 93.5% of cases [33]. The pathogenic character of these cysts has often been questioned. They are widely regarded as the consequence of a very limited involvement (haemorrhage or microinfarction) of the germinal zone [32, 34–37]. Germinolysis, when it is associated with much more extensive cerebral lesions (Figs. 6, 7), has an accordingly poor prognosis.

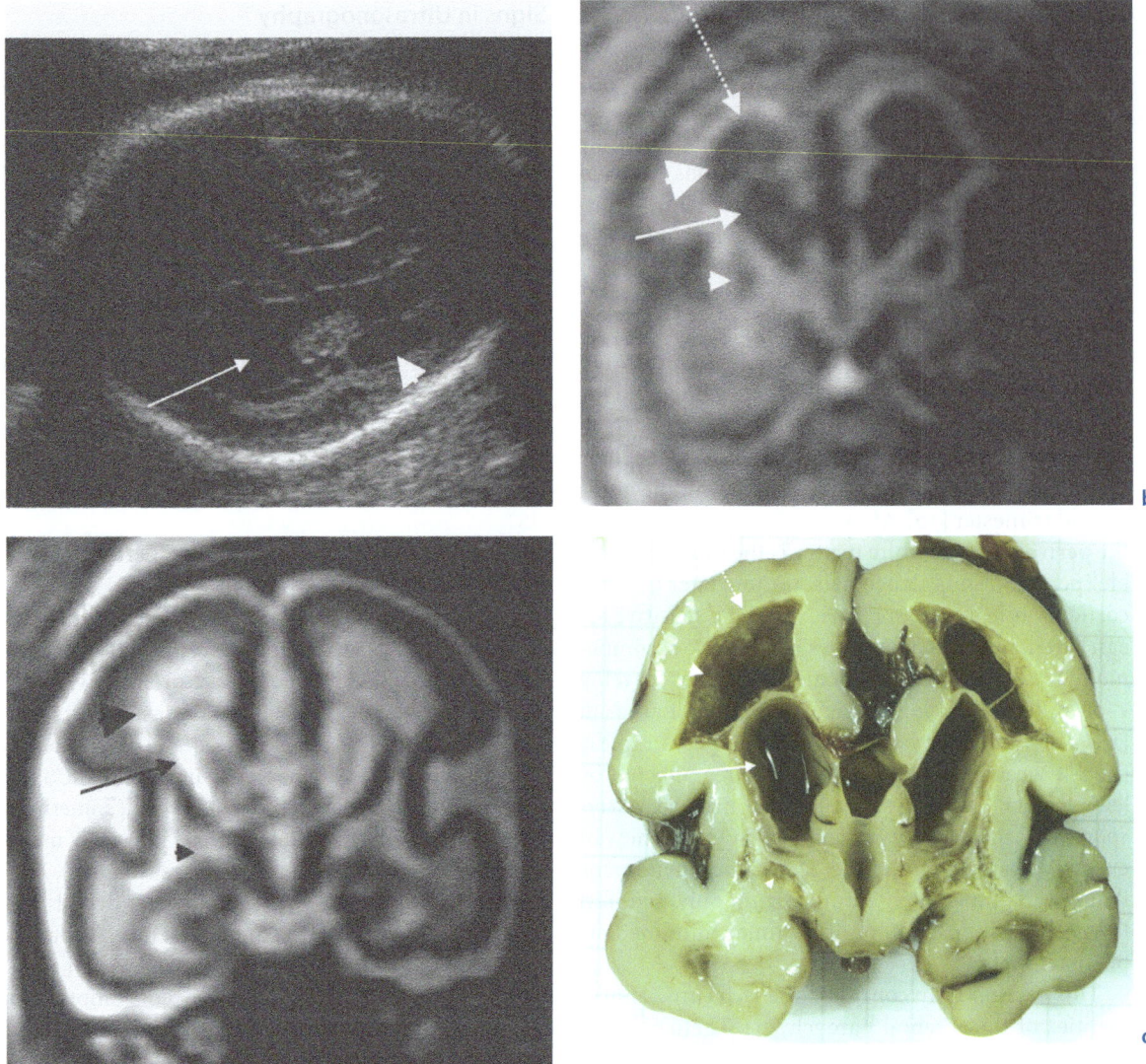

Fig. 5a–d. Diabetic patient at 28 weeks of gestation. Numerous hypoglycaemic episodes during pregnancy, including a recent one with coma. **a** US finds values for biparietal diameter (BPD) and head circumference (HC) to be very much lower than the 10th percentile. The lateral ventricles are dilated (*arrow*). The white mater seems hypoechoic (*large arrowhead*). The hemisphere closest to the probe cannot be analysed. **b, c** T1- (**b**) and T2-weighted (**c**) coronal slices at the level of the frontal horns. The frontal horns are dilated (*arrow*). A white matter abnormality (*arrowhead*) appears next to it in T1 hypo- signal and clear T2 hypersignal. Additionally, there is a T1-hyperintense lining further in the periphery (*dotted arrow*). The lentiform nuclei (*small arrowhead*) are T1 hypointense and T2 hyperintense, which points to necrotic lesions. **d** Fetopathological examination. Coronal slice, macroscopic view. Ventricular dilatation (*arrow*), necrosis with cavitation of the white matter (*arrowhead*) and calcifications in the periphery (*dotted arrow*) (corresponding to the T1-hypersignal) are observed. Also noted are a cerebral atrophy and a necrosis of the basal ganglia (*small arrowhead*)

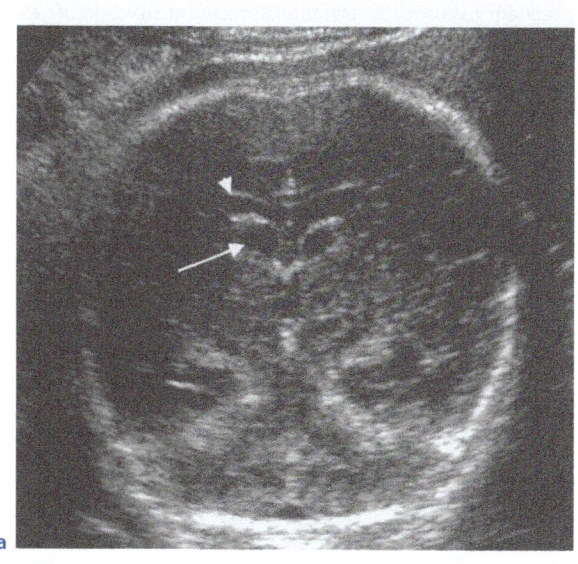

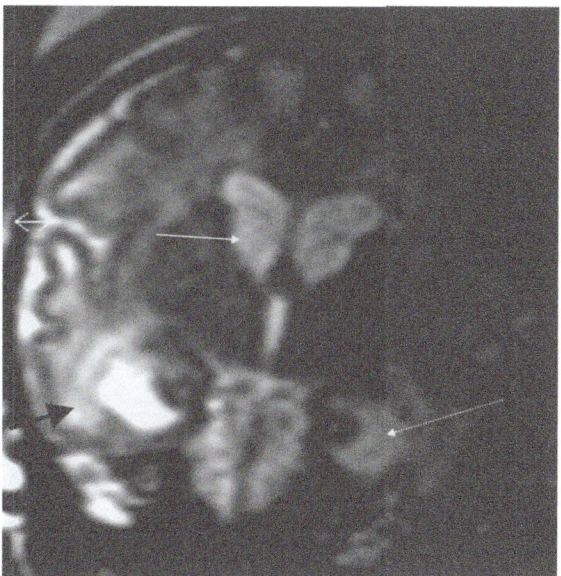

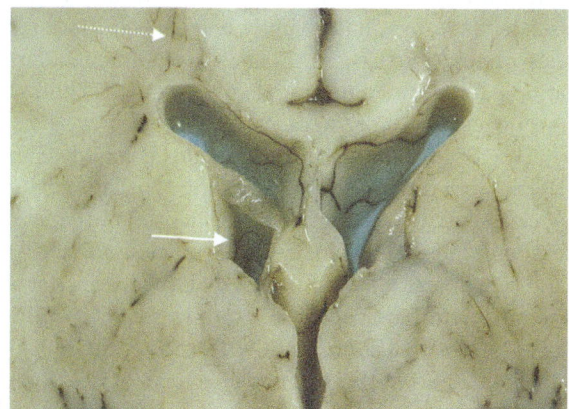

Fig. 6a–c. Germinolysis and parenchymal ischaemia in CMV fetopathy. Fetus at 35 weeks of gestation. **a** US, coronal slice. The bilateral germinolysis (*arrow*) is clearly visible under the frontal horns (*arrowhead*). **b** MRI, T2-weighted coronal slice. The bilateral germinolysis is confirmed (*arrow*). The distinction between germinolysis and frontal horn is less clear-cut than in US. The temporal horns are dilated (*dotted arrow*) and the temporal white matter is very hyperintense (*black arrow*). **c** Feto-pathological examination (termination of pregnancy at 36 weeks of gestation: the fetus displayed other cerebral lesions not shown here). Macroscopic view, coronal slice centred on the frontal horns. The subependymal pseudocysts are clearly visible (*arrow*). There is no haemorrhage around it. A softening of the white matter (*dotted arrow*) is also observed

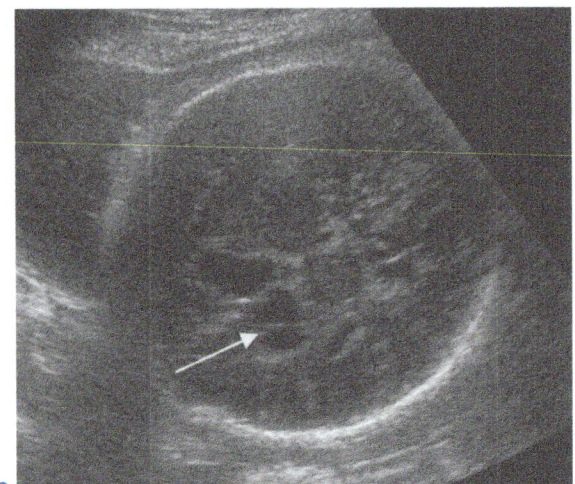

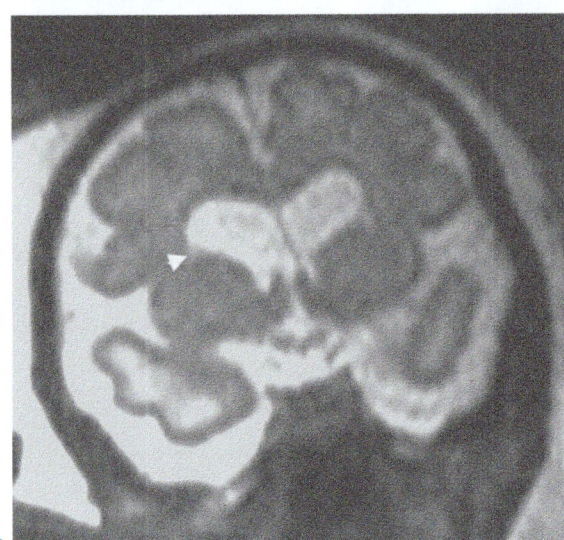

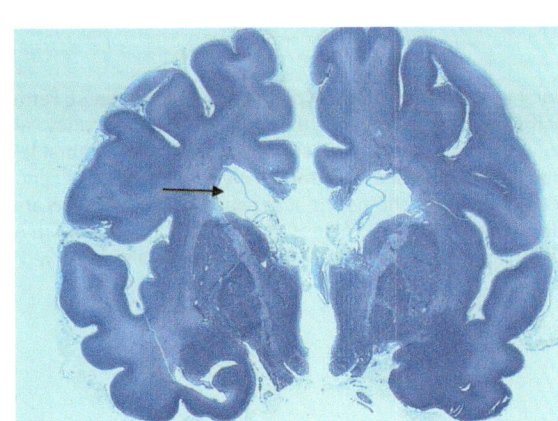

◀ **Fig. 7 a–c.** Old hypoxic and ischaemic cerebral lesions. Normal pregnancy; ventricular dilatation detected at 36 weeks of gestation. **a** US, axial slice. The frontal horns are dilated, with a septum inside the deepest horn. **b** MRI, T2-weighted coronal slice. The frontal horns are dilated, and mildly squared; on their external aspects, a small hyperintense image (*arrowhead*) extends bilaterally into the parenchyma. The right leaf of the septum is not visible. **c** Fetopathological examination (termination of pregnancy at 37 weeks of gestation; numerous cerebral abnormalities not shown here). Coronal histological slice. The septum leaves are ruptured. There are bilateral cavitary lesions (*arrow*) in the germinal zone region (pseudocysts). These extend to the white matter at the level of the external side of the frontal horns (this probably corresponds to the T2 hypersignals observed in MRI). The centrum semiovale, seemingly normal on this slice, contained many foci of softening at the back associated with extensive gliosis

Contribution of MRI

The contribution of MRI to the diagnosis of cerebral ischaemic lesions has recently been studied in a series of seven fetuses [38]. The following considerations were formed on the basis of this article and of our own experience (30 cases).

The diagnosis of ischaemic lesions is based, as in US, on both direct and indirect signs. The latter category essentially consists of abnormalities of the fetal brain biometry in extensive ischaemic lesions (Fig. 5) and ventricular dilatation. Such dilatation, even if it is isolated, and particularly if it grows steadily in the absence of signal abnormalities from the cerebral parenchyma and in the absence of a clear cause of obstructive hydrocephalus, ought to arouse suspicion on the potential presence of diffuse ischaemic lesions, of which ventricular dilatation may be the only stigma (see Chap. 11). A cerebral oedema is another indirect sign. The pattern in MRI is the association of a thin pericerebral space, compared with what is normally observed at the given stage [12], ventricular collapse (the CSF production in the capillaries' endothelium might be reduced where a circulatory disorder is revealed by abnormalities on the umbilical and cerebral Doppler scans), filling of the cisterns in the posterior fossa and, in some rarer cases, a loss of differentiation between the normally T1-hyperintense cortical ribbon and the hypointense adjacent white matter. These four symptoms are each present to diverse extents, and the first three are frequently observed in our experience (85 cases) of fetuses suffering from intrauterine growth retardation, with pathological uterine, cerebral and umbilical Doppler scans (Figs. 8, 9). The prognostic value of these signs has yet to be established. A significant diminution of

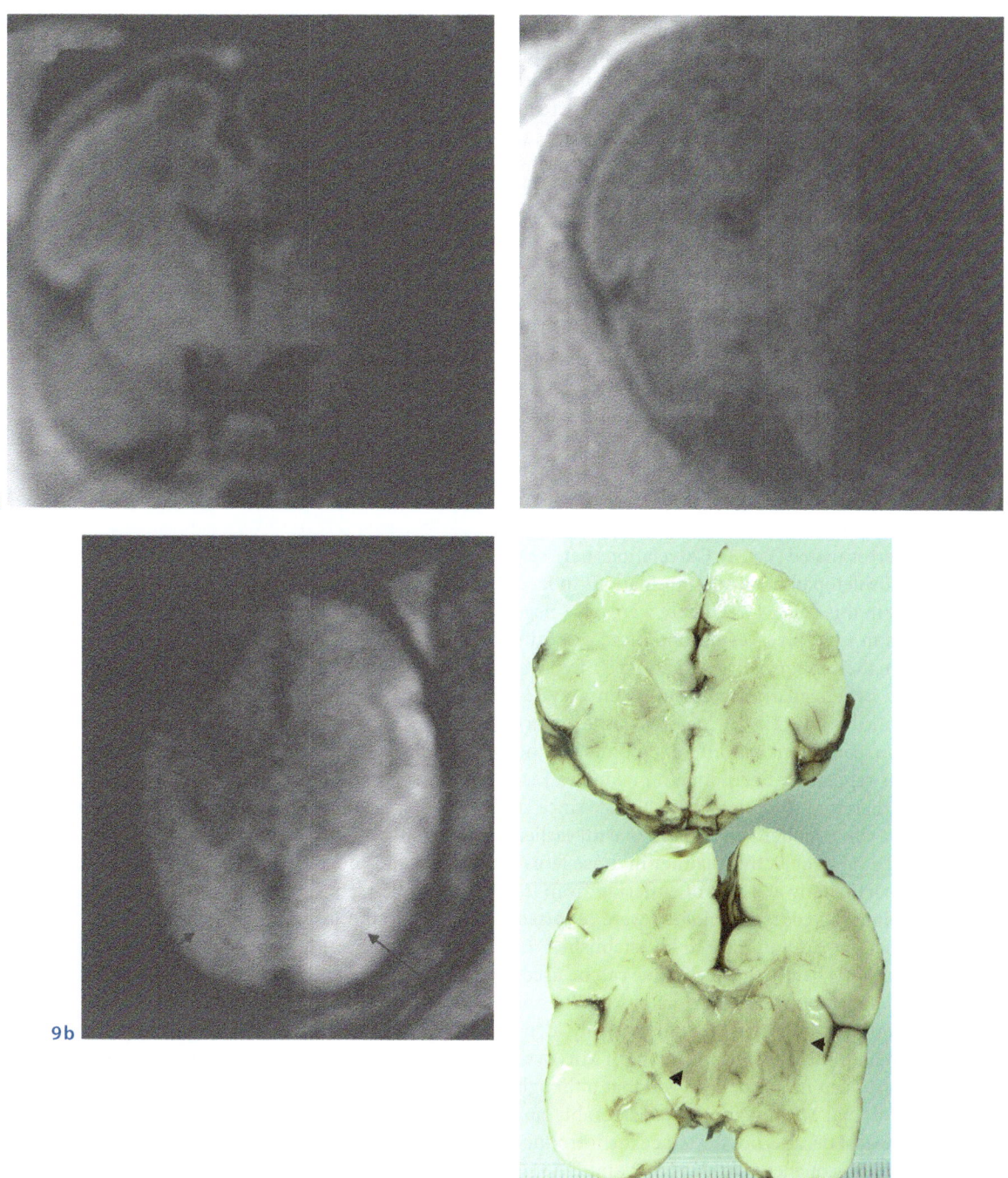

8

9a

9b

9c

Fig. 8. Subacute hypoxic-ischaemic distress. Pre-eclampsia. Severe intrauterine growth retardation, with abnormalities detected on umbilical and cerebral Doppler scans. Examination performed at 29 weeks of gestation. MRI, T1-weighted frontal slice. Thin pericerebral space. The white matter is normally hypointense for the stage. However, a more marked bilateral hyposignal is arguable in the centrum semiovale. In fact, this is probably an artefact, as no abnormality was localized in this spot in fetopathology. Fetal death in utero 6 days after the MRI was done. The fetopathological examination confirms diffuse gliosis in the periventricular white matter made up of large globular astrocytes

Fig. 9 a–c. Chronic and subacute hypoxic-ischaemic distress. Pre-eclampsia. Severe intrauterine growth retardation, with abnormalities detected on umbilical and cerebral Doppler scans. **a, b** MRI done at 28 weeks of gestation, T1-weighted frontal and T2-weighted axial slices. The subarachnoid space is completely absent; the ventricles are collapsed. The white matter is T1 hypointense and markedly T2 hyperintense (*arrows*) in the parieto-occipital regions. Pregnancy was terminated at 29 weeks and 5 days of gestation. **c** Fetopathological examination. Coronal macroscopic view. A diffuse oedema collapses the ventricles and sulci. The parenchyma is diffusely pale, with a shiny, puffed up aspect. The basal ganglia are too clearly visible (*arrowheads*)

the supratentorial biometrical parameters is also noted. In our experience, a decrease in the supra- and infratentorial biometry parameters seems to convey a poor prognosis. In this type of indication, a real-time measurement in MRI of the blood flow in the carotid arteries and the brain without cardiac gating could be useful. This technique is beginning to be used on adult patients [39], but it has not been used on fetuses yet.

The direct signs of ischaemia consist in signal abnormalities in the white matter. The contrast between the lesion and the fetal parenchyma is reduced because of the very high water content of the fetal brain, and because the myelination process is very much incomplete in fetuses [12, 13, 40]. The white matter of fetuses is normally T1 hypointense and T2 hyperintense. Hence, it can be very difficult to detect the small variations in white matter signal when the white matter remains homogeneous. Diffuse glioses may therefore be underestimated (Fig. 8). Correlations between MRI and neurofetopathological examinations indeed showed that in this field as well, there were false-negative results in MRI [41]. Very pronounced and diffuse white matter abnormalities (distinct T1 hyposignal and T2 hypersignal) often result from very severe ischaemic lesions (Fig. 9). Measuring the apparent diffusion coefficient at different points in the brain, as has reportedly been done on neonates [42, 43], would therefore doubtlessly be useful, since it would detect white matter abnormalities at an earlier stage and in a more objective manner in those fetuses that are particularly at a risk of suffering from ischaemic lesions. Of course, standards were reported on a small series [44] and have to be established on larger cohorts [45] before this technique can be used.

The focal or asymmetrical signal abnormalities of the cerebral parenchyma are often more easily identified, which is another certain advantage of MRI over US. One must keep in mind, however, that although the quality of fetal MR images has considerably improved in the last decade, notably since the introduction of ultrafast sequences such as SSFP and HASTE and the homogenization of the field by phased-array coils, the spatial and contrast resolution are still lower on the images obtained than in the examinations done postnatally. Many artefacts remain, whether linked to movements (fetal or maternal), vascular pulsations [maternal, placental (Fig. 10) or fetal] or even with an inhomogeneous field. One must remain careful when interpreting such very focal abnormalities of the cerebral parenchyma, particularly if these are completely isolated.

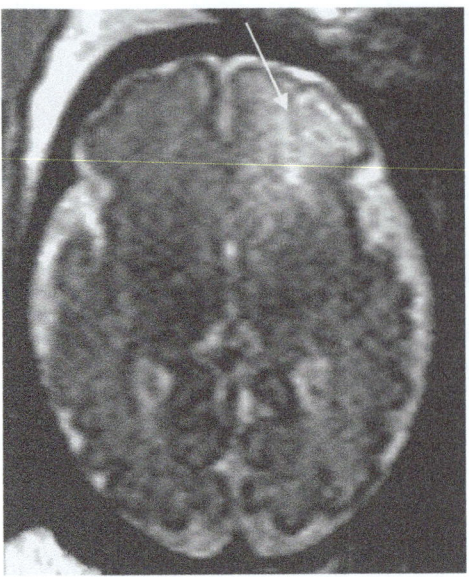

Fig. 10. Placental flow artefact. Fetus at 33 weeks of gestation. T2-weighted axial slice. The left frontal hypersignal (*arrow*) is an artefact caused by the blood flow in placental vessels. It is not visible on slices done in other planes

In this indication, it is absolutely necessary to use T1-, T2- and T2*-weighted sequences. Indeed, in our experience, some ischaemic lesions (confirmed by the neuropathological examination) appear in T1 hypersignal, as what can be seen in neonates [1]. These abnormalities are the lesions resulting from laminar necrosis and some forms of periventricular leucomalacia. In the second type of cases, the T1 hypersignal observed in the absence of haemorrhage is attributed to microcalcifications (Figs. 5, 11). The mechanism of the T1 hypersignal in laminar necrosis is less certain. It might result from the denaturation of some proteins [41]. Other ischaemic lesions appearing in T1 hyposignal are often indistinguishable from the surrounding physiological T1 hyposignal of the fetal white matter.

The focal T2 hypersignals on the cerebral parenchyma are particularly intense when they correspond to cavitary lesions. In most cases, they are located in the white matter and sometimes in the basal ganglia (Fig. 5). Gliosis appears as a less marked hypersignal. The recognition and the precise signification of these hypersignals are delicate questions (Fig. 12). Indeed, similarly to what is observed in preterm neonates [40], detecting a pathological hypersignal within the physiological hypersignal of the white matter can prove difficult. Furthermore, because of the lack of studies on very large cohorts of normal fetuses, the

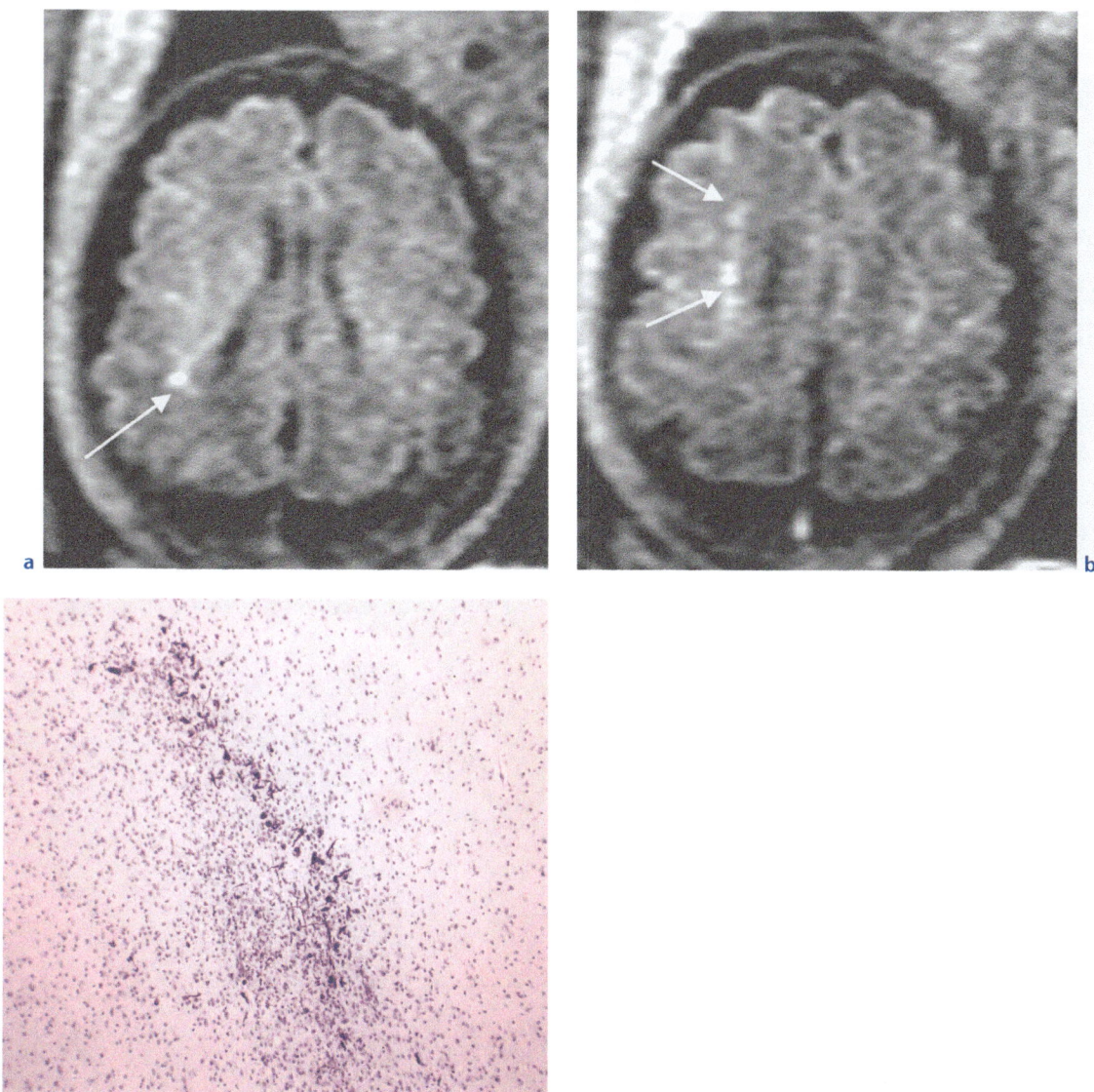

Fig. 11a–c. Calcified leucomalacia. MRI done at 35 weeks of gestation on a fetus with atresia of the proximal small intestine, diminution in limb mobility, amyotrophy and intrauterine growth retardation. **a, b** T1-weighted axial slices at the levels of the lateral ventricles (**a**) and of the centrum semiovale (**b**). Outside the posterior part of the right lateral ventricle and into the right semi-oval centre, the white matter displays punctiform hypersignals (*arrows*) reminiscent of haemorrhagic lesions in this context (but no abnormality is detected in either T2 or T2*), or rather of calcified leucomalacia. **c** Histological slice in front of the atrium. Pattern of calcified leucomalacia

many possible variations of fetal white matter in different areas of the brain and at different stages are not all known at the present time. Just as there are unsolved questions in postnatal examinations regarding the signification of the terminal zones at the level of the fornix, the same debate exists in antenatal examinations concerning other areas of the brain. For example, in our experience, it seems that a T2 hypersignal of the temporal white matter is rather frequently observed in the physiological state.

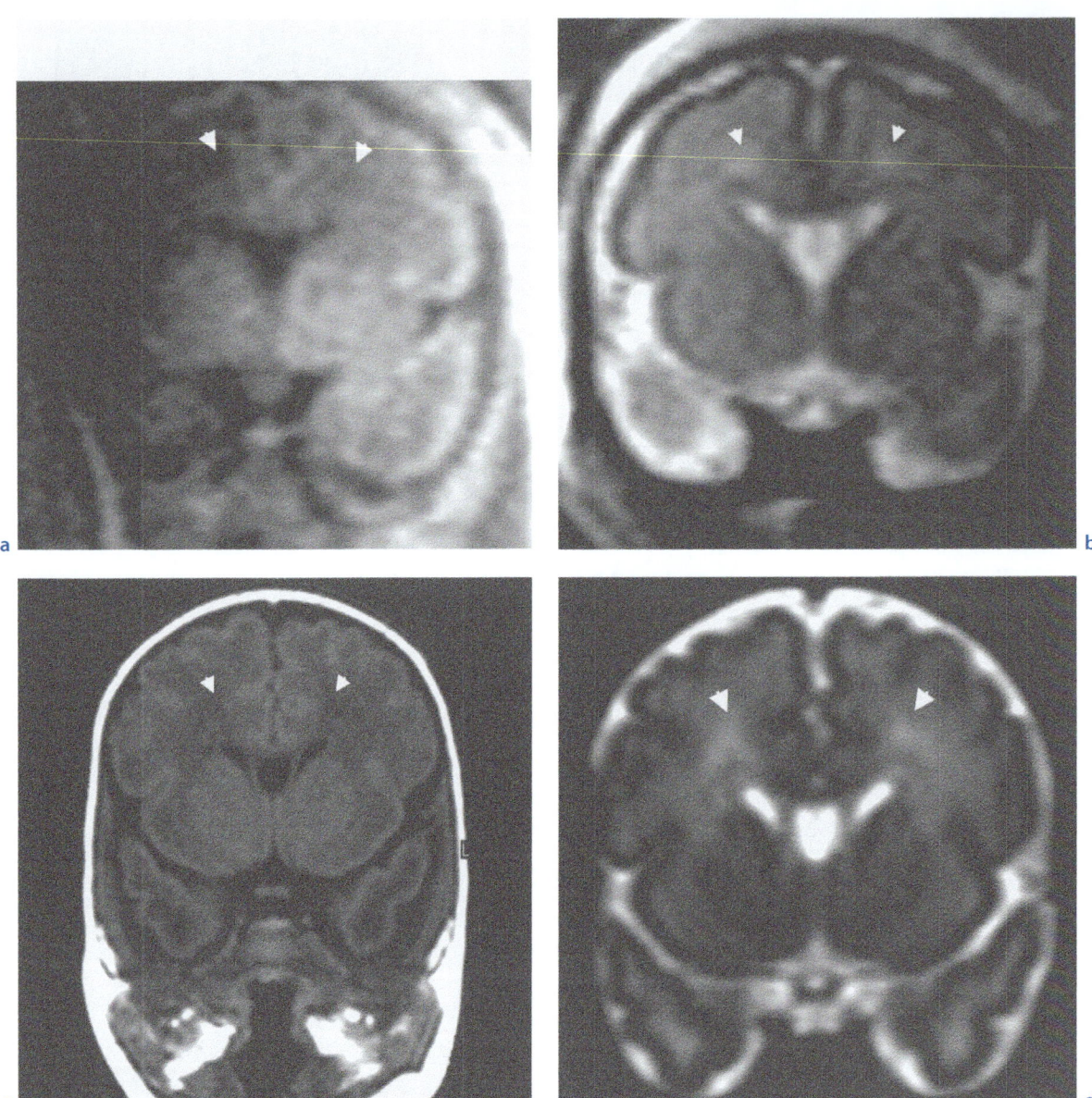

Fig. 12 a–d. Signal abnormalities in the cerebral parenchyma. Fetus at 27 weeks of gestation displaying intrauterine growth retardation in a context of pathological umbilical and cerebral Doppler. **a, b** Antenatal MRI at 27 weeks of gestation, T1- and T2-weighted coronal slices. The MRI is normal, apart from the bilateral T1 hyposignal and T2 hypersignal right above the frontal horns (*arrowheads*). **c, d** Postnatal MRI at 1.5 months of life (birth at 29 weeks of gestation). Signal abnormalities are found again in the white matter of the centrum semiovale (*arrowheads*), right above the frontal horns (T1 hyposignal, T2 hypersignal). These are, given the age and prematurity, considered as physiological. Normal clinical examination at 6 months

Prognosis

Unlike with some rather standardized congenital malformations, it seems quite difficult to suggest a global prognosis for ischaemic and haemorrhagic lesions. Indeed, each case is particular and a number of questions remain concerning the interpretation and the predictive value of the images obtained. Some fundamental principles, extrapolated from the work conducted on cerebral ischaemo-haemorrhagic lesions in neonates, can, however, be reviewed here. Very focal haemorrhages, notably in the germinal matrix and the choroid plexuses, generally have a good prognosis, as do isolated subependymal cysts [34–36]. The degree of ventricular dilatation, especially when dilatation is increasing, has a poor prognostic significance (see Chap. 11). Because the corticospinal tracts are located in the periventricular regions, the most frequent neurological sequelae of periventricular white matter lesions are motor disorders. Since the lower limb axons are more internal than those of the upper limbs, the lower limbs are more frequently involved (spastic diplegia). Visual disorders are also frequent, as the optic radiations are located in the posterior periventricular regions [1]. Generally, these sequelae depend directly on the severity of the involvement, the causal mechanism and the stage at which the parenchymal insult occurs. Before 37 weeks of gestation, a late consequence of ischaemic lesions that has been observed in a significant number of cases is the decrease in the volume of white matter associated with a widening of the lateral ventricles [40].

References

1. Barkovich AJ (2000) Brain and spine injuries in infancy and childhood: In: Barkovich AJ (ed) Congenital malformations of the brain and skull in pediatric neuroimaging. Lippincott Williams & Wilkins, Philadelphia, pp 157–253
2. Rorke LB, Zimmerman RA (1992) Prematurity, postmaturity and destructive lesions un utero. AJNR 13:517–536
3. Langer B, Boudier E, Gasser B, Christmann D, Messer J, Schlaeder G (1997) Antenatal diagnosis of brain damage in the survivor after the second trimester death of a monochorionic monoamniotic co-twin. Fetal Diagn Ther 12:286–291
4. Sibony O, Stempfle N, Luton D, Oury JF, Blot P (1998) In utero fetal cerebral intraparenchymal ischemia diagnosed by nuclear magnetic resonance. Dev Med Child Neurol 40:122–123
5. Vannucci RC (2000) Hypoxic-ischemic encephalopathy. Am J Perinatol 217:113–120
6. Marret S, Zupan V, Gressens P, Lagercrantz H, Evrard P (1998) Les leucomalacies périventriculaires. I – Aspects histologiques et étiopathogéniques. II – Diagnostic, séquelles et neuroprotection. Arch Pédiatr 5:525–545
7. Jammes JL, Gilles FH (1983) Telencephalic development: matrix volume and isocortex and allocortex surface areas. In: Gilles FH, Leviton A, Dooling EC (eds) The developing human brain. John Wright-PSG, Boston, pp 87–93
8. Brisse H, Fallet C, Sebag G, Nessmann C, Blot P, Hassan M (1997) Supratentorial parenchyma in the developing fetal brain: in vitro MR study with histologic comparison. AJNR Am J Neuroradiol 18:1491–1497
9. Canapicchi R, Cioni G, Strigini FAL, Abbruzzese A, Bartalena L, Lencioni G (1998) Prenatal diagnosis of periventricular hemorrhage by fetal brain magnetic resonance imaging. Childs Nerv Syst 14:689–692
10. Fukui K, Morioka T, Nishio S, Mihara F, Nakayama H, Tsukimori K, Fukui M (2001) Fetal germinal matrix and intraventricular haemorrhage diagnosed by MRI. Neuroradiology 43:68–72
11. Simon EM, Goldstein RB, Coakley FV, Filly RA, Broderick KC, Musci TJ, Barkovich AJ (2000) Fast MR imaging of fetal CNS anomalies in utero. AJNR Am J Neuroradiol 21:1688–1698
12. Garel C, Chantrel E, Sebag G, Brisse H, Elmaleh M, Hassan M (2000) Le développement du cerveau fœtal : atlas IRM et biométrie. Sauramps Médical
13. Counsell SJ, Maalouf EF, Fletcher AM, Duggan P, Battin M, Lewis HJ, Herlihy AH, Edwards D, Bydder GM, Rutherford MA (2002) MR imaging assessment of myelination in the very preterm brain.. AJNR Am J Neuroradiol 23:872–881
14. Childs AM, Ramenghi LA, Cornette L, Tanner SF, Arthur RJ, Martinez D, Levene MI (2001) Cerebral maturation in premature infants: quantitative assessment using MR imaging. AJNR Am J Neuroradiol 22:1577–1582
15. Fusch C, Ozdoba C, Kuhn P, Dürig P, Remonda L, Müller C, Kaiser G, Schroth G, Moessinger AC (1997) Perinatal ultrasonography and magnetic resonance imaging findings in congenital hydrocephalus associated with fetal intraventricular hemorrhage. Am J Obstet Gynecol 177:512–518
16. Ali Ahmed SA, Charlier C, Deschamps F, Couture A, Boulot P (1998) Hémorragie intraventriculaire fœtale par contusion cérébrale et résolution spontanée. J Gynecol Obstet Biol Reprod 27:825–828

17. Knuppel RA, Day Salvatore DL, Agarwal R, Leiman S, Sikka A (1994) Documented fetal brain damage resulting from a motor vehicle accident. J Ultrasound Med 13:402–404

18. Green PM, Wilson H, Romaniuk C, May P, Welch CR (1999) Idiopathic intracranial haemorrhage in the fetus. Fetal Diagn Ther 14:275–278

19. Hildebrandt T, Powell T (2002) Repeated antenatal intracranial haemorrhage: magnetic resonance imaging in a fetus with alloimmune thrombocytopenia. Arch Dis Child Fetal Neonat 87:F222–F223

20. Meagher SE, Walker SP, Choong S (2002) Mid-trimester fetal subdural hemorrhage: prenatal diagnosis. Ultrasound Obstet Gynecol 20:296–298

21. Sharony R, Kidron D, Aviram R, Beyth Y, Tepper R (1999) Prenatal diagnosis of fetal cerebellar lesions: a case report and review of the literature. Prenat Diagn 19:1077–1080

22. Reiss I, Gortner L, Möller J, Gehl HB, Baschat AA, Gembruch U (1996) Fetal intracerebral hemorrhage in the second trimester: diagnosis by sonography and magnetic resonance imaging. Ultrasound Obstet Gynecol 7:49–51

23. Achiron R, Hamiel Pinchas O, Reichman B, Heyman Z, Schimmel M, Eidelman A, Mashiach S (1993) Fetal intracranial haemorrhage: clinical significance of in utero ultrasonographic diagnosis. Br J Obstet Gynaecol 100:995–999

24. Kirkinen P, Partanen K, Ryynänen M, Ordén MR (1997) Fetal intracranial hemorrhage. J Reprod Med 42:467–472

25. Barozzino T, Sgro M, Toi A, Akouri H, Wilson S, Yeo E, Blaser S, Chitayat D (1998) Fetal bilateral subdural haemorrhages. Prenatal diagnosis and spontaneous resolution by time of delivery. Prenat Diagn 18:496–503

26. Catanzarite VA, Schrimmer DB, Maida C, Mendoza A (1995) Prenatal sonographic diagnosis of intracranial haemorrhage: report of a case with a sinusoidal fetal heart rate tracing, and review of the literature. Prenat Diagn 15:229–235

27. Batukan C, Holzgreve W, Bubl R, Visca E, Radü EW, Tercanli S (2002) Prenatal diagnosis of an infratentorial subdural hemorrhage: case report. Ultrasound Obstet Gynecol 19:407–409

28. Bradley WG (1994) Hemorrhage and hemorrhagic infections in the brain. Neuroimaging Clin N Am 4:707–732

29. Bordarier C, Robain O (1992) Microgyric and necrotic cortical lesions in twin fetuses: original cerebral damage consecutive to twinning? Brain Dev 14:174–178

30. Castillo M, Mukherji SK (1996) Destructive, ischemic and vascular disorders. In: Imaging of the pediatric head, neck, and spine. Lippincott-Raven, Philadelphia, pp 145–190

31. Everett MF, Shulkin B, Kuhns LR, Donn SM. Intrauterine stroke, cerebral injury and seizures. J Perinatol 1996;16(6):494–497

32. Malinger G, Lev D, Ben Sira L, Kidron D, Tamarkin M, Lerman-Sagie T (2002) Congenital periventricular pseudocysts: prenatal sonographic appearance and clinical implications. Ultrasound Obstet Gynecol 20:447–451

33. Bats AS, Molho M, Senat MV, Paupe A, Bernard JP, Ville Y (2002) Subependymal pseudocysts in the fetal brain: prenatal diagnosis of two cases and review of the literature. Ultrasound Obstet Gynecol 20:502–505

34. Thun-Hohenstein L, Forster I, Künzle C, Martin E, Boltshauser E (1994) Transient bifrontal solitary periventricular cysts in term neonates. Neuroradiology 36:241–244

35. Sudakoff GS, Mitchell DG, Stanley C, Graziani LJ (1991) Frontal periventricular cysts on the first day of life. A one-year clinical follow-up and its significance. J Ultrasound Med 10:25–30

36. Rademaker KJ, De Vries LS, Barth PG (1993) Subependymal pseudocysts: ultrasound diagnosis and findings at follow-up. Acta Paediatr 82:394–399

37. Larroche JC (1972) Sub-ependymal pseudo-cysts in the newborn. Biol Neonate 21:170–183

38. De Laveaucoupet J, Audibert F, Guis F, Rambaud C, Suarez B, Boithias-Guérot C, Musset D (2001) Fetal magnetic resonance imaging (MRI) of ischemic brain injury. Prenat Diagn 21:729–736

39. Wetzel SG, Lee VS, Tan AGS, Heid O, Cha S, Johnson G, Rofsky NM (2001) Real time interactive duplex MR measurements: application in neurovascular imaging. AJR Am J Roentgenol 177:703–707

40. Panigrahy A, Barnes PD, Robertson RL, Back SA, Sleeper LA, Sayre JW, Kinney HC, Volpe JJ (2001) Volumetric brain differences in children with periventricular T2-signal hyperintensities: a grouping by gestational age at birth. AJR Am J Roentgenol 177:695–702

41. Brisse H, Fallet C, Sebag G, Garel C, Elmaleh M, Vuillard E, Blot P, Evrard P, Hassan M (1997) In utero MRI: diagnosis of antenatal brain ischemia (abstract). Pediatr Radiol 27:465

42. Neil JJ, Shiran SI, McKinstry RC, Schefft GL, Snyder AZ, Almli CR, Akbudak E, Aronovitz JA, Miller JP, Lee BCP, Conturo TE (1998) Normal brain in human newborns: apparent diffusion coefficient and diffusion anisotropy measured by using diffusion tensor MR imaging. Radiology 209:57–66

43. Hüppi PS, Maier SE, Peled S, Zientara GP, Barnes PD, Jolesz FA, Volpe JJ (1998) Microstructural development of human newborn cerebral white matter assessed in vivo by diffusion tensor magnetic resonance imaging. Pediatr Res 44:584–590

44. Righini A, Bianchini E, Parazzini C, Gementi P, Ramenghi L, Baldoli C, Nicolini U, Mosca F, Triulzi F (2003) Apparent diffusion coefficient determination in normal fetal brain: a prenatal MR imaging study. AJNR Am J Neuroradiol 24:799–804

45. Bui T, Daire JL, Alberti C, Elmaleh M, Garel C, Luton D, Hassan M, Sebag G (2003) Microstructural development of fetal brain assessed in utero by diffusion tensor imaging. Pediatr Radiol 33:526

Subject Index

The manufacturer's authorised representative in the EU is Springer
Nature Customer Service Centre GmbH, Europaplatz 3, 69115 Heidelberg,
Germany. If you have any concerns regarding our products, please
contact ProductSafety@springernature.com

Printed and bound by CPI Group (UK) Ltd, Croydon, CR0 4YY
28/04/2026
02098462-0003